SURGICAL DEBATES

EDITED BY

ALDEN H. HARKEN, M.D.

Professor and Chairman
Department of Surgery
University of Colorado Health Sciences Center
Denver, Colorado

HANLEY & BELFUS, INC. / Philadelphia

Publisher: HANLEY & BELFUS, INC.
210 S. 13th Street
Philadelphia, PA 19107

SURGICAL DEBATES

ISBN 0-932883-11-7

Last digit is the print number: 9 8 7 6 5 4 3 2 1

CONTENTS

DEBATERS

At the time of the debates, all participants were members of the Department of Surgery, University of Colorado School of Medicine, Denver, Colorado.

B. TIMOTHY BAXTER, M.D.
REGINALD C.W. BELL, M.D.
RAMON BERGUER, M.D.
JAMES M. BROWN, M.D.
LARRY J. BUTLER, M.D.
JODI A. CHAMBERS, M.D.
DEBORAH K. DAVIS, M.D.
JOHN D. EBELING, M.D.
LUKE S. ERDOES, M.D.
MICHAEL A. GROSSO, M.D.
JEFFREY J. GUTMAN, M.D.

CRAIG E. HAUG, M.D.
IRENE R. HORESH, M.D.
ANDREW I. LIGHT, M.D.
ANITA PATT, M.D.
JOSEPH J. PIOTROWSKI, M.D.
JOHN A. RIDGE, M.D., Ph.D.
ANDREW J. SAUERACKER, M.D.
FRANCIS L. SHANNON, M.D.
ALLEN L. TETER, M.D.
THOMAS A. WHITEHILL, M.D.
GLENN J.R. WHITMAN, M.D.

INTRODUCTION

If, in the last few years, you have not discarded a major opinion or acquired a new one, check your pulse—you may be dead.   Burgess (1866–1951)

The purpose of these debates is not only to delineate and rigorously critique controversial issues in clinical surgery but also, more importantly, to demonstrate that a very convincing case may be made for each of two diametrically opposing positions.

Too often, in clinical medicine, we base a diagnosis or therapy upon the experience of our most recent patient (a personal case report) or on a single article. How many times have we all witnessed our colleagues declare: "Have you seen the recent article in . . . ?" and "These authors indicate that you *must*. . . ." Who cares?

The premise of this series of debates is that, as clinicians, we must digest a huge amount of conflicting information in order to develop a responsible conclusion; and an intelligent, articulate advocate can develop a frighteningly credible and persuasive case for *either* side of most clinical questions.[1]

Indeed, for many years in our department we have debated clinical issues every Saturday morning. Residents are randomly assigned a position.[2] The sole bias in these assignments is that the more senior resident may be given the side perceived as being more difficult to defend. The advocates are instructed to present a comprehensive defense of their positions—they are not permitted to equivocate, waffle, or concede. (Thus, portions of the subsequent discussions, taken out of context, may give a dangerously irresponsible impression.)

At the conclusion of each of the most recent 200 debates, each advocate was asked whether he or she *believed* or *was inclined to believe* the position that he or she had just espoused. When positions are randomly assigned, one would anticipate an equal distribution of supporters versus critics. Fifty percent of the advocates should have believed their position and 50 percent should have questioned it. This was *not* the case! Three hundred sixty-two (362) out of 400 resident advocates *believed* the position they had presented. This means that if an inquisitive clinician goes to the library with a preconceived notion, he usually will return with that notion *confirmed*.[2] That's dangerous!

Darwin wrote: " . . . that whenever a published fact, a new observation or thought came across me, which was opposed to my general results, (I strove) to make a memorandum of it without fail; I had found by experience that such facts and thoughts were far more apt to escape from the memory than favorable ones."

This book of debates is presented as a challenge to the reader. Please notice that apparently untenable positions may be cogently defended. Please notice that the same clinical study may be used to support diametrically opposing positions. Please notice also that some of your own most cherished beliefs can be critically assaulted. Ultimately, please begin to criticize yourself openly and freely. That is how one continues to learn. Franklin D. Roosevelt said, "This country [American surgery] needs and, unless I mistake its temper, demands bold, persistent experimentation. It is common sense to take a method and try it. If it fails, admit it frankly and try another. But above all, try something."

If this book can initiate, stimulate, and promote a program of self-examination and self-criticism, together we will have accomplished our mission.

Alden H. Harken, M.D.
Denver, Colorado
December 1987

REFERENCES

1. Harken, A. H.: Surgery as applied physiology. J. Surg. Res., 36:289–293, 1984.
2. Harken A. H.: Presidential Address: Natural Selection in University Surgery. Surgery, 100(2):129–133, 1986.

DEBATE I

Is Physical Diagnosis Obsolete?

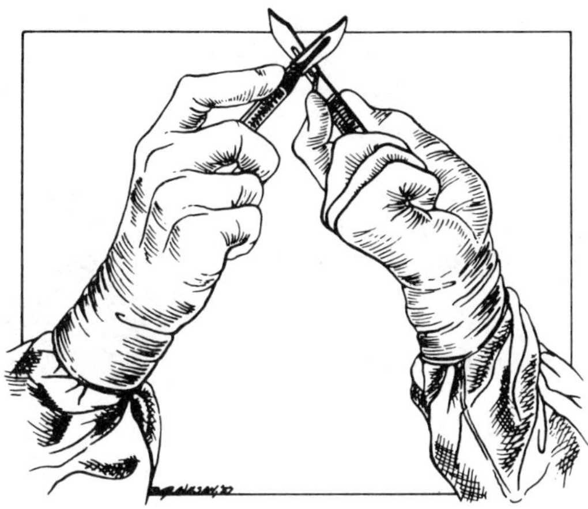

We are in an exciting era of scientific advancement. Radioimmunoassays provide us with techniques of identifying picogram quantities of compounds floating in our patients' blood. Enhanced CT, PET, and MRI scans can now detect, recreate, and image the *milieau interieux* with gratifying precision. Stress radionuclide studies reflect not only anatomy but also organ function.

Do we persist in including physical examination in our diagnostic evaluation for other than sentimental reasons? Perception and identification in physical diagnosis are specific to the examining physician. "A hill and a valley are distinguished by the surrounding landscape." Physical examination is an art form—*not* an objective science.

Dr. Light examines several common surgical diseases to illustrate the inadequacy of physical examination as a rigorously scientific tool worthy of continued inclusion in our diagnostic process. Conversely, Dr. Davis persuasively argues that disease and its physical manifestations have not changed.

Physical examination can be individualized and repeated to provide longitudinal patient-specific data. Physical diagnosis provides a rational springboard from which further invasive, expensive diagnostic procedures may be optimized. Equally important, the history and physical examination establish a sympathetic, caring, and even tactile relationship between the physician and patient. The sensitive physician establishes a compassionate relationship with each patient. Fortunately, medicine remains a very human science. Physical diagnosis and the resultant positive and reinforcing doctor–patient relationship most emphatically are *not* obsolete.

I-A: PHYSICAL DIAGNOSIS IS OBSOLETE

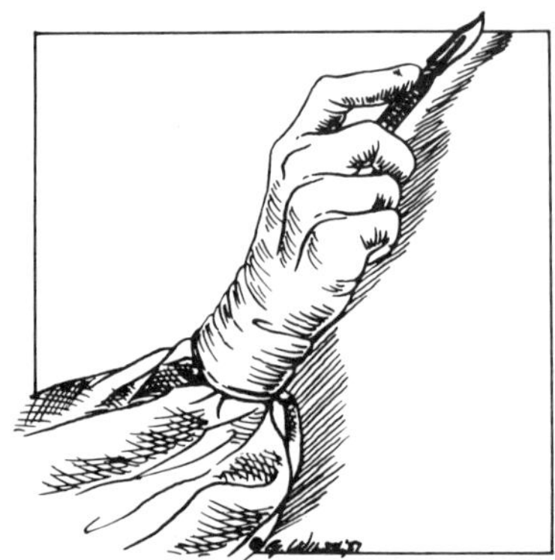

ANDREW I. LIGHT, M.D.

Physical diagnosis is the process of searching for or determining the patient's disease by direct patient examination. The diagnostic process involves four steps:

1. Acquisition of facts (the history and physical examination),
2. Evaluation of facts,
3. Listing of hypotheses (the differential diagnoses), and
4. Choosing between hypotheses (making the diagnosis.).[1]

Step 1 is perhaps the most important, but the subsequent evaluation can only be as good as this data base. The data acquisition process involves the medical history, which furnishes the chronology of symptoms and is purely subjective from the standpoint of both patient and examiner. The physical examination discloses physical signs that, as perceived by the examiner, are manifestations of disease. Laboratory tests and x-ray examinations furnish objective findings. This discussion is based on the physical examination and laboratory tests.

Physical examination involves four skills: inspection, palpation, percussion, and auscultation. Again, these are subjective manifestations of disease as perceived by the examiner. A hill and a valley are distinguished by the surrounding landscape. Perception and identification are specific to the examiner. Physical examination is an art form, *not* an objective science. In today's practice of medicine, is this adequate?

Carcinoma of the breast, abdominal trauma, and deep venous thrombosis are disease states that are encountered frequently in a general surgical practice. Physical examination in these disease processes has many shortcomings. The following discussion will examine these common surgical problems to illustrate the inadequacy of physical examination as a rigorously scientific tool worthy of continued inclusion in our diagnostic process.

Carcinoma of the breast is now the second leading cause of death in women. In the United States, approximately 70,000 new cases occur annually, and about 20,000 women die of this disease each year. Breast self-examination as well as breast examination on routine physicals are important in detecting breast cancer. But, just how good are they when compared to mammography?

Mammography was introduced in the 1950s and gained popularity in the 1960s. It currently is available as both conventional mammography or xeroradiography.

In 1963 a randomized trial was initiated to determine the impact of screening for breast carcinoma.[2] This study continued until 1975 and the results were published in 1977. This was a project of the health insurance plan of greater New York and involved over 62,000 women. The study group received mammography in addition to clinical examination. Control women continued to receive the usual medical care. The findings of the study showed a case fatality rate from mammography of 14 percent, physical examination 41 percent, and combined 32 percent. Also, about 33 percent of the breast carcinomas detected through screening would have been missed without mammography.

Another interesting study was conducted by Malone and colleagues[3] in which 6,238 mammograms were performed, detecting 185 breast cancers. Of these, 62 were occult and constituted one-third of the demonstrable carcinomas. Of importance here is the stage of disease when the carcinoma is detected. The group picked up by xeroradiography had evidence of nodal involvement in 32 percent, while the physically palpable group had 51 percent nodal involvement (Figure 1). Clearly, waiting for palpable disease by physical examination is impractical and perhaps dangerous!

The clinical diagnosis of deep venous thrombosis is highly nonspecific. In 50 percent of the cases, clinical suspicion is not confirmed by objective testing. The common signs and symptoms of deep venous thrombosis are shown in Table I. They include the following: unilateral leg edema, positive Homan's sign, and a palpable cord.[4,5]

Just how good is physical examination in deep venous thrombosis?

McLachlin observed that edema was lacking in 17 percent, local tenderness absent in 59 percent, positive Homan's sign present in only 8 percent, and false positive Homan's sign in 6 percent.[6]

In two studies by Haeger,[7] he clearly shows and documents the shortcomings of physical examination in deep venous thrombosis (DVT). In a retrospective study of 512 patients treated for DVT, only 277, or 54 percent, had positive venograms. In a second study, he prospectively hammers the nails into the coffin of physical examination for DVT. On physical examination, if the patients exhibited four or more signs and symptoms, they were classified as highly suspicious for disease. If they had one to three, they were suspected of disease.

Of 72 patients studied, 40 were classified as highly suspicious and 32 were suspected of having DVT. All patients underwent venography within two hours of admission with the following results: 55 percent in the highly suspicious group and 34 percent in the suspicious group were diagnosed correctly. The discharge diagnoses in patients with negative venograms are shown in Table II.[8] The inescapable conclusion is that a lot of heparin and Coumadin were given to patients with muscle strain or idiopathic leg pain.

Trauma is the number one cause of death in ages up to 44 years. The chronology of management of penetrating abdominal wounds is shown in Table III.[9] Shafton[10] selectively managed patients based on physical examination and diagnostic peritoneal lavage. Just how good is physical examination versus peritoneal lavage?

Two-thirds of patients with stab wounds to the abdomen who had penetration of the peritoneum were watched, and *only* one-half of these wounds caused significant

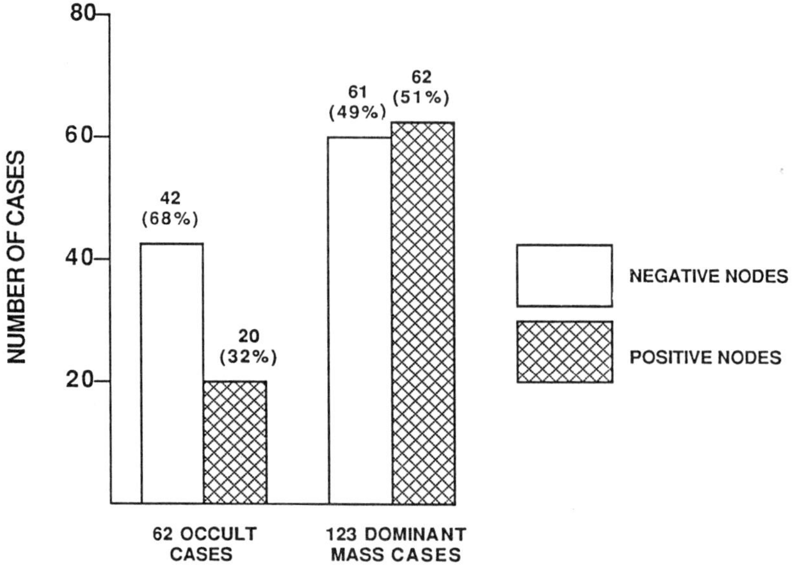

FIGURE 1. Axillary nodes in 185 breast cancers. From Malone, L.J., Frankl, G., Dorazio, R.A., and Winkley, J.H.: Occult breast carcinomas detected by xeroradiography: Clinical considerations. Ann. Surg., 181:134, 1975.

TABLE I. SIGNS AND SYMPTOMS OF DVT*

Spontaneous calf pain
Tenderness to calf palpation
Temperature difference between legs
Swelling of ankle and calf
Dilation of superficial veins
Homan's sign
Lowenberg's sign

*From Shapiro, S: Evidence on screening for breast cancer from a randomized trial. Cancer, 39(6): 2772–2782, 1977.

visceral damage. Gunshot wounds have a higher potential for injury as shown in Table IV.

In a recent article by Thompson and Moore,[11] the management of 300 stab wounds to the abdomen was detailed. The outcome of these patients is shown in Figure 2. In this study, the accuracy of diagnosis by peritoneal lavage was compared with physical examination, and the inadequacy of the physical examination was exhibited (Tables V and VI).

This conclusion is supported by a review of the literature.[11-13] Physical findings correlate with significant abdominal trauma in only 25 to 30 percent of cases, and physical examination bears a significant false positive rate of 15 to 30 percent. The accuracy (or inaccuracy) of physical examination in patients sustaining penetrating abdominal wounds is shown from various studies (Table VI).

The shortcomings of physical examinations are encountered not only in surgical

TABLE II. THE ALTERNATE DIAGNOSIS IN 87 CONSECUTIVE PATIENTS WITH NEGATIVE VENOGRAMS*

DIAGNOSIS **	NO. OF PATIENTS
Muscle strain associated with unaccustomed exercise	21
Direct twisting injury to leg	9
Leg swelling in paralyzed leg	8
Venous reflux	6
Lymphangitis, lymphatic obstruction	6
Muscle tear	5
Baker's cyst	4
Cellulitis	3
Internal abnormality of knee	2
Unknown	23
Total	87

*From Hull, R., Hirsh, J., Sackett, D.L., et al.: Clinical validity of a negative venogram in patients with clinically suspected venous thrombosis. Circulation, 64: 623, 1981.
**Diagnosis made after venography with knowledge of the negative venogram.

TABLE III. PENETRATING ABDOMINAL WOUNDS*

Nonoperative management until late 19th century
1881—J. Marion Sims: Advocates celiotomy
1887—A.S.A.: Routine exploration for GSW
1915—U.S. Military: Mandatory celiotomy
1960—Shafton: Selective management based on PE & DPL

*From Thompson, J.S., Moore, E.E., VanDuzen-Moore, S., et al.: The evolution of abdominal stab wound management. J. Trauma, 20:478–484, 1980.

TABLE IV. STAB WOUNDS VERSUS GUNSHOT WOUNDS: POTENTIAL FOR INJURY*

STAB WOUNDS

⅔ penetrate peritoneum
½ of these cause significant visceral damage

GUNSHOT WOUNDS

80 percent of bullets striking anterior abdomen violate peritoneum
95 percent sustain significant visceral damage

*From Thompson, J.S., Moore, E.E., VanDuzen-Moore, S., et al.: The evolution of abdominal stab wound management. J. Trauma, 20:478, 1980; pp. 478–484. Moore, E.E. and Marx, J.A.: Penetrating abdominal wounds. Rationale for exploratory laparotomy. J.A.M.A., 253:2705, 1985; pp. 2705–2708.

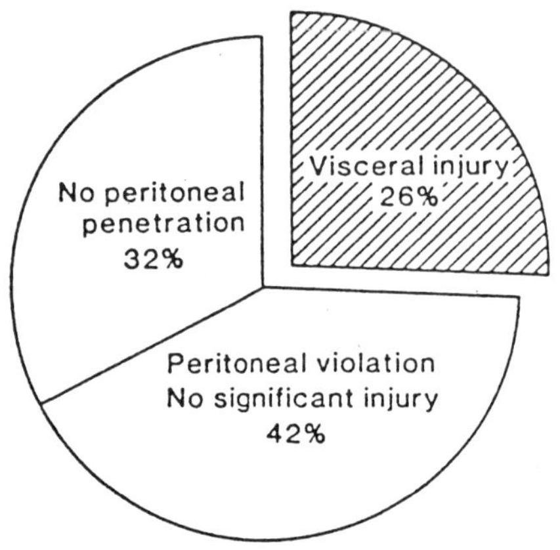

FIGURE 2. Outcome of 300 patients sustaining abdominal stab wounds. From Thompson, J.S., Moore, E.E., VanDuzen-Moore, S., et al.: The evolution of abdominal stab wound management. J. Trauma, 20:481, 1980.

TABLE V. ACCURACY OF OBSERVATION VERSUS DPL IN STAB WOUNDS*

	UNNECESSARY LAPAROTOMY	MORBIDITY
Observation	15%	17%
DPL	4%	9%

*From Thompson, J.S., Moore, E.E., VanDuzen-Moore, S., et al.: The evolution of abdominal stab wound management. J. Trauma, 20:478–484, 1980.

TABLE VI. ACCURACY OF PHYSICAL EXAMINATION IN PENETRATING ABDOMINAL WOUNDS*

	FALSE (+)	FALSE (−)
Bull and Mathewson	18	23
Thal	14	36
Thompson, Moore	36	
Perry	26	
Olsen	21	43

*From Thompson, J.S., Moore, E.E., VanDuzen-Moore, S., et al.: The evolution of abdominal stab wound management. J. Trauma, 20:478–484, 1980.

practice but also in other specialties. Gynecologists rely on amniocentesis for diagnosis of fetal abnormalities and Pap smear for early detection of cervical carcinoma. Neurologists now rely on MRI and CT scans of the head as well as spinal tap for diagnosis of various neurologic diseases. Internists and pulmonologists rely on chest x-ray examinations and endoscopy to support their clinical suspicions. This supports the adage that "the chest is meant to be seen and not heard."

Physical diagnosis is a discipline that is taught early in the medical school years. However, the physical examination has many shortcomings. In the technologically advanced era of medicine of the 1980s, physical examination is becoming increasingly obsolete. Although it should not be forgotten, physical examination should be used as an adjunct to the more sensitive and specific laboratory tests that have become available.

REFERENCES

1. DeGowin, E.L. and DeGowin, R.L.: Bedside Diagnostic Examination, 3d ed. New York, MacMillan Publishing Company, Inc., 1976.
2. Shapiro, S.: Evidence on screening for breast cancer from a randomized trial. Cancer, 39(6): 2772-2782, 1977.
3. Malone, L.J., Frankl, G., Dorazio, R.A., and Winkley, J.H.: Occult breast carcinomas detected by xeroradiography: Clinical considerations. Ann. Surg., 181: 133-136, 1975.
4. Hull, R.D. and Hirsh, J.: Diagnostic techniques in venous thrombosis. In Surgery of the Veins. New York, Grune and Stratton, 1985, pp. 47-71.
5. Gallus, A.S., Hirsh, J., Hull, R., and vanAken, W.G.: Diagnosis of venous thromboembolism. Semin. Thromb. Hemost. 2: 203-231, 1976.
6. McLachlin, J., Richards, T., and Paterson, J.C.: An evaluation of clinical signs in the diagnosis of venous thrombosis. Arch. Surg., 85: 738-744, 1962.
7. Haeger, K.: Problems of acute deep venous thrombosis. The interpretation of signs and symptoms. Angiology, 20: 219-223, 1969.
8. Hull, R., Hirsh, J., Sackett, D.L., et al.: Clinical validity of a negative venogram in patients with clinically suspected venous thrombosis. Circulation, 64: 622-625, 1981.
9. Moore, E.E. and Marx, J.A.: Penetrating abdominal wounds. Rationale for exploratory laparotomy. J.A.M.A., 253: 2705-2708, 1985.
10. Shafton, G.W.: Indications for operation in abdominal trauma. Am J. Surg., 99: 657-664, 1960.
11. Thompson, J.S., Moore, E.E., VanDuzen-Moore, S., et al.: The evolution of abdominal stab wound management. J. Trauma, 20: 478-484, 1980.
12. Olsen, W.R. and Hildreth, D.H.: Abdominal paracentesis and peritoneal lavage in blunt abdominal trauma. J. Trauma, 11: 824-829, 1971.
13. Rodriquez, A., DuPriest, R.W., and Shatney, C.H.: Recognition of intraabdominal injury in blunt trauma victims. A prospective study comparing physical examination with peritoneal lavage. Am. Surg., 48: 456-459, 1982.

I-B: PHYSICAL DIAGNOSIS IS NOT OBSOLETE

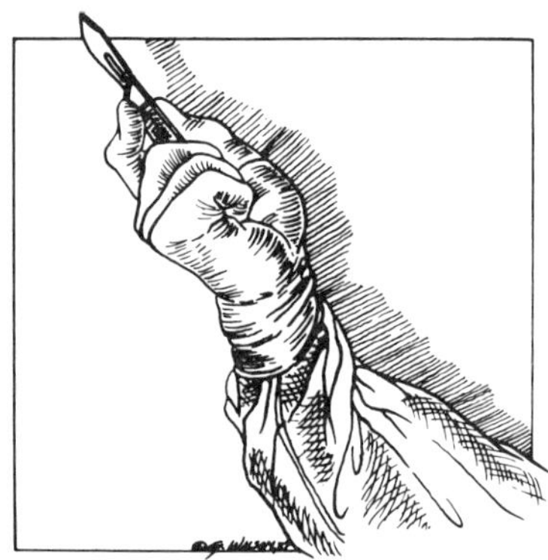

DEBORAH K. DAVIS, M.D.

Despite the technological advances of the last two decades, physical diagnosis is not obsolete. There are those who would say, "Why listen to the chest when you can get a chest x-ray? Why feel the abdomen when upper GI, ultrasound, MRI, and CT scan are available? No patient should enter the hospital without a urinalysis, SMA 12, EKG, chest x-ray, and one of three radiologic diagnostic studies."

Physical diagnosis is not obsolete. Obsolete is, according to Webster's, " . . . fallen into disuse, out of date, imperfectly developed." First of all, physical diagnosis has not fallen into disuse. We use it every day, every clinic visit, every admission, and not just because it is required by medical records and the Joint Commission on Hospital Accreditation. It is not out of date.

Disease and its physical manifestations have not changed. The description of thyroid disease, its signs, and its symptoms are no different now from what they were in 1909 when Kocher won the Nobel Prize for his treatise on the subject. Physical diagnosis may be imperfectly developed because it is subjectively limited by the training, alertness, and compulsiveness of the examiner. However, interviewing and examining a patient provide an impression based on the clinical evidence and the past experience of the doctor—an impression that is a gestalt, more than the sum of the parts.

Is this the art of medicine—to decide on the diagnosis and then spend thousands of dollars on tests that merely confirm that initial impression and make it appear that medicine is always scientific?

Sherlock Holmes said that " . . . on meeting a fellow mortal, learn at a glance to distinguish the history of the man and the trade or profession to which he belongs. By a man's fingernails, by his coat sleeve, by his boot, by his trouser knees, by the callosities of his fingers and thumb, by the expression, by his shirt cuffs. By each of these things, a man's calling is plainly revealed."

I ran across an interesting article by a British physician who claimed that he could make a diagnosis aided by an inspection of the patient's shoes and the odors and stains of his clothing. I am not advocating that we all should be like Sherlock Holmes. There is a place for the use of laboratory tests and other investigative methods, but we need to recognize that the key is to use history and physical examination to differentiate those patients with disease from those without disease and to guide our laboratory and radiologic examinations accordingly.

Physical diagnosis is cheap. It can be performed multiple times a day without extra charge. It may be rapid. The trauma patient can be evaluated rapidly by a quick examination, treatment can be prescribed quickly, and further studies can be directed accordingly. It is innocuous to the patient and it is wonderfully effective. No x-rays have replaced a hand on the abdomen to diagnose peritonitis with the resultant need for immediate surgical attention.

For those who say that physical diagnosis is obsolete, what is the alternative? The alternative to physical diagnosis is mandatory, serial, laboratory, radiologic, and interventional screening. In contrast, this approach to finding disease would not be cheap, rapid, innocuous, or effective.

The opposition states that physical diagnosis is obsolete because it is too crude, that we cannot detect disease—for example, cancer of the pancreas—by physical examination before it is too late to cure the patient. What we need to do is to detect it at an early stage when it is treatable. The problem hinges on the prevalence of disease. Let's go over a few basic statistical principles.

In 100 patients with disease X,[1] using a test that has a sensitivity of 65 percent and a specificity of 90 percent, 65 patients will have a positive test and 35 patients will have a negative test. If another 100 patients without the disease receive the same test, with the same sensitivity and specificity, 10 patients will have a positive test and 90 patients will have a negative test. If the prevalence of disease X is 5 percent, then for every 1,000 people, 50 patients will have the disease and 950 patients will have no disease. Sixty-five percent of the 50 patients with disease—or 33 patients with disease—will have a positive test. Ten percent of the 950 patients without disease—or 95 patients with no disease—will have a positive test. The total of 33 + 95 gives 128 patients both with and without disease who have a positive test; however, 95 of the 128—or 75 percent—positive tests occur in patients without disease. If the prevalence is 1 percent, 94 percent of positive testing will occur in patients without disease. If the sensitivity of the test is increased to 90 percent from 65 percent, the change is minimal; then only 91 percent rather than 94 percent of positive tests will be in patients without disease.

The problem with routine screening in asymptomatic patients is the prevalence of disease. However, history and physical examination can increase effectively detection of the prevalence of disease in a tested population by identifying those at risk and finding those with minimal suggestive symptoms or questionable findings on examination. If test X is thus used in these patients, the likelihood of finding disease is higher; and, therefore, the test is more valuable, predictive, and cost effective.

However, there are some diseases that have a high enough prevalence in the population that a routine screening is required to find those patients with disease who cannot be diagnosed by routine history and physical examination.

The three best examples are colon cancer, breast cancer, and lung cancer. However, let me make three statements.

For breast cancer, I will concede that mammography is very effective in identifying women with cancer that is not obvious on physical examination. However, the long-term results of our current screening methods in terms of overall survival and recurrences in patients treated at an early stage are still to be seen.

For colon cancer, a study by Bolt[2] showed that, despite the use of barium enema, colonoscopy, or sigmoidoscopy, a simple stool guaiac on routine physical examina-

TABLE I.   RATING OF TESTS FOR COLORECTAL CANCER*

PROCEDURE	PATIENT ACCEPTANCE (COMPLIANCE)	SENSITIVITY	SPECIFICITY	COST†	SAFETY‡ (INVASIVENESS)	TOTAL
Colon radiography	2	4	4	2	3	15
Colonoscopy	1	5	5	1	2	13
Sigmoidoscopy	2	3	3	3	4	15
Flexible sigmoidoscopy	3	3	4	3	4	17
Colon washings and cytology	2	1	2	2	4	11
Immunosurveillance	5	1	2	2	5	15
Testing for occult blood in stool	4	4	3	5	5	21

*Numbers 1 to 5 = poor to good.
†Cost 1 to 5 = most to least expensive.
‡Safety 1 to 5 = least safe to most safe, or most invasive (1) to least invasive (5).
*From Bolt, R.J.: Evaluation of screening tests for colorectal cancer. Primary Care, 7:683–689, 1980.

tion is the best way to screen for colon carcinoma (Table I).

For lung cancer, in a study by Collen and colleagues,[3] patients at high risk for lung cancer—in other words, male smokers more than 45 years of age—were screened with serial sputum cytology. They found that within those patients who were subsequently found to have carcinoma of the lung there was an increased thoracotomy rate and an increased resectability rate, but there was *no change* in overall survival compared with patients found by symptoms and changes on physical examination or routine chest x-ray.

Criteria for screening for disease must be: (1) the disease must result in significant morbidity or mortality; (2) there should be effective treatment for the disease; (3) the disease must have an asymptomatic period; (4) early detection must make a difference in prognosis; (5) the screening test should be accurate, simple, and acceptable to the population; and (6) the prevalence should be sufficient to justify screening costs and follow-up.[4]

The study by Sandler[5] showed that the history and physical examination was of diagnostic value in 83 percent of 630 patients and of value in patient management in 63 percent of patients. Routine laboratory tests were only of diagnostic value in 5 percent of patients and of management value in 9 percent of patients. Other special tests were of diagnostic value in 18 percent of patients and of management value in 24 percent of patients (Table II).

Another study by Hampton and colleagues[6] showed that 82.5 percent of 80 patients were diagnosed correctly by history alone. In 30 percent of these patients, the physical examination merely confirmed the diagnosis. In less than 10 percent, laboratory studies were required to determine the diagnosis. In 8 percent, laboratory tests were helpful in diagnosis or management only. In 90 percent of patients overall, the management could be confirmed on history and physical examination alone (Table III).

In conclusion, history and physical examination are the best screens for disease.

TABLE II. DIAGNOSTIC AND MANAGEMENT VALUES*

630-PATIENT SERIES		
	DIAGNOSTIC	MANAGEMENT
History, physical	83%	63%
Routine labs	5%	9%
Special tests	18%	24%

*From Sandler, G.: Costs of unnecessary tests. Br. Med. J., 6181:21–24, 1979.

TABLE III. DIAGNOSTIC ACCURACY*

80 PATIENTS

82.5 percent—Correctly diagnosed after history alone
30 percent—Physical-confirmed diagnosis
<10 percent—Laboratory required to confirm diagnosis
8 percent—Laboratory tests helpful in diagnosis or management
90 percent—Predict management on history and physical alone

*From Hampton, J.R., Harrison, M.J.G., Mitchell, J.R.A., et al.: Relative contributions of history-taking, physical examination, and laboratory investigation to diagnosis and management of medical outpatients. Br. Med. J., 2: 486–489, 1975.

They direct the use of other more probing tests and maintain the flexibility of medicine. Perhaps just as important, the history and physical examination establish a sympathetic, caring, and even tactile relationship between the physician and the patient. We live in an exciting age of nuclear, bioengineering, and computer advancement. The sensitive physician, however, establishes a compassionate relationship with each patient. The history and physical examination not only serve to bond that unique relationship but also serve to establish a foundation upon which further diagnosis and eventual therapy may be directed appropriately.

Fortunately, medicine remains a *very human* science. The physical examination and the resultant positive and reinforcing doctor-patient relationship most emphatically are not obsolete.

REFERENCES

1. Rose, S.D.: The periodic health examination. Primary Care, 7:653–665, 1980.
2. Bolt, R.J.: Evaluation of screening tests for colorectal cancer. Primary Care, 7:683–689, 1980.
3. Collen, M.F., Feldman, R., Siegelaub, A.B., and Crawford, D.: Dollar cost per positive test for automated multiphasic screening. N. Engl. J. Med., 283:459–463, 1970.
4. Riegelman, R.K.: The dogged physical examination in the era of the C.A.T. Primary Care, 7:625–635, 1980.
5. Sandler, G.: Costs of unnecessary tests. Br. Med. J., 2:21–24, 1979.
6. Hampton, J.R., Harrison, M.J.G., Mitchell, J.R.A., et al.: Relative contributions of history-taking, physical examination, and laboratory investigation to diagnosis and management of medical outpatients. Br. Med. J., 2:486–489, 1975.

DEBATE II

Is Gastric Cancer Curable?

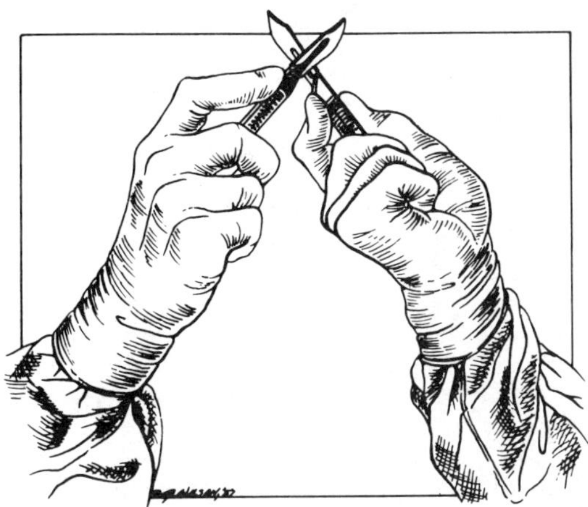

Cancer is the domain of the surgeon. More than 60 percent of all cancer that is cured is cured surgically. Surgery is invasive. Radical surgery is of necessity more invasive. In any therapeutic program, the potential risks and benefits must be weighed.

Halstedian principles dictate that cancer begins locally, spreads regionally, and eventually metastasizes widely. Any discussion of cancer prognosis must rigorously delineate the extent of disease being treated. Assuming a monotonously sequential, concentric spread of disease, histologic staging probably is relatively precise at the time of surgery. No current test, however, assesses the "biological aggression" of a tumor. Is gastric cancer a homogeneous entity?

Similarly, assume that two groups of 100 patients have gastric cancer and both will live four years. Additionally, assume that two *equal* therapies are initiated, one at one year (Group A) and one at three years (Group B). Again, assume the therapeutic value of the two therapies is *not* different. This exercise will indicate a huge, statistically significant benefit from the therapy provided to Group A patients.

Is "early" gastric cancer different from "late" gastric cancer? Are Japanese and American gastric cancers different? If there were 20,000 new cases of gastric cancer in 1985, why are there *no* prospective, randomized studies evaluating therapy?

Perhaps I am fickle, but I find the observation compelling that the survival from curative resections from gastric cancer is sufficiently rare that in any surgical series survival figures that include "curative" resections of 10 percent at five years are *not* distinguishable from those from series of patients undergoing palliative resections alone. Conversely, (1) if all patients without distant disease are explored, and (2) if nodes that would "upstage" a patient from Stage II to Stage III are biopsied, then a palliative procedure may be performed on patients with Stage III or IV disease. An extended total gastrectomy performed on patients with Stage I and II disease should *double* the 5-year survival.

I want to believe that gastric cancer is curable—I believe that an extended gastrectomy is what I would want for Stage I and II disease.

II-A: GASTRIC CANCER IS NOT CURABLE

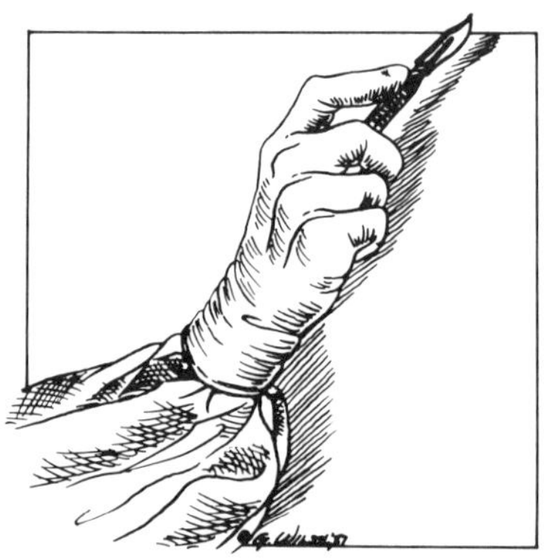

GLENN J.R. WHITMAN, M.D.

In 1985 there were approximately 25,000 new cases of gastric cancer and 14–15,000 deaths resulting from this disease.[1] Despite the tremendous experience medicine has had with this disease during this past century, evidence suggests that we are no better at treating this disease now than we were 30 years ago.[2] Fortunately, its incidence has declined from 30–38/100,000 of population in 1930 to 5–10/100,000 of population in 1980. It is the purpose of this discussion to convince doctors—and surgeons in particular—that surgery directed at curing gastric cancer is at best palliative and at worst a gross misdirection of energy, time, and expenditure for those patients with this dreadful problem.

Staging of gastric cancer has been based on gross appearance as well as on macroscopic features. In 1972 the American Joint Committee on Staging and End Results adopted a TNM classification that provided the basis for the current staging scheme (Table I).[3] This classification takes into consideration size of the lesion, level of nodal involvement, and presence or absence of distant metastases. Although this system improved the uniform staging of gastric cancer, a more simplified version will be used for this discussion: Stage O, I, II—early disease without nodal metastases; Stage III—N_1, N_2 nodes without visceral metastases; Stage IV—N_3 nodes or visceral metastases. This classification is based on the fact that the prognosis of gastric cancer is based almost solely on the presence or absence of nodal involvement: Stages I and

TABLE I. STAGE GROUPING OF CARCINOMA OF THE STOMACH*

Stage 0	Tis, N_0M_0
Stage I	T_1, N_0, M_0
Stage II	T_2, T_3; N_0, M_0
Stage III	T_1–T_3; N_1, N_2; M_0
	T_{4a}, N_0–N_2; M_0
Stage IV	T_1–T_3; N_3, M_0
	T_{4b}, any N, M_0
	Any T, and N, M_1

*From American Joint Committee on Cancer: *Manual for Staging Cancer,* 1983, p. 69.

II refer to cases without nodal involvement, Stage III with nodal involvement, and Stage IV with distant metastases.

In a review of his own personal series of 478 patients with gastric cancer seen between 1950 and 1972 at the Cleveland Clinic, Hoerr[4] revealed an aggressive approach to all gastric cancers, never assuming inoperability. His operability rate was 95 percent with an associated 10 percent mortality. Of the 460 patients in his series undergoing surgery, only one-third underwent curative resections. Hoerr found the following:

Stage	Number (%)	5-year Survivors (%)
I	82 (16)	67
II	59 (11)	23
III	28 (6)	11
Total	169	42 (N=72)

We see a combined survival rate for the 27 percent in Stages I and II (no positive nodes) of less than 50 percent. Furthermore, in spite of the 42 percent 5-year survival for the 169 patients undergoing resection for cure, another 12 percent recurred at ten years. It is important that, in this surgical series in which the referred cases had an operability rate of 95 percent, only 27 percent had negative nodes, with a less than 50 percent 5-year survival. If one considers that this series was selected from only surgical candidates, the population seen by the referral sources must have been significantly larger than that seen by Hoerr. The overall 5-year survival for the population at risk then would not be 15 percent but would be significantly less than that.

In another retrospective study, Bizer[5] reviewed the experience of 171 patients who were seen by his surgical service between 1972 and 1976. One hundred percent of patients underwent laparotomy with a 14 percent mortality. The overall 5-year survival in this surgical series was only 10 percent.

Of the 51 patients (29 percent) who were Stages I and II (no positive nodes), the 5-year survival was only 30 percent. Stage II patients had a 2 percent 5-year survival, and no Stage IV patient lived five years.

Again, as in Hoerr's series, of the less than one-third of patients who had negative nodes, there was only a 30 percent 5-year survival. Furthermore, this figure does not take into consideration the 10 to 15 percent recurrence rate between 5 and 10 years.

Finally, Adashek and colleagues[2] reviewed the UCLA experience of over 500 patients with gastric cancer who were seen between 1956 and 1975. In this series, 74 percent of patients seen by the surgical service underwent laparotomy with a 13 percent mortality. The overall 5-year survival was 13 percent. As seen in the previous two studies, only 26 percent of those operated upon were considered resections for cure. Although stage of disease is not given, 40 percent of those curative resections had negative nodes with only a 44 percent 5-year survival. Of the 60 percent with positive nodes, only 25 percent lived five years.

One criticism of all of these studies is that perhaps the correct operation was not done; i.e., conceivably the surgery was not sufficiently radical. Absolutely no randomized study exists that addresses this question. A review of applicable literature provides only circumstantial evidence; but, as seen below, the more radical resections do not fare better and probably fare worse.

Extent of Resection
(5-year Survivors)

	Subtotal (%)	Total (%)
Adashek[2]	40	0
Buchholtz[6]	17	16
Hoerr[4]	50	17
Longmire[7]	30	18

The issue of improving survival with increasingly radical surgery suffers from the lack of a randomized trial.

However, Papachristou and colleagues[8] provide compelling evidence that gastric cancer is not a localized disease. Eight patients who underwent a subtotal gastrectomy for Stages I and II gastric cancer and then died in the immediate postoperative period underwent autopsy. Absolutely no evidence of gastric cancer was found pathologically. However, as we have seen above, this is the identical group that has a greater than 50 to 60 percent 5-year mortality. Clearly, this is a strong argument that gastric cancer is not localized but rather is a microscopically systemic disease even in its earliest clinical stages.

To be complete, one must consider another presentation of gastric cancer seen predominantly in Japan. Referred to as "early gastric cancer," it is defined as cancer confined to the gastric mucosa or submucosa regardless of size or presence of lymph node metastases. Though its name implies early discovery, this is probably a misnomer. More correctly, it should be called *curable gastric cancer* for its biology is benign compared to the "advanced gastric cancer" discussed previously, better called *incurable gastric cancer.*

In a review by Coit and Brennan,[3] the incidence of early gastric cancer is at worst 40 percent in Japan while comprising only 5 to 15 percent of gastric cancer patients in the United States. As opposed to a resectability for cure rate of 25 to 30 percent as seen with advanced gastric cancer, virtually all early gastric cancers can be resected for cure.

Kodama and colleagues[9] report that in Stages I and II disease, their 5-year survival was greater than 90 percent; and, in patients with positive nodes, 40 percent survival was achieved. However, Isidore Cohen, Jr., M.D., comments that:

It seems likely that the carcinoma of the stomach they are treating is either a different disease than that which the majority of others are treating, or that they are finding it so much earlier, it is almost the same thing as another disease.[9]

Claude E. Welch, M.D., reiterates that:

Many individuals have stressed the differences between cancer of the stomach in Japan and in the United States, and conclusions drawn in one country will not necessarily be valid for others.[9]

If cancer of the stomach is resectable, it would make sense that adjuvant chemotherapy along with surgery should be of benefit. Several prospective, randomized trials examining this question have been performed. No significant effect has been established for thioTEPA, floxuridine, or mitomycin.

However, the gastrointestinal study group[10] did find the addition of 5-FU and methyl-CCNU to approach a significance in improving survival time (control vs. treated, 33 months mean survival vs. 48 months; p < 0.03). In the first year, there was no survival advantage, but at four years there was a 20 percent improvement in survival. However, in a study using a similar protocol, no impact was found.[3] One must conclude that, for adjuvant therapy for gastric cancer, there is no uniformly accepted role for chemotherapy.

In view of the above studies, which review recent results with gastric cancer, a summary of the course of a group of patients with gastric cancer is as follows:

Results of Surgical Therapy

N = 100 patients referred for surgery
90 operable lesions
80 survivors of surgery
30 patients resected for cure
5 patients of the 12 with negative lymph nodes who will survive five years
5 patients of the 18 with positive lymph nodes who will survive five years
Total: 10 5-year survivors

As slight as this survival might be, the argument for the surgical therapy of gastric cancer still revolves around a 0 percent survival without surgery. But is this in fact the case?

Perhaps the most revealing study on the natural history of gastric cancer is by Longmire and colleagues.[7] Figure 1 and Table II summarize the results pertinent to this question. Between 1957 and 1968, over 600 patients with gastric cancer were followed. Surgical therapy was standardized as much as possible. Although one purpose of the study was to determine the benefit of thioTEPA as adjuvant chemotherapy, another purpose was to analyze the data for subsets that might relate to prognosis. Results showed that, of the 254 patients receiving palliative surgery with evidence of residual cancer tissue, 5 percent of the control group and 8 percent of the thioTEPA-treated group survived five years. Clearly, this rivals the survival data for curative resections.

In conclusion, the results of surgery for gastric cancer as seen in the United States (excluding early gastric cancer) are abysmal. In preselected surgical series, the 5-year survival is no bettter than 10 percent, with another 10 to 15 percent recurrence rate between 5 and 10 years. Though no prospective, randomized studies exist, more radical surgery does not appear to be of benefit. Furthermore, adjuvant chemotherapy, most notably 5-FU with methyl-CCNU, has no proven benefit. Perhaps the most important fact to be considered is that the survival from curative resections is so rare that

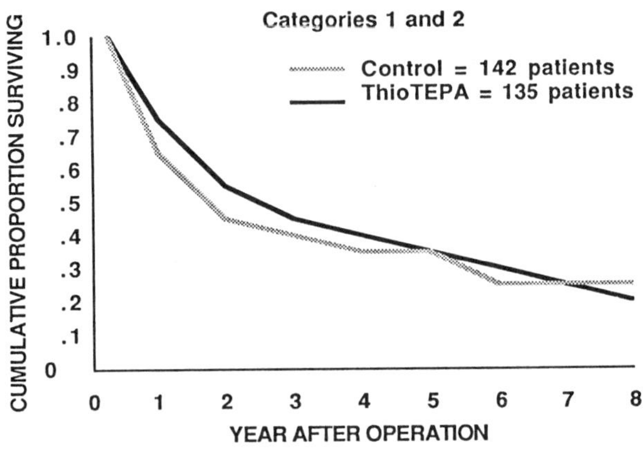

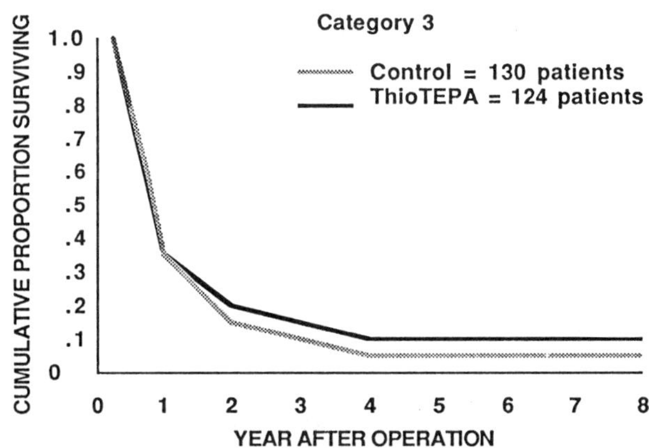

FIGURE 1. Survival curves for all patients by category and control and thioTEPA groups (excluding 30-day deaths). From Longmire, W.P., Kuzma, J.W., and Dixon, W.J.: The use of triethylenethiophosphoramide as an adjuvant to the surgical treatment of gastric cancer. Ann. Surg., 167:304, 1968.

in any given surgical series survival figures that include "curative" resections of 10 percent at five years are not distinguishable from those in patients undergoing palliative resections alone. It appears that curative surgical attempts have no influence and are in vain.

REFERENCES

1. A Cancer Journal for Clinicians, 35(1):26-27, 1985
2. Adashek, K., Sanger, J., and Longmire, W. P.: Cancer of the stomach. Ann. Surg., 189:6-10, 1979.

TABLE II. SURVIVAL RATES BY CATEGORY, CONTROL AND thioTEPA GROUPS AND OTHER VARIABLES (EXCLUDING 30-DAY DEATHS)*

	CATEGORY 1 & 2		CATEGORY 3		ALL CATEGORIES	
	CONTROL	ThioTEPA	CONTROL	ThioTEPA	CONTROL	ThioTEPA
ONE YEAR SURVIVAL						
Male	0.71	0.76	0.33	0.38	0.54	0.58
Female	0.62	0.76	0.47	0.38	0.53	0.56
Without concomitant diseases	0.79	0.70	0.39	0.39	0.63	0.56
With concomitant diseases	0.65	0.77*	0.37	0.38	0.51	0.58
Without complications	0.69	0.82*	0.38	0.41	0.54	0.62
With complications	0.64	0.68	0.37	0.33	0.51	0.52
Without positive lymph nodes	0.75	0.89*	0.54	0.52	0.71	0.76
With positive lymph nodes	0.63	0.66	0.35	0.34	0.46	0.49
Without serosal involvement	0.76	0.88	0.57	0.39	0.71	0.75
With serosal involvement	0.65	0.68	0.35	0.38	0.48	0.51
Without other organs removed	0.78	0.86	0.38	0.40	0.56	0.61
With other organs removed	0.60	0.66	0.38	0.33	0.51	0.54
Without recurrence	0.89	0.85	0.59	0.78	0.81	0.83
With recurrence	0.52	0.67	0.33	0.31	0.41	0.45
THREE YEAR SURVIVAL						
Male	0.42	0.46	0.11	0.13	0.28	0.31
Female	0.41	0.49	0.09	0.12	0.23	0.29
Without concomitant diseases	0.39	0.36	0.04	0.18	0.25	0.28
With concomitant diseases	0.42	0.50	0.11	0.11	0.27	0.31
Without complications	0.42	0.53	0.09	0.16	0.26	0.35
With complications	0.40	0.40	0.12	0.08	0.26	0.25
Without positive lymph nodes	0.53	0.75	0.15	0.34	0.46	0.61
With positive lymph nodes	0.35	0.27	0.10	0.07	0.20	0.16
Without serosal involvement	0.53	0.65	0.07	0.11	0.43	0.51
With serosal involvement	0.35	0.36	0.10	0.13	0.22	0.23
Without other organs removed	0.54	0.55	0.07	0.10	0.28	0.32
With other organs removed	0.31	0.39	0.15	0.12	0.24	0.29
Without recurrence	0.79	0.73	0.41	0.67	0.69	0.71
With recurrence	0.12	0.22	0.04	0.04	0.07	0.11
FIVE YEAR SURVIVAL						
Male	0.33	0.31	0.06	0.12	0.21	0.23
Female	0.31	0.40	0.04	0.00	0.16	0.19
Without concomitant diseases	0.36	0.18	0.04	0.09	0.23	0.14
With concomitant diseases	0.31	0.39	0.05	0.07	0.18	0.24
Without complications	0.32	0.38	0.03	0.11	0.18	0.24
With complications	0.31	0.30	0.09	0.04	0.20	0.18
Without positive lymph nodes	0.39	0.54	0.15	0.23	0.35	0.44
With positive lymph nodes	0.29	0.19	0.04	0.03	0.14	0.11
Without serosal involvement	0.41	0.45	0.07	0.11	0.33	0.36
With serosal involvement	0.28	0.27	0.05	0.07	0.15	0.16
Without other organs removed	0.40	0.36	0.03	0.08	0.20	0.21
With other organs removed	0.25	0.31	0.08	0.07	0.19	0.22
Without recurrence	0.66	0.65	0.32	0.54	0.57	0.63
With recurrence	0.06	0.04	0.00	0.00	0.03	0.02
EIGHT YEAR SURVIVAL						
Male	0.26	0.25	0.06	0.12	0.17	0.19
Female	0.19	0.31	0.04	0.00	0.10	0.15
Without concomitant diseases	0.29	0.11	0.04	0.09	0.19	0.10
With concomitant diseases	0.21	0.33	0.05	0.07	0.13	0.21

*From Longmire, W.P., Kuzma, J.W., and Dixon, W.J.: The use of triethylenethiophosphoramide as an adjuvant to the surgical treatment of gastric cancer. Ann. Surg., 167:307, 1968.

3. Coit, D. G. and Brennan, M. F.: Gastric cancer. In Surgical Treatment of Digestive Diseases. F. G. Moody, L. C. Carey, R. S. Jones, et al. (eds.). Chicago, Yearbook Medical Publishers, 1986, pp. 239-256.

4. Hoerr, S. O.: Prognosis for carcinoma of the stomach. Surg. Gynecol. Obstet., 137:205-209, 1973.

5. Bizer, L. S.: Adenocarcinoma of the stomach: Current results of treatment. Cancer, 51:743-745, 1983.

6. Buchholtz, T. W., Welch, C. E., and Malt, R. A.: Clinical correlates of resectability and survival in gastric carcinoma. Ann. Surg., 188:711-715, 1978.

7. Longmire, W. P., Kuzma, J. W., and Dixon, W. J.: The use of triethylenethiophosphoramide as an adjuvant to the surgical treatment of gastric cancer. Ann. Surg., 167:293-312, 1968.

8. Papachristou, D. N. and Fortner, J. G.: Is gastric cancer generalized at the time of surgery? J. Surg. Oncol., 18:27-29, 1981.

9. Kodama, Y., Sugimachi, K., Soejima, K., et al.: Growth patterns and prognosis in early gastric cancer. World J. Surg., 5:241-248, 1981.

10. Gastrointestinal Study Group. Controlled trial of adjuvant chemotherapy following curative resection for gastric cancer. Cancer, 49:1116-1122, 1982.

II-B: GASTRIC CANCER IS CURABLE

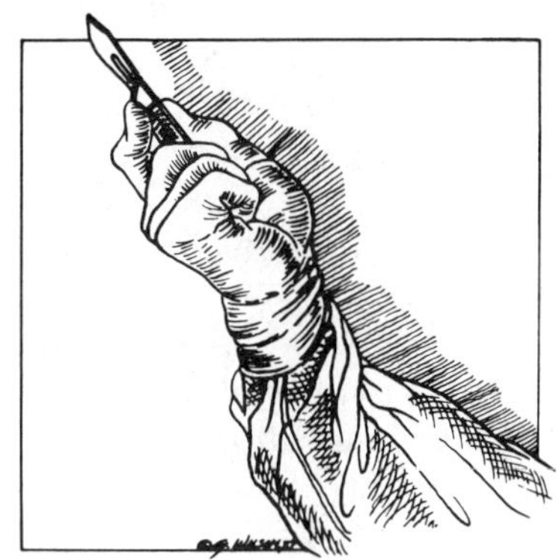

JOHN A. RIDGE, M.D., Ph.D.

Each year in the United States there are some 25,000 new cases of gastric cancer and some 14,300 deaths. Thus gastric cancer ranks fifth in cancer-causing mortality. Sixty percent of the victims are men, and 70 percent are from "lower" socioeconomic groups. There is no known association with tobacco or alcohol use.

More than 90 percent of gastric malignancies are adenocarcinomas, more than 70 percent are ulcerative, and most tumors develop in the antrum. The adenocarcinomas spread rapidly to regional nodes. They involve not only the perigastric nodes but also nodes of the porta hepatis, celiac, pancreatic, splenic hilar, and transverse mesocolon.

Current approaches to gastric cancer offer dismal results. In a collected review of 19,000 patients[1] (comprising 11 series), the 5-year survivals range from 5 to 17 percent. In fact, in seven of the 11 reports, the 5-year survival is less than 10 percent (Table I).

In the analysis of treatment and survival for any malignancy, it is important to elaborate a staging system. Other staging protocols have been used, but the TNM staging method described by Kennedy[2] will be used throughout this discussion. All referenced results were originally reported using it, with the exception of the Japanese work, which I have reinterpreted. T refers to the primary tumor. T1 disease is *limited to the mucosa and/or submucosa.* T2 disease extends *to and/or into the serosa.* T3 disease *penetrates the serosa.* T4 tumors extend to *non-gastric tissue.*

The staging with respect to nodal involvement is particularly important to this discussion. NO disease obviously means that *no nodes* are involved. N1 means that *gastric lymph nodes within 3 centimeters* of the tumor are involved. N2 nodes are *more*

TABLE I.   COLLECTED REVIEW OF 19,000 PATIENTS*

5-year survivals range from 5 to 17 percent in 11 series
5-year survival is less than 10 percent in 7 of the 11 reports

*From Dupont, J., Lee, J., Burton, G., et al.: Adenocarcinoma of the stomach: Review of 1,497 cases. Cancer, 41:941-947, 1978.

than 3 centimeters from the tumor (including the opposite curve). N3 lesions involve *regional non-gastric* nodes.

If there is metastatic disease, then the cancer is M1.

Thus, early gastric cancer is T1, NO-N3, MO. Stage I disease is T1-T3, NO, MO. Stage II disease is T4, NO or T1-T4, N1, MO. If the tumor is N2, MO, then it is Stage III; and it is Stage IV with any M1. There is an inverse correlation between stage and survival.

However, there is a dramatic weakness in the staging system.[3] Patients who died within a month after curative resection for gastric cancer were autopsied. None of eight patients who were Stage I or Stage II had any residual tumor. However, 10 of 13 (70 percent) of Stage III patients had residual tumor—typically as lung or liver metastases (Table II). This is a significant difference, and an important one. This study means that, as far as surgical treatment is concerned, the staging system is inadequate. The majority of patients in Stage II—and this means all those with nodes on the contralateral curve or more than 3 centimeters from the primary—already have metastatic disease. Unfortunately, in the United States today, 70 percent of patients have Stage III or IV gastric cancers at presentation. Such advanced cancers are not amenable to surgery—a local-regional therapy.

Surgery can remove the primary tumor to prevent obstruction. We can obtain tumor-free margins around the cancer. We can remove nodes that are likely to be involved with the disease. However, surgical therapy is *regional*, and tumor-free margins cannot be secured on concurrent but unrecognized lung metastases. In 70 percent of Stage III patients (those who appear to have only regional nodes involved), the cancer already has spread too far for removal.

In fact, for curative resection to have any impact on gastric cancer survival at all, operations must be able to cure node-positive cancers. If this is true, then radical resections should work better than limited operations. In addition, one must perform big procedures with low enough mortality and morbidity to justify surgical attack.

Fortunately, node involvement does not mean that gastric cancer is incurable. Fifteen percent of early gastric cancers have positive nodes; and the 5-year survival with N1 lesions is 85 percent, in contrast to 95 percent for NO tumors (Table III).[4] Early gastric cancer is not special—if you observe the lesion without treatment, the 5-year survival is only 65 percent. It becomes "late" gastric cancer! Hence, we have confidence that operations can cure gastric cancer, even if it has spread beyond the stomach.

Given that an operation can cure more advanced cancers, which should we choose? The usual procedure performed in the United States is the *subtotal gastrec-*

**TABLE II.   WEAKNESS OF THIS STAGING
(EARLY AUTOPSY)***

Stage I-II patients	0/8 residual disease
Stage III patients	10/13 residual disease
This difference is significant (p < 0.01)	

*From Papachristou, D. and Fortner, J.: Is gastric cancer generalized at the time of surgery? J. Surg. Oncol., 18:27–29, 1981.

TABLE III. OPERATIONS CAN CURE
NODE-POSITIVE CANCERS*

Early gastric cancer
15 percent have positive nodes (N1-N2)

5-year survival in NO lesions is 95 percent after resection

5-year survival in N1 lesions is 85 percent after resection

*From Murakami, T.: Early cancer of the stomach. World J. Surg.,
3(6):685–692, 1979.

tomy, which involves resection of the appropriate portion of the stomach, contiguous viscus, and both omenta. I recommend the *extended total gastrectomy,* which entails resection of the entire stomach, the distal esophagus, the first part of the duodenum, the spleen, both omenta, the distal pancreas, and the celiac nodes. This is a big operation! Is it of any benefit?

Even without consideration of survival, the extended total gastrectomy offers better palliation than does subtotal gastrectomy. The local recurrence rate drops from 33 percent to 18 percent (a significant difference) if the big procedure is used.

More importantly, the extended total gastrectomy cures "late" gastric cancer as long as the disease remains confined to the region of the stomach. Table IV compares the results of operations for Stages I and II gastric cancer at a single institution, Memorial Hospital in New York.[5] It is important to remember that these do not represent the results of a randomized trial. However, in all parts of the stomach, the extended total gastrectomy offers 2.5- to 5-fold higher survival than the subtotal gastrectomy. In most cases, the differences are significant. The results for antral lesions (admittedly, only 11 extended total resections were performed for antral gastric cancer) are particularly impressive.

In results from the personal series of a single surgeon, Kodama[6] has performed more than 400 operations for gastric cancer (Table V). He engaged in traditional subtotal gastrectomies until 1963 and then changed his therapy to extended subtotal gastrectomies involving meticulous lymph node dissections. In patients whose primary lesion extended to the serosa, the 5-year survival for extended dissection was 45 percent (in contrast to 18 percent after traditional subtotal gastrectomy). This difference is significant. In patients with involved lymph nodes, the 5-year survival of extended subtotal gastrectomy was 39 percent, while that for subtotal gastrectomy was

TABLE IV. EXTENDED RESECTIONS REDUCE
LOCAL RECURRENCE*

RESECTION	RECURRENCE
Extended total	18 percent (17/93)
Subtotal	33 percent (26/79)
This difference is significant (p < 0.05)	

*From Papachristou, D. and Fortner, J.: Local recurrence of gastric adenocarcinomas after gastrectomy. J. Surg. Oncol., 18:47–53, 1981.

TABLE V.   BIGGER OPERATIONS CAN CURE BIGGER CANCERS*

5-YEAR SURVIVALS FOR TUMORS AFTER RESECTION

Site	Extended	Subtotal	p
Serosa	45 percent (113/251)	18 percent (33/179)	< 0.001
Nodes	39 percent (95/245)**	18 percent (32/181)	< 0.001

*Adapted from Kodama, Y., Sugimachi, K., Soejima, K., et al.: Evaluation of extensive lymph node dissection for carcinoma of the stomach. World J. Surg., 5:243, 1981.
**EGC n = 23

18 percent. Again, this is a significant difference. It is noteworthy that only 23 patients with involved nodes (less than 10 percent) had early gastric cancer. In fact, some of the 5-year survivors actually had N2 node involvement. In other words, the extended resection cured Stage III gastric cancers.

Surgical procedures of such magnitude are justified only if they can be performed with low mortality. In fact, they are safe in the hands of experienced surgeons. Between 1970 and 1975 at Memorial Hospital, the extended total gastrectomy was performed with an 8.5 percent mortality, while at Vanderbilt University between 1960 and 1983 the operative mortality was 9.6 percent. At these institutions the mortality for "ordinary" subtotal gastrectomy was entirely comparable. In Kodama's personal series of extended subtotal gastrectomies (between 1964 and 1972), more than 240 operations were performed with only 1.7 percent mortality.[6-8]

From these data one may conclude that operations do cure patients with positive lymph nodes (in early gastric cancer, Stage I and Stage II). Extended resections increase the frequency of 5-year survivors (200–300 percent). The extended resections can be performed without added mortality (less than 10 percent for subtotal gastrectomy or for the much more aggressive extended total gastrectomy).

Hence, there are distinguishable management paradigms for gastric cancer. Of 100 patients with gastric cancer, 70 will have distant disease (Stage II or Stage IV cancers). There will be four 5-years survivors. If subtotal gastrectomies are performed on the remaining 30 patients (with 20 percent 5-year survival), then a total of 10 patients will survive five years. In fact, these are the survival figures currently obtained in the United States.

In contrast, if extended gastrectomy is performed, then the same four individuals with Stage III and Stage IV cancer will be alive after five years. However, one may anticipate a 5-year survival—or 60 percent—for the 30 patients who present with Stage I and Stage II tumors. Twenty-two patients will live for five years. The number of "cured" patients will be doubled (Table VI).[8-10]

These statistics suggest an approach to the surgical management of patients with gastric cancer. All patients without distant disease should be explored. Nodes that would "upstage" a patient from Stage II to Stage III should be biopsied. The principles of cancer surgery are not abrogated by this biopsy: If the nodes are involved, then the cancer is Stage III (and incurable). Palliative procedures can be performed for patients who prove to have Stage III or Stage IV disease at laparotomy. If the patient proves to

TABLE VI. EXTENDED RESECTIONS THAT CAN CURE "LATE" CANCERS*

5-YEAR SURVIVALS FOR STAGES I AND II			
Site	Extended Total	Subtotal	p
Fundus	68 percent	13 percent	< 0.01
Cardia	83 percent	16 percent	< 0.03
Midstomach	42 percent	17 percent	NS
Antrum	100 percent	37 percent	< 0.02
	n = 147	n = 114	

*From Shiu, M., Papachristou, D., Kosloff, C., et al.: Selection of operative procedure for adenocarcinoma of the midstomach. Ann. Surg., 192:730-737, 1980; Papachristou, D. and Fortner, J.: Adenocarcinoma of the gastric cardia—Choice of gastrectomy. Ann. Surg., 192:58-64, 1980; Papachristou, D. and Fortner, J.: Selection of gastrectomy for adenocarcinoma arising in the gastric fundus. J. Surg. Oncol., 21:165-169, 1982.

have Stage I or Stage II gastric cancer after exploration (and staging lymph node biopsy), then extended total gastrectomy should be performed.

Gastric cancer can be cured.

REFERENCES

1. Dupont J., Lee, J., Burton, G., et al.: Adenocarcinoma of the stomach: Review of 1,497 cases. Cancer, 41:941-947, 1978.
2. Kennedy, B.: TNM classification for stomach cancer. Cancer, 26:971-983, 1970.
3. Papachristou, D. N. and Fortner, J. G.: Is gastric cancer generalized at the time of surgery? J. Surg. Oncol., 18:27-29, 1981.
4. Murakami, T.: Early cancer of the stomach. World J. Surg., 3(6):685-692, 1979.
5. Papachristou, D. and Fortner, J.: Local recurrence of gastric adenocarcinomas after gastrectomy. J. Surg. Oncol., 18:47-53, 1981.
6. Kodama, Y., Sugimachi, K., Soejima, K., et al.: Evaluation of extensive lymph node dissection for carcinoma of the stomach. World J. Surg., 5:241-248, 1981.
7. Scott, W., Adkins, R., and Sawyers, J.: Results of an aggressive surgical approach to gastric carcinoma during a twenty-three year period. Surgery, 97:55-59, 1985.
8. Shiu, M., Papachristou, D., Kosloff, C., et al.: Selection of operative procedure for adenocarcinoma of the midstomach. Ann. Surg., 192:730-737, 1980.
9. Papachristou, D. and Fortner, J.: Adenocarcinoma of the gastric cardia—Choice of gastrectomy. Ann. Surg., 192:58-64, 1980.
10. Papachristou, D. and Fortner, J.: Selection of gastrectomy for adenocarcinoma arising in the gastric fundus. J. Surg. Oncol., 21:165-169, 1982.

DEBATE III

Should Rectal Adenocarcinoma Be Treated by Abdominoperineal Resection or Fulguration?

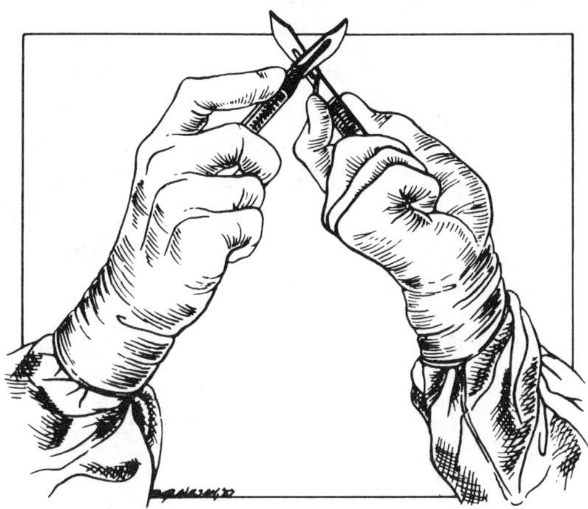

Responsible surgeons continually search for less invasive methods of curing cancer. The following discussion illustrates one of the fundamental questions in modern surgery: Is cancer a local or a systemic disease?

As most of us believe, cancer begins with a single cell, and that cell divides unchecked. Initial spread is to regional nodes. Distant spread is late. Halstedian principles suggest that a period exists during which the entire neoplastic process may be encompassed within a surgical resection. If the surgical excision is bigger or earlier, the likelihood of cure should be increased.

Big surgery, however, may result in big complications. This observation has resulted in a decrease in the popularity of radical mastectomy in favor of more limited breast resection. Similarly, pneumonectomy for cancer essentially has been retired in favor of lobectomy or even wedge resection.

Can local fulguration of rectal cancer possibly result in control comparable to abdominoperineal resection of the tumor, rectum, and adjacent nodes? Drs. Saueracker and Brown argue that a limited, local procedure (fulguration) must comprise cancer control. Although definitive and complete tumor excision requires a more extensive procedure, operative mortality for AP resection has plummeted from the 41 percent originally cited by Miles to recent reports of 1.7 percent. The primary responsibility of the surgical oncologist is control of cancer. The trivial reduction in morbidity associated with a limited procedure that merely skims (or burns) the surface of a tumor that could be cured by en bloc resection is not warranted.

Conversely, Dr. Baxter points to the colostomized, impotent, incontinent, and ungrateful patient who has weathered an abdominoperineal resection and argues that this patient's 5- and 10-year survivals are not different from those of the patient initially treated locally.

If cancer does develop in a primary site, is there an interval during which viable tumor has spread to but is contained in adjacent nodes? Ultimately, is regional lymphadenectomy therapeutic or diagnostic (please see separate Debate on this issue)? Dr. Baxter cites studies indicating that tumor cells do not even decelerate as they pass through regional nodes.

In order to compare two surgical procedures, we must analyze comparable groups of patients. Surgeons do not argue that patients with Dukes Stage C (N-2 disease) lesions have a poor survival. Fulguration, however, prevents stratification. In this regard, must we resign ourselves to comparing baskets of apples and oranges? Dr. Baxter thinks not. He believes that over 90 percent of patients with rectal adenocarcinoma will derive no survival benefit by undergoing an AP resection but will be exposed to the additional morbidity and mortality associated with this operation. When fulguration alone is performed, survival is comparable to abdominoperineal resection. Initial fulguration does not adversely affect survival if AP resection is subsequently performed.

III-A: ABDOMINOPERINEAL RESECTION FOR RECTAL ADENOCARCINOMA

ANDREW J. SAUERACKER, M.D.
JAMES M. BROWN, M.D.

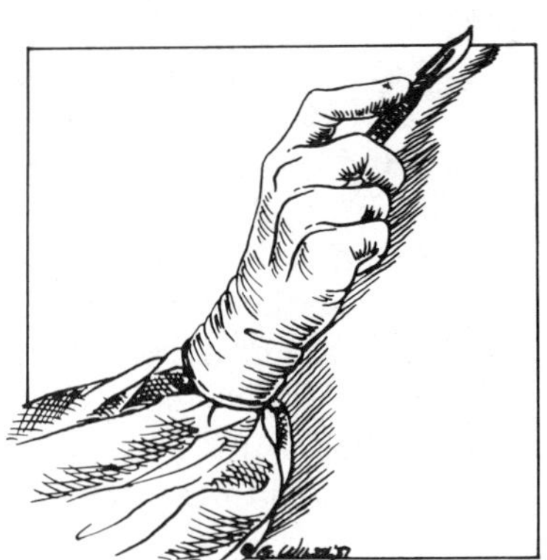

The abdominoperineal resection remains the gold standard for the treatment of low rectal cancer. The ensuing discussion will cover pertinent aspects of rectal cancer, the technique, results, and complications of the AP resection, and, finally, an interpretation of the flaws of local therapy (of which fulguration, or electrodesiccation, is only one aspect).

Colorectal cancer is the second most common visceral cancer in the United States. Rectal cancers comprise 30 to 40 percent of colorectal tumors. In 1985 an estimated 42,000 new cases of rectal cancer were diagnosed with an estimated 8,300 deaths.

A strict histologic definition of rectal cancer needs to be emphasized. The World Health Organization requires invasive penetration on the muscularis mucosa (into submucosa). Anything less should be termed "adenoma" with cellular atypia or dysplasia. The terms "cacinoma *in situ*" or "superficial carcinoma" should be avoided.[1] The key point is that metastatic disease does not occur in the absence of submucosal invasion. In weighing the subsequent discussion, you are urged to pay particular attention to the lesions treated by fulguration, as most series include many noncancerous adenomas. The overwhelming majority of rectal cancers are adenocarcinomas. Again, studies comparing treatment modalities for rectal cancer must be limited to the treatment of adenocarcinomas alone.

Rectal cancer tends to progress in an orderly fashion. So-called horizontal growth produces annular lesions that eventually constrict bowel lumen. More importantly, vertical growth results in bowel wall invasion. Below the peritoneal reflection (about 10 cm from the anus), bowel wall penetration into the mesorectum occurs. Lateral spread along the distribution of the middle hemorrhoidal vessels or upward spread along the distribution of the superior hemorrhoidal vessels then occurs. Distal growth in bowel wall or mesorectum is rare, except in advanced disease with proximal lymphatic obstruction.[2] Hematogenous dissemination into the portal or systemic circulation is possible, although the vast majority of distant matastases are first seen in the liver.

The visualized size of the primary tumor is a poor predictor of extent of disease. Palpable evidence of bowel wall mobility or fixation is a better indicator of depth of penetration, and depth of penetration does correlate with lymph node status.[3] Histologic grade (degree of differentiation) is much less significant than disease stage.

The prognosis for patients with rectal cancer is closely related to the depth of penetration and presence or absence of regional lymph node metastases. This is the basis of the Dukes staging system as described in 1940: Stage A tumor limited to submucosa, no nodal metastases; Stage B tumor invading the muscular layer, no nodal metastases; and Stage C tumor of any depth with nodal metastases. A subsequently added Stage D included tumors with distant metastases.

Multiple series since then show remarkably similar 5-year survival rates—90 percent for A lesions, 60 percent for B lesions, 30 percent for C lesions, and near 0 percent for D lesions.[4] Few recurrences are noted past five years. Obviously, staging information (and thus prognosis) can be provided only by an en bloc resection of the primary lesion with its regional node-bearing tissue.

The abdominoperineal resection was popularized by Miles in 1908.[5] With few modifications, this is the procedure performed today for those rectal cancers not amenable to resection with primary reanastomosis. It involves removal of the anorectum with its mesorectum and the so-called "zone of upward spread" to near the origin of the inferior mesenteric artery. Generally utilizing two surgical teams, a permanent end sigmoid colostomy is created and the perineum closed.

With the advent of the EEA stapler and the realization that the distal bowel wall margin can be less than the traditional 5 cm, many midrectal lesions formerly treated by AP resection are now resected with sphincter preservation.[6] Additional technical controversies include preservation or sacrifice of the left colic artery, management of the pelvic and perineal wounds, and extent of the pelvic lymphadenectomy. Preoperative chemotherapy and/or radiation therapy may be of benefit in selected cases.

The abdominoperineal resection remains a formidable operation, although operative mortality figures have plummeted to the 2 to 5 percent range from Miles' original 41 percent. Morbidity remains high—approximately 40 to 60 percent. Urologic, perineal, and stomal complications account for the majority of complications.[4]

The results of a recent retrospective review from Boston published by Rosen and colleagues[4] reveal typical 5- and 10-year survival figures based on Dukes stage in their 200 patients. Operative mortality was 1.7 percent; morbidity was 60 percent. Local recurrence occurred in 10 percent (all Stage B or C); distant recurrence occurred in 33 percent (all Dukes stages represented). Median time to recurrence tended to be shorter for more advanced lesions, but median time from recurrence to death was relatively consistent. This kind of follow-up information is often lacking for patients treated by local means.

Proponents of local therapy (including fulguration) point to similar survival rates with far less morbidity. However, as previously mentioned, the lesions dealt with in this manner often are poorly characterized and may include noncancerous adenomas in up to 50 percent of cases.[7] Also, anal and atypical rectal tumors may make up as much as 15 percent of cases.[8] Because the Dukes classification cannot be identified in locally treated cases, comparisons of 5-year survivals are not possible or valid. Finally, even in institutions where local therapy is encouraged, only a small fraction of patients with rectal cancer (3 to 12 percent) are treated in this fashion.[9, 10, 11]

TABLE I. STUDIES SUPPORTING FULGURATION

Hoekstra, et al.[13]	Cancer, 1985
Madden and Kandalaft[12]	Surg. Gynecol. Obstet., 1983
Hughes, et al.[14]	Dis. Colon Rectum, 1982
Crile & Turnbull[15]	Surg. Gynecol. Obstet., 1972
Madden & Kandalaft[7]	Am. J. Surg., 1971

Table I depicts a group of studies in which the operative mortality in patients treated with AP resection is indicated. Though Madden and Kandalaft[12] claim that an operative mortality of 10 percent exists in the United States for AP resection, in their paper supporting fulguration the average shown as of 1974 is 7.7 percent, with two studies creating a large upward shift in this percentage. Surely, in 1987 operative mortality is less than 7.7 percent.

Let's do some calculations. Assume 7 percent operative mortality and 50 percent presentation with positive nodes. Of patients with positive nodes, one-third will live five years. Of 100 patients, seven will die of operation. Seventeen of the 50 with positive nodes will live five years. This is a positive balance of 10 patients whose disease would have gone unseen, unresected, and untreated if they had been fulgurated.

Permit us to critique several of the studies supporting fulguration. The paper by Hoekstra and colleagues[13] acknowledges the following selection criteria:

1. 2-10 cm in rectum from anal orifice,
2. lesions must be less than one-third circumference of rectal wall,
3. lesions must show exophytic or polypoid growth,
4. no evidence of bowel wall infiltration by tumor on physical examination,
5. no palpable adenopathy, and
6. tumor or node well differentiated by biopsy prior to procedure.

This select group of patients cannot properly be compared to all patients with rectal cancer treated by resection.

The study by Madden and Kandalaft[12] reports in favor of fulguration. They studied 204 patients treated with fulguration for rectal cancer and reported a 77 percent overall 5-year survival. This compares to an overall survival rate of 50 percent for rectal cancer patients treated by resection. This initially seems good; again, patient selection may have played a role. *Excluded* from this study were high rectal lesions that could not be encompassed safely by fulguration, anterior wall tumors in females, and invasive circumferential lesions. Though these exclusions account for a minority of patients, the patient selection criteria alone cast doubt on any comparison made.

Furthermore, the fulguration complication rate in Madden and Kandalaft's group was 23.5 percent with no mortality (Table II). Fifty percent of complications involved hemorrhage requiring transfusion or operative hemostasis. The average number of fulguration sessions was four, with as many as 13 sessions. Also, in looking at survival at five years for those lesions greater than 3 cm in size, the percentage drops to 57.

Hughes and colleagues[14] showed a 92 percent, 5-year disease-free survival for patients selected with exophytic or polypoid rectal cancers. Thirty-seven of 39

TABLE II.   COMPLICATIONS OF FULGURATION*
MORBIDITY STUDY 204 PATIENTS

COMPLICATION	Pts.	%
Bleeding**	33***	16.1
Perforation	2	0.9
Rectovag. Fist.	4	1.9
Pul. Emb.	1	0.5
Fem. Art. Throm.	1	0.5
Rec. Stricture	5	2.4
Rectal Prolapse	2	0.9
Total	48	23.5

*From Madden, J.L. and Kandalaft: Electrocoagulation as a primary curative method in the treatment of carcinoma of the rectum Surg. Gynecol. Obstet., 157:166, 1983.
**Stopped spont.: 16 (48.9%)
   Bl. trans.: 16 (48.9%)
***69% of pts. with complications bled.

patients had well- or moderately well-differentiated carcinoma proven by biopsy. Hughes found only a 33 percent 5-year disease-free survival in patients with ulcerative lesions.

Crile and Turnbull[15] studied 226 patients treated with fulguration and 62 patients treated with AP resection. They *excluded* high rectal lesions, ulcerating annular lesions, and anterior wall lesions ending toward the vagina. In the fulguration group, the average tumor size was 3.1 cm, whereas in the AP resection group, average tumor size was 4.8 cm. Even though the resected patients seemed to have more advanced disease, their 5-year survival compared favorably—57 percent for fulguration versus 52 percent for AP resection.

A specific concession is made in the case of the pedunculated adenoma with focally invasive well-differentiated carcinoma confined to the polyp's head and without evidence of lymphatic or vascular invasion. Local excision, by whatever means, is curative in these usual cases.[10, 11]

To conclude, based on a rational interpretation of current literature, the abdominoperineal resection remains the definitive treatment for applicable rectal cancers. Lesser therapy, such as fulguration, while appealing in some restricted cases, has numerous drawbacks. Chief among them is the insecurity engendered by a form of treatment that may be merely skimming (or burning) the surface of a tumor that could be cured by an en bloc resection. Because no prospective, randomized studies comparing these types of treatment exist and no reliable means of preoperative stratification of patients with rectal cancer exist, any comparison of local therapy to standard surgical therapy is rendered invalid.

REFERENCES

1. Hermanek, P.: Evolution and pathology of rectal cancer. World J. Surg., 6:502-509, 1982.
2. Hojo, K., Koyama, Y., and Moriya, Y.: Lymphatic spread and its prognostic value in patients with rectal cancer. Am. J. Surg., 144:350-354, 1982.

3. Wolmark, N., Fisher, E. R., Wieand, H. S., et al.: The relationship of depth of penetration and tumor size to the number of positive nodes in Dukes C colorectal cancer. Cancer, 53:2707-2712, 1984.

4. Rosen, L., Veidenheimer, M. C., Coller, J. A., and Corman, M. L.: Mortality, morbidity, and patterns of recurrence after abdominoperineal resection for cancer of the rectum. Dis. Colon Rectum, 25(3):202-208, 1982.

5. Miles, W. E.: A method of performing abdominoperineal excision for carcinoma of the rectum and of the terminal portion of the pelvic colon. Lancet, 2:1812-1813, 1908.

6. Mettlin, C., Mittelman, A., Natarajan, N., et al.: Trends in the United States for the management of adenocarcinoma of the rectum. Surg. Gynecol. Obstet., 153:701-706, 1981.

7. Madden, J. and Kandalaft, S.: Clinical evaluation of electrocoagulation in the treatment of cancer of the rectum. Am. J. Surg., 122:347, 1971.

8. Stearns, M. W., Jr., Sternberg, S. S., and DeCosse, J. J.: Treatment alternatives: Localized rectal cancer. Cancer, 54:2691-2694, 1984.

9. Gingold, B. S., Mitty, W. F., Jr., and Tadros, M.: Importance of patient selection in local treatment of carcinoma of the rectum. Am. J. Surg., 145:293-296, 1983.

10. Whiteway, J., Nicholls, R. J., annd Morson, B. C.: The role of surgical local excision in the treatment of local rectal cancer. Br. J. Surg., 72:694-697, 1985.

11. Killingback, M. J.: Indications for local excision of rectal cancer. Br. J. Surg., 72(Suppl):s54-s58, 1985.

12. Madden, J. L. and Kandalaft, S. I.: Electrocoagulation as a primary curative method in the treatment of carcinoma of the rectum. Surg. Gynecol. Obstet., 157:164-179, 1983.

13. Hoekstra, H. J., Verschueren, R. C. J., Oldhoff, J., and VanDerPloeg, E.: Palliative and curative electrocoagulation for rectal cancer: Experience and results. Cancer, 55:210-213, 1985.

14. Hughes, E. P., Jr., Veidenheimer, M. C., Corman, M. L., and Coller, J. A.: Electrocoagulation of rectal cancer. Dis. Colon Rectum, 25:215-218, 1982.

15. Crile, G., Jr., and Turnbull, R. B., Jr.: The role of electrocoagulation in the treatment of carcinoma of the rectum. Surg. Gynecol. Obstet., 135:391-396, 1972.

III-B: FULGURATION OF RECTAL ADENOCARCINOMA

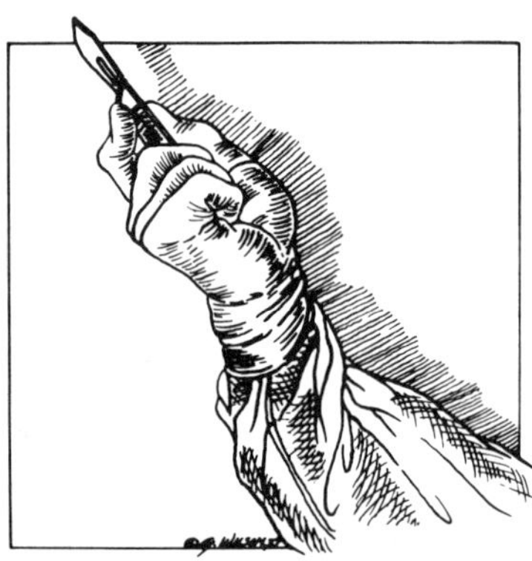

B. TIMOTHY BAXTER, M.D.

Fulguration of rectal adenocarcinoma is an operation requiring the same skills and experience as abdominoperineal resection and, when performed as such, yields comparable cure rates. Unlike abdominoperineal resection where the colostomized, impotent, incontinent ingrate may be referred postoperatively to the medical or radiation oncologist, a high degree of commitment with close follow-up is required following fulguration of rectal adenocarcinoma. However, with GI, bladder, and sexual function intact, these grateful patients are much easier to follow.

Over 100 years ago, Byrne[1] stated what Wanebo[2] and other investigators more recently have demonstrated—that miserable results can be anticipated when fulguration is carried out in the office setting with the same attention as that given to wart removal. Because patients undergoing fulguration tend to be older with more associated diseases, a thorough preoperative evaluation is necessary. Regional or general anesthesia is required for adequate relaxation and exposure. Mechanical bowel prep is necessary, and suction and good lighting make the operating room a necessity. Follow-up is on a monthly basis for six months with repeat fulguration for any sign of recurrence or residual disease. Although 20 percent of patients will be cured with a single treatment, an average of three sessions may be required to effect cure.

Morbidity is consistent in the three series shown in Table I.[3-6] These studies involve over 300 patients. Seventy percent of the morbidity consists of minor postoperative bleeding, and stricture and fistula are rare complications.

Mortality also is consistent from one series to the next as shown in the four studies in Table I. These studies involve over 300 patients. There were two deaths related to postoperative cardiovascular complications. This mortality is extremely low considering the ages and associated diseases of patients who often are relegated to this form of treatment.

In 1987, abdominoperineal resection is the procedure of choice for treating rectal adenocarcinoma in all but the extremely high-risk patient. To the tearful patient learning of the need for permanent colostomy, we reassure him or her. Then we reassure ourselves: He or she is old, and it is really not that big a deal. Besides, Bob Hope has a colostomy and look at him. Why should such patients be concerned about

TABLE I. FULGURATION: MORBIDITY AND MORTALITY

MORBIDITY

Eisenstat[3]	20.5%
Hughes[4]	22.0%
Madden[5]	23.5%

MORTALITY

Eisenstat[3]	1.5%
Hughes[4]	0%
Madden[5]	0%
Crile[6]	0%

[3]Eisenstat, et al.: Am. J. Surg., 143:127–132, 1982.
[4]Hughes, et al.: Dis. Colon Rectum, 25:215–218, 1982.
[5]Madden and Kandalaft: Surg. Gynecol. Obstet., 157:164–179, 1983.
[6]Crile and Turnbull: Surg. Gynecol. Obstet., 135:391–396, 1972.

having sex anyway? They have cancer to worry about.

Morbidity from AP resection is the rule, not the exception, with major complications related to sepsis and bleeding. The studies shown in Table II[7-9] are representative and include over 400 patients. The average hospital stay is three weeks in most series.

Five to 15 percent of patients will die from the operation. Although there are some small series reporting mortality of less than 5 percent, 12 percent is the mortality rate noted by Gazzaniga and colleagues[12] in the community hospital; and Dwight and colleagues[13] reported the same mortality rate of 12 percent in a survey of 23 VA hospitals. Over 1,000 patients were involved in the four studies shown in Table III.[13]

Since there really is no question that fulguration properly done can control local disease, what really is at issue is the benefit of pelvic lymphadenectomy. By virtue of our training as surgeons, we are also anatomists. With this orientation, it is not surprising that we cling to the tenants of Virchow and Halsted. They considered lymph nodes to be barriers to tumor spread and cure was effected only when every last tumor cell had been removed. Not only is this concept outdated and oversimplified, but also it is wrong.

Fisher and Fisher[14] have demonstrated that radiolabeled tumor cells hardly slow down as they pass through lymph nodes to exit efferent lymphatics and also venous channels. Furthermore, these cells emerge unscathed, viable, and ready for implantation. This information is corroborated in a study by Pressman and colleagues,[15] who

TABLE II. MORBIDITY FOLLOWING AP RESECTION

Colcock[7]	58.3%
Cohn[8]	70.0%
Salvati[9]	72.0%

[7]Colcock and Jarpa: Dis. Colon Rectum, 1:90–96, 1958.
[8]Fitzgibbons, et al.: Am. J. Surg., 134:624–629, 1977.
[9]Salvati and Rubin: Am. J. Surg., 132:583–586, 1976.

TABLE III. OPERATIVE MORTALITY FOLLOWING AP RESECTION

Gilbertsen[10]	9.8%
Burke[11]	6.0%
Gazzaniga[12]	12.5%
Dwight[13]	12.0%

[10]Gilbertsen: Arch. Surg., 80:135–143, 1960.
[11]Welch and Burke: N. Engl. J. Med., 266:211–219, 1962.
[12]Gazzaniga, et al.: Am. J. Surg., 120:62–65, 1970.
[13]Dwight, et al.: Am. J. Surg., 129:93–103, 1972.

showed that tumor cells could exit lymph nodes by hematogenous route because of lymphaticovenous shunts.

If lymph nodes were barriers to tumor spread, then one would expect improved survival from extended lymphadenectomy. Grinnell[16] extended his resection to include hypogastric nodes and found that this had prognostic significance but no therapeutic benefit. He had zero survivors with positive hypogastric nodes in three years. Stearns[17] compared standard abdominoperineal resection to more radical abdominal-pelvic lymphadenectomy without any significant improvements in 5-year survival. Although the title of a paper by Enker and colleagues, "Enhanced Survival with Wide Anatomic Section," sounds promising, the results were not.[18] In fact, modifications of all types of the Miles' standard AP resections have not changed survival over the past 70 years.

Dukes and Bussey[19] correlated lymph node status with prognosis. They also demonstrated another interesting finding. When tumor was found in lymph nodes at the cut margins of the surgical specimens (and, therefore, in individuals who were left with disease), the patients did not all go on to die. In fact, one in seven was disease-free at five years. Although we would like to think that our resection cured the patient, the complex relationship between tumor and host is the predominant factor. The role of lymphadenectomy in effecting this balance between tumor and host is unclear. When primary tumor is obliterated by excision or fulguration, the additional benefit of pelvic lymphadenectomy is not known. Yet, we advocate this morbid procedure as the standard of care.

If you are alert enough at this point to think this makes little sense, then you are right.

What results can be achieved by fulguration alone? Jackman[20] was impressed with the results he and Wittoesh obtained with fulguration recommended for 252 patients referred for palliation only. Patients were offered fulguration as a primary means of treating rectal adenocarcinoma that was at least 2 cm in size and had no evidence of fixation or associated palpable adenopathy. Polyps and adenomas were excluded, and all lesions were biopsy-proven adenocarcinoma. Two hundred eleven patients followed the recommendation for fulguration; and 203, or 96.2 percent, were free of disease at 8- to 18-year follow-up, or at the time of death from intercurrent disease. Eight patients failed this therapy and died of cancer after treatment. Forty-one patients underwent AP resection despite their recommendations, and only one had positive lymph nodes (Table IV). Jackman showed that fulguration in these select patients was comparable to or better than results anticipated for Dukes A or B lesions treated by AP resections.

TABLE IV.   RESULTS IN 252 SELECTED PATIENTS*

211—Fulguration
    203 without disease at 8 years
       8 died from disease

41—AP Resection
    40 of 41 Dukes A or B
     1 of 41 Dukes C

*From Jackman, R.J.: Conservative management of selected patients with carcinoma of the rectum. Dis. Colon Rectum, 4:429–434, 1961.

Salvati and Rubin[9] published their experience with fulguration and AP resection. There were 47 patients in each group, with 13 crossing over from the fulguration to the abdominoperineal resection group. Patients in the fulguration group were older, and yet survival was not different over a similar follow-up period. Of these patients who crossed over to the AP resection group, survival also was no different from either of the two groups. Their conclusions were that no survival advantage was noted in the AP resection group, postoperative morbidity and mortality were much higher in the AP resection group, and failure of fulguration followed by AP resection did not adversely affect survival.

Crile and Turnbull[6] also were encouraged by results of conservative treatment. As a result, they recommended and performed fulguration in 62 patients as primary therapy. During this same period, 226 patients underwent AP resection. All patients had biopsy-proven carcinoma. Adenomas and polyps were excluded. Eight patients initially treated by fulguration crossed over into the abdominoperineal resection group, and seven of the eight had Dukes A or B lesions at the time of surgery. Patients in the fuguration group were older and had smaller tumors, although there is no known correlation between tumor size and lymph node involvement. More patients lived five years after conservative treatment despite advanced age. Twelve patients died as a result of resection, nine in the immediate postoperative period; and three late postoperative deaths occurred (Table V).

Patients from both groups then were matched for tumor size and age. A comparison of 5-year survival within the 46 matched pairs showed no difference—52 percent for the AP resection group and 57 percent for the fulguration group. Crile con-

TABLE V.   AP RESECTION VERSUS FULGURATION*

	AP RESECTION	FULGURATION
Number	226	62
Age	61	67
Size	4.8 cm	3.1 cm
5-year survival	46%	68%
Postoperative mortality	9 (3)	0
5-year disease free	52%	57%

*Modified from Crile, G. and Turnbull, R.B.: The role of electrocoagulation in the treatment of carcinoma of the rectum. Surg. Gynecol. Obstet., 135:391–396, 1972.

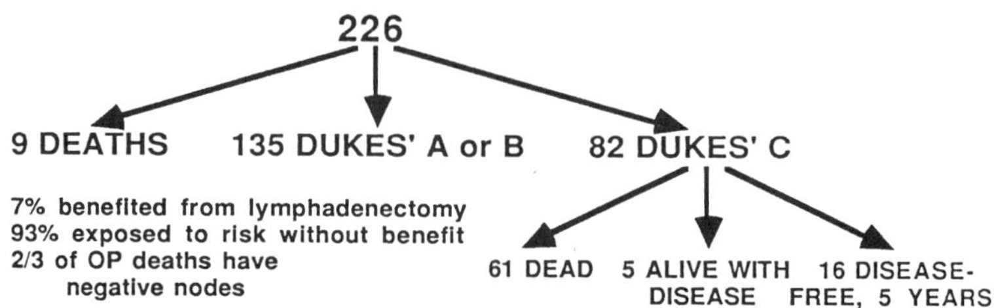

FIGURE 1. AP resection. From Crile, G. and Turnbull, R.B.: The role of electrocoagulation in the treatment of carcinoma of the rectum. Surg. Gynecol. Obstet., 135:391–396, 1972.

cluded that no survival benefit was found by AP resection, and no harm was done by initial treatment with fulguration.

Patients undergoing AP resection were analyzed further. Of the 226 patients, there were nine immediate postoperative deaths, 135 with Dukes A or B lesions, and 82 with Dukes C lesions. Of the 82 with Dukes C lesions, 61 were dead at five years, five are alive with disease, and 16 were disease free at five years. Given these numbers, only 7 percent of the patients benefited from pelvic lymphadenectomy, while 93 percent were exposed to the risk without benefit. Two-thirds of the operative deaths had negative nodes (Figure 1).

The largest series of patients undergoing fulguration was that studied by Madden.[5] This landmark study covered a 20-year period with follow-up from five to 27 years. Two hundred four patients were treated by fulguration for rectal carcinoma. There were 156 patients in the treatment-for-cure group and 48 patients referred for palliation because of inoperability related mainly to cardiovascular disease. Eight patients were lost to follow-up, but only two of those were lost before the 5-year follow-up period was complete. Therefore, 99 percent of the patients were followed for at least five years or until death. All age groups were included, including 8 percent below the age of 50 and 47.4 percent between the ages of 50 and 70. Tumor size also was variable, but the majority of the tumors were large, between 3 and 8 cm. Twenty-two and one-half (22.5) percent of the patients had complications—mainly they were related to postoperative bleeding that occurs predictably on the sixth to ninth day and usually resolves on its own. Rectovaginal fistula occurred in four patients, one of whom was symptomatic while three had no symptoms. Rectal stricture was uncommon and was treated without the need for colostomy in all four patients in whom it occurred. Perforation above the peritoneum occurred in two patients, and one required colostomy.

The author used fulguration in a series of patients as a primary mode of therapy. When one includes the 48 patients referred for palliation, this represents a high-risk group, many of whom were refused surgery. Despite this, the overall disease-free survival at five years with 99 percent follow-up was 56 percent. This is comparable to any large series for AP resection (Table VI).

In conclusion, the benefit of pelvic lymphadenectomy has yet to be proven. Over 90 percent of patients with rectal adenocarcinoma will derive no survival benefit by undergoing AP resection and yet will be exposed to the morbidity and mortality

TABLE VI.   DEFINITIVE FOLLOW-UP STUDY*

204 PATIENTS: 5–27 YEARS			
	OPER.	INOPER.	TOTAL
No. pts.	156 (76.5%)	48 (23.5%)	204 (100.0%)
Alive 5 yrs.	111 (71.2%)	20 (41.7%)	131 (64.2%)
Free of disease	97 (62.2%)	17 (35.4%)	114** (55.9%)

*From Madden, J.L. and Kandalaft, S.I.: Electrocoagulation as a primary curative method in the treatment of carcinoma of the rectum. Surg. Gynecol. Obstet., 157:169, 1983.
**3 (2.7%) recurr. > 5 yrs.—Loc. 1
Dist. 2 (brain, liver & lung)

associated with this operation. When fulguration alone is used, survival is comparable to abdominoperineal resection. Initial attempts to treat by fulguration do not adversely affect survival if abdominoperineal resection is then performed.

REFERENCES

1. Byrne, J.: Electro-cautery. In Uterine Surgery. New York, William Wood & Company, 1873.
2. Wanebo, H. S. and Quan, S. H.: Failures of electrocoagulation of primary carcinoma of the rectum. Surg. Gynecol. Obstet., 138:174-176, 1974.
3. Eisenstat, T. E., Deak, S. T., Rubin, R. J., Salvati, E. P., and Greco, R. C.: Five-year survival in patients with carcinoma of the rectum treated by electrocoagulation. Am. J. Surg., 143:127-132, 1982.
4. Hughes, E. P., Viedenheimer, M. C., Corman, M. L., and Coller, J. A.: Electrocoagulation of rectal cancer. Dis. Colon Rectum, 25:215-218, 1982.
5. Madden, J. L. and Kandalaft, S. I.: Electrocoagulation as a primary curative method in the treatment of carcinoma of the rectum. Surg. Gynecol. Obstet., 157:164-179, 1983.
6. Crile, G. and Turnbull, R. B.: The role of electrocoagulation in the treatment of carcinoma of the rectum. Surg. Gynecol. Obstet., 135:391-396, 1972.
7. Colcock, B. P. and Jarpa, S.: Complication of abdominoperineal resection. Dis. Colon Rectum, 1:90-96, 1958.
8. Fitzgibbons, R. J., Harkrider, W. W., and Cohn, I.: Review of abdominoperineal resection for cancer. Am. J. Surg, 134:624-629, 1977.
9. Salvati, E. P. and Rubin, R. J.: Electrocoagulation as primary therapy for rectal carcinoma. Am. J. Surg., 132:583-586, 1976.
10. Gilbertsen, V. A.: Adenocarcinoma of the rectum: A fifteen-year evaluation of the results of curative therapy. Arch. Surg., 80:135-143, 1960.
11. Welch, C. E. and Burke, J. F.: Carcinoma of the colon and rectum. N. Engl. J. Med., 266:211-219, 1962.
12. Gazzaniga, A. B., Munster, A. M., and Ross, F. P.: Adenocarcinoma of the colon and rectum: Results of therapy in a community hospital. Am. J. Surg., 120:62-65, 1970.
13. Dwight, R. W., Higgins, G. A., Roswit, B., LeVeen, H. A., and Keehn, R. J.: Preoperative radiation and surgery for cancer of sigmoid colon rectum. Am. J. Surg., 129:93-103, 1972.
14. Fisher, B. and Fisher, E. R.: Barrier function of lymph node to tumor cells and erythrocytes. Cancer, 20:1907-1913, 1967.
15. Pressman, J. J., Simon, M. B., Hand, K., and Miller, J.: Passage of fluids, cells, and bacteria via direct communications between lymph nodes and veins. Surg. Gynecol. Obstet., 115:204-214, 1962.

16. Grinnell, R. S.: Results of ligation of the inferior mesenteric artery at the aorta in resections of carcinoma of descending and sigmoid colon and rectum. Surg. Gynecol. Obstet., 120:1031-1036, 1965.
17. Stearns, M. W.: Abdominoperineal resection for cancer of the rectum. Dis. Colon Rectum, 17:612-616, 1974.
18. Enker, W. E., Laffer, U., and Brock, G. E.: Enhanced survival in patients with colon and rectal cancer is based on wide anatomic resection. Ann. Surg., 190:350-357, 1979.
19. Dukes, C. E. and Bussey, J. R.: The spread of rectal cancer and its effect on prognosis. Br. J. Cancer, 12:309-320, 1958.
20. Jackman, R. J.: Conservative management of selected patients with carcinoma of the rectum. Dis. Colon Rectum, 4:429-434, 1961.

DEBATE IV

Splenectomy vs. Splenorrhaphy

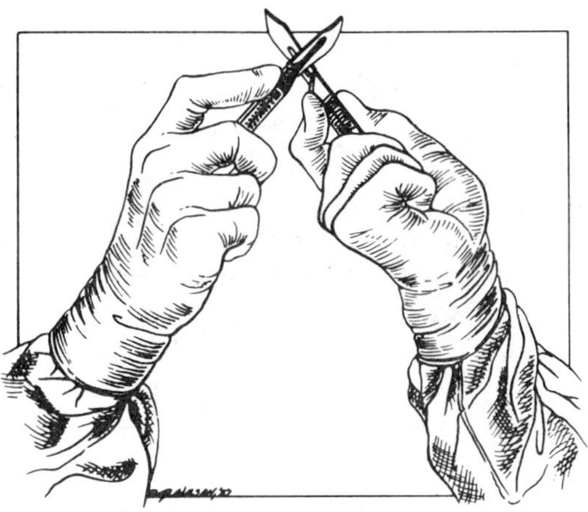

The spleen is a commonly traumatized organ. To what length should the responsible surgeon go in order to salvage the spleen by splenorrhaphy? Splenectomy is definitive, expeditious, and obviates the risk of post-splenorrhaphy rebleeding. At what point in the multiply injured trauma patient do the added risks of splenorrhaphy outweigh the risk of the asplenic state?

Does the spleen have significant immunologic function? Both advocates agree that the spleen controls the circulation of immune cells and is pivotal in initially processing antigenic material. The spleen is a large volume, slow filtration system that permits unopsonized, encapsulated organisms to be trapped, thus buying time until the immune system can be activated. Dr. Haug points out that, if the spleen has significant function, this value should be exhibited only in young, previously non-immunized patients.

Drs. Piotrowski and Haug both cite series by Moore and Feliciano to make diametrically opposite points. Drs. Piotrowski and Haug have reviewed the surgical literature conscientiously, and they not only disagree on the relative value of splenectomy vs. splenorrhaphy but also disagree on the importance of splenic auto-transplantation, vaccination, and prophylactic antibodies.

Gertrude Stein said: ''A difference, to be a difference, must make a difference.'' In examining the controversy concerning splenectomy vs. splenorrhaphy, does it?

IV-A: SPLENORRHAPHY IS APPROPRIATE IN TRAUMA

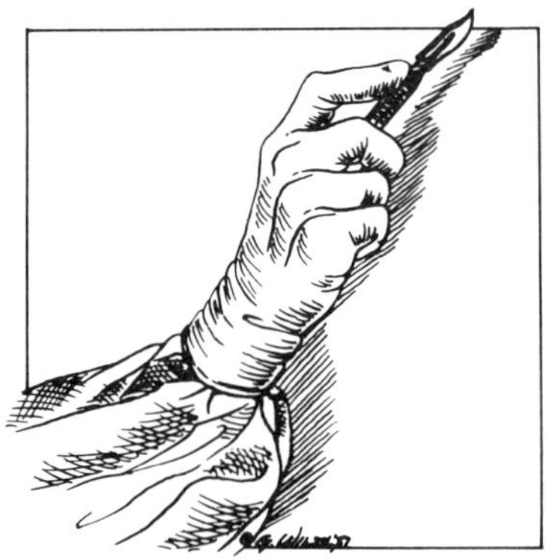

JOSEPH J. PIOTROWSKI, M.D.

Hippocrates described the spleen as "an organ of mystery"; we have since learned a great deal about its immune function. The spleen consists of white and red pulp. Arteries enter the splenic tissue and branch out into the white pulp, which consists of a periarterial lymphoid sheath and adjoining follicles. At this point, the arteriole enters into the red pulp, first entering Billroth's cords and then the venous sinuses. The spleen receives 5 percent of the cardiac output. Approximately 90 percent of this blood flow enters the sinuses directly. These venous sinuses coalesce to form the venous outflow from the spleen. As a blood pool, the spleen acts only as a small reserve in man. There is less than 5 percent of the total red cell mass present in the spleen. There is no real granulocyte pool. There is, however, a significant platelet pool in the normal spleen.

IMMUNE CELL TRAFFIC

The most important function of the spleen is in immune surveillance. The spleen contains approximately 25 percent of the T-lymphocyte and 15 percent of the B-lymphocyte pool. The antigenic functions of the spleen are related to its unique anatomical arrangement and are referred to as the immune cell traffic.

As the blood passes through the spleen, the plasma and leukocytes are skimmed from this solution into the white pulp. In this area, the B- and T-cells remain together in T-dependent areas for several hours. Approximately one to six hours later, the B-cells migrate to the follicles. T-lymphocytes return to the red pulp and thereby to the circulation. If, however, these T-lymphocytes are activated by antigen, they remain in these areas much longer. Red cells generally remain in the arterial system at this point. As the plasma and leukocytes are skimmed, the hematocrit progressively increases in this fluid until it passes into Billroth's cords. At this point, the red cells are forced to squeeze through slits in the endothelium in order to enter the venous sinuses. During this process, various appendages, such as Howell-Jolly bodies, are amputated. Decreased oxygen and glucose in these areas stress these red cells and also make them less deformable. Therefore, this is a process by which the spleen is utilized to cull out damaged red cells. The spleen also acts in phagocytosis of circulating particulate matter. This occurs via fixed macrophages and includes foreign material and defective red cells.

PRIMARY RESPONSE

Antigenic material is delivered to the spleen and is trapped by follicular dendritic cells, which are a nonlymphoid-type cell present in the spleen. These cells process and present antigen to the B-cells. This evokes a primary response. The B-cells are either stimulated to differentiate into plasma cells and produce IgM, or they are stimulated to produce memory cells which, at a later time upon secondary exposure to an antigen, differentiate into plasma cells which produce IgG. In all of these cases, T-cells are important in facilitating both the stimulation of undifferentiated B-cells and in producing antibody from the plasma cells.

IMMUNE DEFICITS FROM SPLENECTOMY

The best way to detect the immune functions of the spleen in humans is to compare the patients who have had their spleens removed with patients who have not. DiPadova and colleagues[1] reported on 30 patients, 15 spenectomized and 15 controls, who had no previous immunization with Pneumovax. They isolated their blood lymphocytes and stimulated these lymphocytes with pokeweed mitogen, a nonspecific stimulator of lymphocytes. The splenectomized patients were unable to secrete antipneumococcal capsular protein of the IgM class. Normals were all able to secrete this antibody. Therefore, they showed an impaired primary response in splenectomized patients at the cellular level.

In a separate study, DiPadova and colleagues[2] reported on 10 patients, five splenectomized and five controls. Before immunization, these patients had no spontaneous secretion of antipolysaccharide capsular protein IgG. Seven days after Pneumovax, antipolysaccharide IgG could be detected in the serum of both groups. By 21 days, these had again returned to baseline and no spontaneous antibody was noted. With the addition of pokeweed mitogen to these lymphocytes, the control group was able again to secrete the IgG antibody, whereas in the splenectomized patients there was no secretion. In other words, an impaired secondary response was detected in splenectomized patients at the cellular level.

Sieber and colleagues[3] reported on 12 patients and also noted the absence of B-lymphocytes able to secrete IgG in response to pokeweed mitogen. They also reconstituted serum with T- and B-cells from controls and revealed that, in addition to the B-cell defect that previously had been elucidated by DiPadova, a T-cell defect was noted in these patients. They, therefore, documented both a B- and T-cell defect at the cellular level in splenectomized patients.

Drew and colleagues[4] reported on 33 patients who had splenectomies secondary to trauma. They also noted an increased IgG in unstimulated lymphocyte cultures from splenectomized patients and a deficient response to pokeweed mitogen. Of interest was that several of these patients had splenosis documented in liver-spleen scan. This was categorized into three different groups in which there was little or no splenosis, moderate splenosis, and significant splenosis. In the patients with significant splenosis, the total amount of splenic tissue, as estimated by liver-spleen scan, was equivalent to the original amount of tissue in a normal unsplenectomized patient. There was no correlation between the amount of splenosis and the correction of the immune deficit; i.e., splenosis or disorganized splenic tissue does not correct the immunologic defect at the cellular level.

Gill and colleagues[5] reported on 32 splenectomized patients for trauma. They documented a defective monocyte-dependent cellular cytotoxicity in these patients. The monocyte is a precursor of the tissue macrophage, so this is another immunologic defect noted in splenectomized patients.

Therefore, immune defects noted in splenectomized patients are:

1. an impaired primary response,
2. an impaired secondary response,
3. impaired T-cell function,
4. deficits not correctable by unorganized splenic tissue, and
5. defective monocyte function.

There also is noted to be decreased tuftsin in these patients; however, this defect is correctable by adding splenic tissue.

OVERWHELMING POSTSPLENECTOMY INFECTION (OPSI)

Why are all these deficits important? King and Schumaker[6] first reported on a syndrome eventually known as overwhelming postsplenectomy infection in five children with hereditary spherocytosis. Half of these cases were caused by pneumococcus; the rest were caused by various combinations of organisms, including H. influenzae and meningococci. Most cases appear to occur within three years of surgery. Sherman[7] reviewed 1,100 children who had splenectomies, and 29 of these patients developed OPSI. The mortality rate in these 29 patients was 25 percent. O'Neil and McDonald[8] reported on 256 patients. Approximately 74 percent of these patients had splenectomies due to trauma. Their death rate from OPSI was 50 percent.

Since the spleen does have important immune functions and is important in the prevention of OPSI, how safe is it to save the spleen? Feliciano and colleagues[9] reported on 326 patients, half of whom had splenectomies and half had splenorrhaphies. They had no rebleeding rates, and they did not mention an incidence of OPSI. However, the complication rate for splenectomy was 21 percent and 12 percent for splenorrhaphy. These figures are not comparable since the patients with splenectomy were patients who had other associated organ injuries. Moore and colleagues[10] reported on 200 trauma patients with splenic injuries. They reported a 42 percent splenorrhaphy rate. Again, in these patients, mortality and complication rates were not comparable. However, what is comparable is the fact that in the splenectomy group there was a 2 percent incidence of OPSI despite splenic implants and only a 4 percent incidence of rebleeding in the splenorrhaphy group. All of the patients that rebled were reoperated and none suffered from this reoperation other than the increased hospital stay. Therefore, the proper comparison is between a 2 percent OPSI rate and a 4 percent rebleeding rate. OPSI has a 50 percent mortality versus no mortality for rebleeding.

SPLENIC SUBSTITUTES

What if we had to take the spleen out anyway? Is there a reasonable substitute for the spleen? Scher and colleagues[11] reported on splenic implantation in rats and showed that there was no increased clearance of pneumococcal bacteria. Other investigators with negative animal results include Schwartz and colleagues,[12] Tesluk and Thomas,[13] Weiss and colleagues,[14] and Oakes and colleagues.[15] The only investigators who have shown positive results in the animal studies are Livingston and colleagues.[16] In this study, the pneumococcus was given via the respiratory route. Lau and colleagues[17] showed that splenectomy results in impaired bactericidal activity of the pulmonary alveolar macrophage, which is partially corrected via splenic implants.

Therefore, all these animal studies have shown is that implanting splenic tissue may increase resistance via the respiratory route; however, the problem in OPSI is the overwhelming bacterial septicemia present. The clearance of bacteria is not improved by implantation of splenic tissue.

Vaccination with pneumococcus also is not completely effective. There are many case reports of patients who had received Pneumovax who still succumbed to OPSI. In addition, pneumococcus only makes up 50 percent of the organisms in the syndrome of OPSI.

Therefore, in summary:

1. The spleen is a unique organ for processing material and in controlling the circulation of immune cells.
2. Impaired immune responses after splenectomy occur at the cellular level.
3. These deficiencies are not correctable by disorganized splenic tissue.
4. OPSI is a real entity, although rare.
5. Splenic salvage is safe in selected patients.
6. Pneumovax and splenic re-implantation are poor substitutes but are as yet undefined in the human system.

REFERENCES

1. DiPadova, F., Durig, M., Harder, F., DiPadova, C., and Zanussi, C.: Impaired antipneumococcal antibody production in patients without spleens. Br. Med. J., 290:14–16, 1985.
2. DiPadova, F., Durig, M., Wadstrom, J., and Harder, F.: Role of spleen in immune response to polyvalent pneumococcal vaccine. Br. Med. J., 287:1829–1832, 1983.
3. Sieber, G., Breyer, H.G., Herrmann, F., and Riehl, H.: Abnormalities of B-cell activation and immunoregulation in splenectomized patients. Immunobiol., 169:263–271, 1985.
4. Drew, P.A., Kiroff, G.K., Ferrante, A., and Cohen, R.C.: Alterations in immunoglobulin synthesis by peripheral blood mononuclear cells from splenectomized patients with and without splenic regrowth. J. Immunol., 132:191–196, 1984.

5. Gill, P.G., DeYoung, N.J., Kiroff, G.K., Leppard, P.I., and McLennan, G.: Monocyte antibody-dependent cellular cytotoxicity in splenectomized subjects. J. Immunol., 132: 1244–1248, 1984.
6. King, H. and Schumacker, H.B.: Splenic studies: I. Susceptibility to infection after splenectomy performed in infancy. Ann. Surg., 136:239, 1952.
7. Sherman, R.: Perspectives in management of trauma to the spleen. (1979 Presidential Address, American Association for the Surgery of Trauma). J. Trauma, 20:1–13, 1981.
8. O'Neil, B.J. and McDonald, J.C.: The risk of sepsis in the asplenic adult. Ann. Surg., 194:775–778, 1981.
9. Feliciano, D.V., Bitondo, C.G., Mattox, K.L., et al.: A four-year experience with splenectomy versus splenorrhaphy. Ann. Surg., 201:568–575, 1985.
10. Moore, F.A., Moore, E.E., Moore, G.E., and Millikan, J.S.: Risk of splenic salvage after trauma. Am. J. Surg., 148:800–805, 1984.
11. Scher, K.S., Wroczynski, A.R., and Scott-Conner, C.: Intraperitoneal splenic implants do not alter clearance of pneumococcal bacteremia. Am. Surg., 51:269–271, 1985.
12. Schwartz, A.D., Goldthorn, J.F., Winselstein, J.A., and Seift, A.J.: Lack of protective effect of autotransplanted splenic tissue to pneumococcal challenge. Blood, 51:475–478, 1978.
13. Tesluk, G.C. and Thomas C.G.: Prevention of postsplenectomy pneumococcal sepsis in rats. Surg. Forum, 30:35–37, 1979.
14. Weiss, J.M., Rusate, F.E., and Steward, E.: Splenic autotransplant function in experimental bacteremia. Surg. Forum, 30:30–32, 1979.
15. Oakes, D.D., Froehlich, J.P., and Charles, C.: Intraportal splenic autotransplantation in rat: Feasibility and effectiveness. J. Surg. Res., 32:7–14, 1982.
16. Livingston, C.D., Levine, B.A., and Sirives, K.R.: Site of splenic autotransplantation affects protection from sepsis. Am. J. Surg., 146:734–747, 1983.
17. Lau, H.T., Hardy, M.A., and Altman, R.P.: Decreased pulmonary alveolar bactericidal activity in splenectomized rats. J. Surg. Res., 34:568–571, 1983.

IV-B: SPLENECTOMY IS APPROPRIATE IN TRAUMA

CRAIG E. HAUG, M.D.

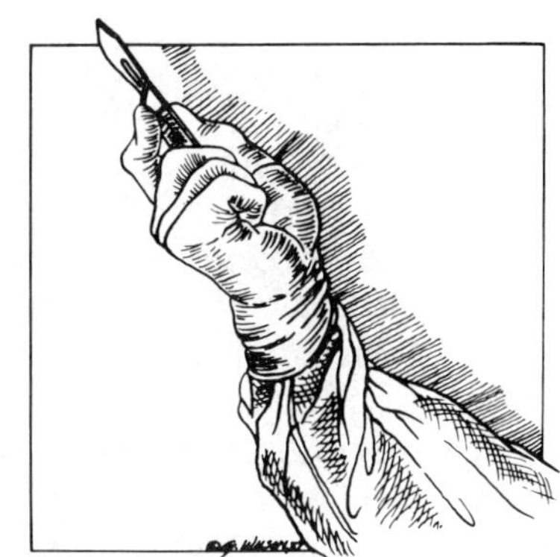

In 1678, the town surgeon of Colberg performed the first total splenectomy for trauma. He did this against the advice of colleagues who emphasized that the authorities had taught that no one could live without the spleen. By the early 20th century, splenectomy was the standard practice for traumatic rupture.

There were several reasons for this. Firstly, the mortality from traumatic rupture without operation was 90 to 100 percent. Secondly, the many early reports of survival after splenectomy spread the belief that the spleen was not necessary for life. Thirdly, it was thought that the spleen could not be repaired safely.

However, over the last 25 years, the recognition of the spleen's immunologic role, along with the evolution of hemostatic and resectional techniques, has caused a dramatic reversal in this attitude.

It seems clear that children, particularly children with hematologic disease, are at excess risk of postsplenectomy sepsis or overwhelming postsplenectomy infection (OPSI) if they undergo splenectomy. The issue, it seems to me, centers around whether the same increased risk can be extrapolated to the population of otherwise healthy adults who undergo splenectomy for trauma and trauma alone. It has taken about 50 years to recognize that the risk in children and in adults is still more anecdotal than statistical, which means the risk must be very small. This is a tough standard against which any new therapy must be measured, which brings up my second point.

Even if there is a very small but finite increased risk of OPSI in normal adults after splenectomy, there must be a point at which the added risks of splenorrhaphy outweigh the risk of the asplenic state. Most would agree that splenectomy is usually more expeditious and technically easier than splenorrhaphy when splenectomy is performed properly. It may be that, in all but the simplest of splenorrhaphies, the morbidity and mortality of added blood loss, OR time, and postoperative rebleeding exceed that of OPSI.

The third area I will discuss is that of autotransplantation of splenic tissue after splenectomy. There is a lot of good evidence to indicate that autotransplantation works and, along with vaccination and antibiotic prophylaxis, might nullify this very small risk of OPSI, assuming OPSI even exists.

SPLENECTOMY

Background.   The spleen is the most common intraabdominal organ injured in blunt trauma and is the second most commonly injured intraabdominal organ overall. Splenectomy for trauma accounts for 10 to 15 percent of all splenectomies performed in several large series.

Mortality and Morbidity of Splenectomy.   More patients have complications or die after splenectomy than splenorrhaphy. However, directly comparing the morbidity and mortality of splenectomy versus splenorrhaphy in published studies is invalid as splenectomy patients are (1) more severely injured and (2) splenectomy in some patients is performed only after time and blood are lost trying and failing to perform a satisfactory splenorrhaphy. In the study of Feliciano and colleagues,[1] very few splenorrhaphies were done in the rarified atmosphere of grades 4 and 5 splenic injuries—the most severe. Associated injuries were greater among splenectomy patients as well. There is no study that takes patients with equal injuries and randomizes them to either splenectomy or splenorrhaphy.

Function of the Spleen.   The spleen is not necessary for life, but it does have several immune functions. Besides serving as an immunologic factory, the spleen is a large-volume, slow-filtration system that permits unopsonized encapsulated organisms to be trapped, thus buying time until the immune system can get cranked up. For this reason, it may be more important in younger people when there is no prior immunity. Adults are more likely to have prior immunity and a quicker response to infection, making trapping by the spleen less crucial.

OPSI

Background.   Overwhelming postsplenectomy infection, or OPSI, presents dramatically and can be clearly distinguished from ordinary instances of septicemia by its abrupt onset, florid bacteremia, fulminant course, and high mortality. The pneumococcus is the most common organism (50 percent), but other encapsulated bacteria also have been reported. These characteristics are important to keep in mind, as they distinguish OPSI from simple pneumonia and from perioperative sepsis, which have been found by Malangoni and colleagues[2] to be a function of injury severity, not type of operation. Unclear definition of OPSI has been responsible for much of the confusion surrounding this whole issue.

Risk of OPSI in Children.   Although there were rumblings in the literature, it was not until a 1973 review by Singer[3] that the splenorrhaphy bandwagon really started rolling. The subgroup of 688 patients (mostly children) splenectomized for trauma had the lowest reported incidence and mortality—1.4 percent and 0.58 percent, respectively (Table I). This, according to Singer, represented a 58-fold increased risk of death from sepsis.

Risk of OPSI in Adults.   Now how does this relate to adults? Most reports of OPSI in adults have been case reports and, therefore, are of no use in determining incidence. However, they are of use in exaggerating the magnitude of the problem in the collective surgical consciousness.

TABLE I.   INCIDENCE OF POSTSPLENECTOMY SEPSIS*

REASON FOR SPLENECTOMY	NUMBER OF PATIENTS	NUMBER OF PATIENTS WITH SEPSIS	NUMBER OF FATALITIES FROM SEPSIS	INCREASED RISK OF DEATH FROM SEPSIS
Trauma	688	10 (1.4%)	4 (0.58%)	58
Incidental to operation	233	5 (2.1%)	2 (0.86%)	86
ITP	489	10 (2.0%)	7 (1.43%)	140
Hereditary spherocytosis	850	30 (3.5%)	19 (2.23%)	220
Acquired hemolytic anemia	67	5 (7.5%)	2 (2.90%)	290
Portal hypertension	221	18 (8.2%)	13 (5.90%)	590
Primary anemia	70	6 (8.5%)	5 (7.01%)	700
Reticuloendothelial disease	69	8 (11.5%)	7 (10.10%)	1000
Thalassemia	109	27 (24.8%)	12 (11.00%)	1100
Totals	2796	119 (4.2%)	71 (2.50%)	

*Modified from Singer, D.B.: Postsplenectomy sepsis. Perspect. Pediatr. Pathol., 1:288, 1973.

One of the studies most often cited to demonstrate increased risk of OPSI in adults splenectomized for trauma is that of Robinette and Fraumeni.[4] These authors reported six cases of fatal pneumonia occurring during 20 years of follow-up of 740 American servicemen who had undergone splenectomy during World War II. There were no cases of pneumonia in a matched comparison group drawn from the same population. However, fatal pneumonia is not necessarily identical to fulminant postsplenectomy sepsis. Also, these authors failed to discern whether pneumonia was what brought these veterans to the hospital in the first place or whether it was only the terminal event.

Further, the incidence of both cirrhosis and heart disease was increased in the splenectomy group compared with controls; either disease may have increased the concomitant risk of pneumonia. Curiously, splenectomized veterans had a lower risk of developing cancer—in fact, less than one-half the risk of lung cancer. So, if you have your spleen out, at least as a result of war trauma, although you are more likely to develop pneumonia, you are at least compensated by protection from cancer.

Other pitfalls are studies that (1) have combined experience of adults with many different indications for splenectomy, (2) have not specified the age of the patient at the time of splenectomy, or (3) have not provided a precise definition of OPSI. The following are some of the more recent and better studies in the literature. For each study, the number of patients followed up, the follow-up time in years and patient-years, the percent of OPSI, and the percent of mortality are listed.

The first six studies provided data on follow-up time (Table II). Combining only these in Total #1 gives an absolute risk of OPSI of 0.22 percent and a 0 percent mortality for almost 900 patients. Adding in the Moore and Feliciano data, which include a 61-year old cirrhotic who died of overwhelming pneumococcal pneumonia five months postoperatively, brings the risk and mortality up to 0.26 percent and 0.09 percent, or, to round up, about 0.3 percent and 0.1 percent, respectively. Translated, this means that for every 1,000 splenectomies done, three patients will get OPSI and one will die from it. Admittedly, the calculations are imperfect. For example, follow-up

TABLE II. RISK OF OPSI

	No. Pt's F/U	F/U (yrs)	F/U (Pt-yrs)	%OPSI	% MORTALITY
1. O'Neal & McDonald, Ann Surg, 1981	128	3.75	480	0	0
2. Standage & Goss, Am J Surg, 1982	64	6.3	405	0	0
3. Schwartz, JAMA, 1982	48	—	300	1/48 (2.1%)	0
4. Sekikawa & Shatney, Am J Surg, 1983	242	4.4	1,046	0	0
5. Malangoni & Condon, Surgery, 1984	140	8.5	1,190	0	0
6. Ragsdale & Hamit, Am Surg, 1984	274	9.5	2,511	1/274 (0.34%)	0
TOTAL #1	896	—	5,932	2/896 (0.22%)	0
7. Moore, Am J Surg, 1984	93	—	—	1/93 (1.1%)	1/93 (1.1%)
8. Feliciano, Ann Surg, 1985	169	—	—	0	0
TOTAL #2	1,158	—	—	3/1,158 (0.26%)	1/1,158 (0.09%)
				0.3%	0.1%

is incomplete, especially in the Moore and Feliciano studies. Nevertheless, I believe these figures give a rough idea of the kind of very small level of absolute risk we are talking about.

Now the question is: Is this risk any different from in the general population? What is the relative risk? Actually, the best way to look at incidence is in terms of patient-years since the length of follow-up is factored in. Total #1 (Table II) shows the combined results of those studies that provided information about length of follow-up. There were two cases of OPSI/5,932 patient-years and a mortality of 0 percent.

Two cases/5,932 patient-years equals 34/100,000 patient-years. Using the pessimistic figure of 50 percent mortality (rather than the actual 0 percent), there would be 17 deaths per 100,000 patient-years. Comparing this with the mortality rate for septicemia in the United States, 3.3 per 100,000 population per year gives a relative risk of about five, not 58. Considering that the mortality in adults may be significantly less than 50 percent, death caused by fulminant sepsis after splenectomy for trauma in adults may be consistent with the general population rate; but insufficient data are available to define the relative risk more exactly. The built-in, unavoidable range of uncertainty in the whole chain of calculations probably exceeds this small difference.

But, even if a relative risk of five compared to the general population is correct, or even 58 as Singer claimed for children, what does that mean? Is splenectomy the cause? Maybe not, in that the general population is not an appropriate comparison group. Patients who need a splenectomy for trauma are not representative of the population as a whole. They

1. have sustained some type of trauma,
2. have undergone an operative procedure, and
3. are self-selected as more accident prone and probably more drink prone.

It might be that this group, with or without their spleens, is going to have a higher incidence of pneumonia. So, while an association might exist between splenectomy and pneumonia, or any number of things, interpreting whether this association implies a cause-and-effect relationship is another matter. In this respect, a better comparison group might have been a group of patients who underwent laparotomy for trauma but had some other injury besides splenic. Such a group might *also* have a relative risk of five or 58 for OPSI compared to the general population. No such study exists.

Finally, the question is really not even whether the risk of sepsis is increased after splenectomy. Even if it is, the real question is whether this increased risk exceeds the risks of splenorrhaphy. Any surgical response to a 0.1 percent mortality risk clearly must involve even a smaller risk. Are the risks of splenorrhaphy sufficiently low and its presumed benefit sufficiently great?

SPLENORRHAPHY

Leon Morgenstern has been an advocate of splenorrhaphy from as early as the 1950s. Now, in the 1980s, he warns: "Splenic salvage increases the length of operating time, results in greater blood loss, and requires more exacting technique than total splenectomy. The aura of success is now too pervasive; it is now time for cautious appraisal."[5]

Definition and Techniques. Splenorrhaphy implies salvage of some spleen attached to its native blood supply. This is accomplished in several ways depending on the severity of injury, and it can be technically demanding. Several studies indicate that with experience a 50 percent salvage rate can be achieved.

Potential Complications. The concept of splenic salvage is not new—it has been repopularized with the increased awareness of the spleen's immunologic role. Operations for splenic conservation were abandoned in favor of total splenectomy, according to Morgenstern, because an increasing number of complications of conservative procedures were accumulating at the same time the operation of splenectomy was becoming increasingly safe.

Studies. Combining the results of several large series gives an incidence of rebleeding of five patients out of 306 splenorrhaphies performed, or 1.6 percent. Four out of the five required reoperation and splenectomy. Of note is that 2/19, or 11 percent, of patients undergoing partial resection rebled in a study by Moore and colleagues.[6] They concluded that " . . . these bleeding episodes confirm that technical complications will no doubt occur as more complex injuries are approached."

If the risk of OPSI is 0.3 percent (i.e., 3/1,000 or 1/330 patients splenectomized for trauma), then it may be that one has to save about 300 spleens without a single complication to justify a serious complication associated with the effort of saving one. The series of splenorrhaphy patients had a 1.6 percent rebleed rate, which means not one but five patients/300 had a serious complication. Four of them had to return to the operating room for splenectomy. Only 0.1 percent, or 1/1,000, of splenectomy patients will die from OPSI. At the rate of five rebleeds/306 patients undergoing splenorrhaphy, there will be approximately 17/1,000 overall and potentially over 100 rebleeds among 1,000 complicated splenorrhaphies using the figure of 11 percent presented by Moore and associates. It is not hard to imagine one or more of these patients dying either as a result of the rebleed itself or of the second operation. However, with only 306 patients, the splenorrhaphy numbers are still too small to compare mortality rates. Remember, among the first 900 splenectomy patients in the series cited (Table II), there was not a single death secondary to OPSI.

Besides the risk of rebleeding, doing a splenorrhaphy does not necessarily eliminate the risk of OPSI. Firstly, there is evidence that at least one-third to one-half of the spleen represents a critical mass that must be left if immunologic protection is to be preserved. Secondly, splenic artery ligation, one splenorrhaphy technique, was found to result in reduced splenic blood flow and delayed pneumococcal clearance in rabbits. It was concluded that, in addition to a critical mass, there is a critical blood flow and that splenic artery ligation to preserve an injured spleen cannot be assured to give protection from sepsis.

FACTORS TO DECREASE THE RISK OF OPSI

Now, let us explore other strategies besides splenorrhaphy used to minimize the risk of OPSI, although these probably have more relevance to higher risk groups, such as children and patients with intercurrent reticuloendothelial disease. These strategies include autotransplantation, vaccination, and prophylactic antibiotics.

Autotransplantation.   One possible explanation for the low incidence of OPSI among trauma patients was proposed by Pearson and colleagues.[7] They found splenosis, or the seeding of splenic tissue into the peritoneum, to be common after splenectomy for trauma as opposed to splenectomy for hematologic disease. Splenic activity was assessed by examination of the percentage of abnormal or pitted RBCs. One percent pitted red cells is normal versus an average of 20 percent in children splenectomized for hematologic disease. Fifty-nine percent of patients (13/22) after a trauma splenectomy had a significantly low or normal percentage of pitted RBCs, suggesting return of splenic function. They concluded that splenosis, or this showing of splenic fragments, is common in trauma patients and might account for their low frequency of OPSI.

Likhite[8] showed that depression of opsonin and leukokinin (tuftsin) activity observed in splenectomized animals could be avoided after ectopic (SC) autotransplantation of splenic tissue. Others have shown return of antibody response to immunization after autotransplantation.

However, while indices of splenic function are fine, what about the ultimate impact? Does autotransplantation decrease mortality after bacterial challenge? Early animal studies on mortality have been many and their results confusing, showing in different studies variously full, partial, or no protective effect of the autotransplanted tissue.

One possible explanation is that bolus intravenous or intraperitoneal challenge (usually used in these studies) may be a poor model. If one considers OPSI in the human, it usually follows a mild respiratory infection, not a massive IV inoculum. Since more organisms causing postsplenectomy sepsis are respiratory tract pathogens, it would seem that pulmonary bacterial challenge would more closely resemble the clinical setting of postsplenectomy sepsis.

There are several studies that support this concept. Moxon and Schwartz[9] found that all sham-operated controls and autotransplanted rats survived after intranasal challenge, whereas 70 percent of asplenic rats died. The excess deaths among asplenic rats were significant (p < .003). They suggested that previous animal studies that used IV inoculation may have underestimated the potential protective role of splenic autotransplantation.

Livingston and colleagues[10] also emphasized the importance of the method of challenge. In this experiment, the animals were challenged via the respiratory tract 12 weeks after autotransplantation; and no significant difference was found in mortality between the rats with mesenteric autotransplants compared to controls. Both groups had a significantly lower mortality than that of asplenic rats (p < .05).

There are several studies that demonstrate that lung defenses are weakened by splenectomy and can be reconstituted by autotransplantation.[9-11] Shennib and associates[11] demonstrated the deterioration of pulmonary alveolar macrophage (PAM) activity in young asplenic rats compared to autotransplanted rats. This difference was significant (p < .001). This effect of splenic tissue on the pulmonary alveolar macrophage conceivably could be mediated by the opsonins and tuftsin, which are known to stimulate macrophage activity, are deficient in splenectomized animals, and are restored after autotransplantation. Interestingly, weakened lung defense following splenectomy disappeared as the rat matured, which parallels the susceptibility pattern to OPSI in the human. This lends further support to the idea that pulmonary bacterial challenge more closely resembles the clinical setting of postsplenectomy sepsis.

There are only four studies that looked at autotransplantation in the human: Patel and colleagues,[12] Kusminsky and colleagues,[13] Nielsen and colleagues,[14] and Moore and colleagues.[6] Altogether they comprise 70 patients. Most of the patients received the equivalent of one-third of the spleen in an omental pouch. All patients studied demonstrated some evidence of splenic function such as technetium uptake and removal of Howell-Jolly bodies, as well as normalization of C3, IgM, and platelet values. Each study noted autotransplantation to be simple and safe.

It is difficult to show that autotransplantation has any impact on OPSI incidence or mortality in humans because of the rarity of OPSI and the small number of patients autotransplanted to date. There is significant animal and human data showing histologic splenic regeneration, as well as evidence of splenic function in terms of removal of worn out RBCs, technetium upake, and restoration of a number of immunological functions including opsonin and tuftsin activity as well as antibody response to IV immunization. In animal studies, mortality is normalized if challenge does not bypass the lung.

Other Prophylaxis. Other methods of prophylaxis include vaccination and prophylactic antibiotics. Since both Pneumovax and penicillin focus on the pneumococcus, the organism responsible for OPSI in 50 percent of cases, each can at best protect the patient against 40 to 50 percent of all causes of OPSI, although potentially other vaccines could be added in the future. Antibiotic prophylaxis probably should be restricted to high-risk groups.

RECAPITULATION

As Robert Frost declared, " . . . truth keeps going in and out of fashion." Splenectomy rides such a pendulum. At first it was considered a death sentence; then it was ubiquitous; now it is almost a crime. I have pointed out a number of reasons why this should not be the case.

1. It cannot be rigorously determined on a statistical basis that the risk of postsplenectomy sepsis in adult trauma patients exceeds the risk in the general population.
2. This does not mean there is no added risk. It does mean that the added risk, if it exists, must be very, very small.
3. Splenorrhaphy exposes the patient to a risk of rebleeding and relaparotomy exceeding the risk of postsplenectomy sepsis in this population.
4. Based on available data, splenectomy, not splenorrhaphy, may be the safest treatment of traumatic rupture of the spleen in the normal adult. The importance of splenic salvage for prevention of postsplenectomy sepsis has been overemphasized, and expeditious splenectomy remains the procedure of choice for patients with a ruptured spleen.
5. In the future, as results on improved prophylaxis against postsplenectomy sepsis on the one hand and more complicated splenorrhaphies on the other hand are added to the equation, the pendulum can be expected to swing back once again to splenectomy.

REFERENCES

1. Feliciano, D.V., Bitondo, C.G., Mattox, K.L., et al.: A four-year experience with splenectomy versus splenorrhaphy. Ann. Surg., 201(5):568–575, 1985.
2. Malangoni, M.A., Dillon, L.D., Klamer, T.W., and Condon, R.E.: Factors influencing the risk of early and late serious infection in adults after splenectomy for trauma. Surgery, 96:775–783, 1984.
3. Singer, D.B.: Postsplenectomy sepsis. Perspect. Pediatr. Pathol., 1:285–311, 1973.
4. Robinette, C.D. and Fraumeni, J.F., Jr.: Splenectomy and subsequent mortality in veterans of the 1939–1945 war. Lancet, 2:127, 1977.
5. Morgenstern, L.: Let the preserver of spleens beware. (Editorial) Surg. Gynecol. Obstet., 154:81, 1982.
6. Moore, F.A., Moore, E.E., Moore, G.E., and Millikan, J.S.: Risk of splenic salvage after trauma: Analysis of 200 adults. Am. J. Surg., 148:800–805, 1984.
7. Pearson, H.A., Johnston, D., Smith, K.A., and Touloukian, R.J.: The born-again spleen. N. Engl. J. Med., 298:1389–1392, 1978.

8. Likhite, V.V.: Opsonin and leukopenic gamma-globulin in chronically splenectomized rats with and without heterotopic autotransplanted splenic tissue. Nature, 253(5494):742–744, 1975.

9. Moxon, E.R. and Schwartz, A.D.: Heterotopic splenic autotransplantation in the prevention of Haemophilus influenzae meningitis and fatal sepsis in Sprague-Dawley rats. Blood, 56:842–845, 1980.

10. Livingston, C.D., Levine, B.A., and Sirinek, K.R.: Improved survival rate for intraperitoneal autotransplantation of the spleen following pneumococcal pneumonia. Surg. Gynecol. Obstet., 156:761–766, 1983.

11. Shennib, H., Chiu, R.C.J., and Mulder, D.S.: The effects of splenectomy and splenic implantation on alveolar macrophage function. J. Trauma, 23(1):7–12, 1983.

12. Patel, J., Williams, J.S., Shmigel, B., and Hinshaw, J.R.: Preservation of splenic function by autotransplantation of traumatized spleen in man. Surgery, 90:683, 1981.

13. Kusminsky, R.E., Chang, H.H., Hossino, H., et al.: An omental implantation technique for salvage of the spleen. Surg. Gynecol. Obstet., 155:407–408, 1982.

14. Nielsen, J. L., Sakso, P., Sorensen, F. H., and Hansen, H. H.: Demonstration of splenic functions following splenectomy and autologous spleen implantation. Acta Chir. Scand., 150(6):469–473, 1984.

DEBATE V

Is Regional Lymphadenectomy in Cancer Therapeutic or Only Diagnostic?

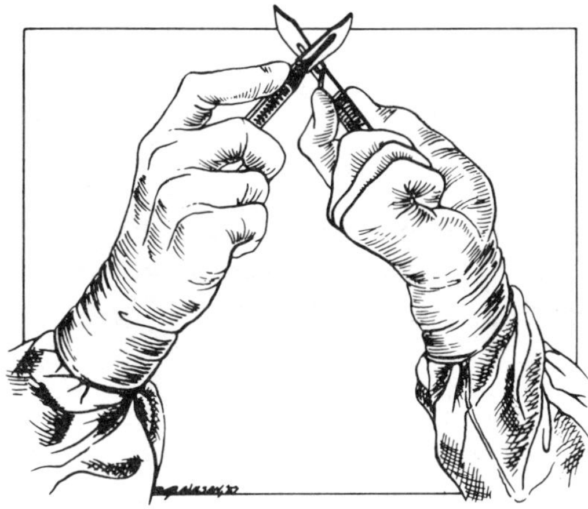

The value of regional lymphadenectomy in surgical oncology addresses a fundamental issue in the nature of cancer. The malignant process begins with the unchecked reproduction of a single cell. In its late stages, cancer spreads widely with the ultimate death of the host. Is there a significant intermediate, or transitional, phase during which time the tumor has spread beyond the bound of the primary site but remains corralled within regional lymph nodes? The concept of direct extension is the premise upon which the classical "en bloc dissection" is based.

Critics of regional nodal function expose lymph nodes as porous fingers but characteristically do not mention the startling frequency of early (apparently limited) neoplastic nodal involvement. Surely lymph nodes feature prominently in the host's immune response.

When large groups of patients encompassing Stages I–IV neoplastic disease are lumped together, any potential benefit of regional lymphadenectomy is submerged. Lymph node resection would not be expected to benefit patients with local (Stage I) disease. Similarly, local-regional surgical extirpation would not be expected to control Stages III and IV disease.

Drs. Grosso and Erdoes, and Ridge have examined the same surgical studies of the same concerns (melanoma, stomach, and breast) in the same manner. Their arguments present unassailable data. They critically review these data in a logical fashion. They derive conclusions based on these data. They represent these conclusions persuasively. Why are these conclusions diametrically opposed? How can they disagree?

V-A: REGIONAL LYMPH NODE DISSECTION IS ONLY DIAGNOSTIC

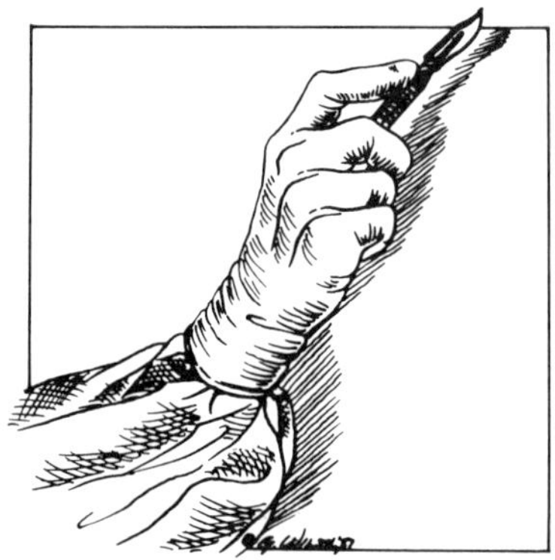

MICHAEL A. GROSSO, M.D.
LUKE S. ERDOES, M.D.

Regional lymph node dissection is only diagnostic. This can be borne out by the literature. There are five important points that support the notion that regional lymph node dissection has no place as a surgically therapeutic deterrent in the management of patients with cancer. These five points are as follows:

1. Lymph node filter function is *poor.*
2. Prophylactic lymph node dissection *does not improve* cure rates in many tumors.
3. Lymph node metastases can be *dissociated from survival* in many tumors.
4. Occult quiescent lymph node metastases are present for years in many tumors and have *no bearing on survival.*
5. Regional lymph node dissection has a high incidence of *complications.*

REGIONAL LYMPH NODE FUNCTION

Regional lymph nodes are important in the initiation of immunity, although some studies indicate that weak antigenic tumors have their growth inhibited by the regional lymph nodes.

Fisher and Fisher[1] found that bacteria, erythrocytes, and labeled tumor cells passed readily through lymph nodes. Additionally, they found that these metastatic cancer cells, having passed through lymph nodes, were viable and capable of growth. Pressman and colleagues[2] found that multiple afferent, lymphaticovenous shunts existed within and about the lymph node. Multiple anatomic and pathologic studies additionally have shown the presence of circulating tumor cells bypassing regional lymph nodes.

Tumor cell filtering by lymph nodes also may be affected by local inflammation or prior damage to the regional lymph nodes or the lymphatics. It is also important to realize that it may be the primary tumor biology that dictates spread as opposed to any innate capacity of the lymph nodes as a filter. It also has been shown in several instances that tumor spread is allowed in an area of local anergy by removing regional lymph nodes. By removing the regional defense system, that is, the regional lymph nodes, tumor spread may occur unabated; and systemic immunity may be insufficient to halt this growth.

The conclusion is that regional lymph nodes allow both afferent and efferent passage of *viable* tumor cells and are not effective "cancer" filters.

PROPHYLATIC LYMPH NODE DISSECTION DOES NOT IMPROVE SURVIVAL

Melanoma. In a prospective, randomized study, Veronesi and colleagues[3] presented 267 patients with excision of tumor and immediate dissection of the regional lymph nodes. A second group of 286 patients underwent excision of the local melanoma with dissection of regional lymph nodes only at the time of palpable involvement. They found that there was an equal percentage of lymph node metastases in both groups. However, there was no difference in survival between the two groups when analyzed according to site, diameter, or Clark-Breslow levels.

A similar study by Sim and colleagues[4] found that there was no significant effect on length of survival or interval to distant metastases with immediate lymph node dissection. This was a prospective, randomized study with 173 patients. Of these patients, 63 underwent no dissection of the regional lymph nodes, 56 underwent delayed dissection of the regional lymph nodes, and 54 underwent immediate dissection of the regional lymph nodes. Again, dissection had no significant effect on length of survival or interval to appearance of distant metastases.

Additional studies by Day and colleagues,[5] Eldh and colleagues,[6] and Cady and colleagues[7] all found in a retrospective fashion that regional lymphadenectomy had no influence on survival. Survival is unaffected by regional lymphadenectomy in melanoma.

Breast Cancer. Fisher and colleagues[8] published a study comparing radical mastectomy with alternative treatments for primary breast carcinoma in a prospective, randomized study. Patients underwent either radical mastectomy, total mastectomy with postoperative x-ray therapy to the regional lymph nodes, or total mastectomy alone. The 3-year mortality was similar among the three groups, indicating no effect of regional lymph node ablation or excision on survival.

Crile[9] published a study consisting of 501 patients undergoing radical mastectomy in one-half of the group and simple mastectomy with late excision of palpable nodes in the remaining half. The 5-year survival in those patients with positive nodes was identical in the two groups.

The Cancer Research Trial[10] conducted a prospective, randomized study that included over 2,200 patients. This group compared simple mastectomy to simple mastectomy plus local radiation therapy to the regional lymph nodes in both Stage I and Stage II disease. They found that local recurrence was significantly greater without local radiotherapy but that the 5-year survival was identical with or without local therapy.

The National Surgical Adjuvant Breast Project trial studied 1,665 patients.[11] It was found that local-regional control was somewhat better with local therapy, but the 5-year relapse-free survival rate was not significantly different. This study looked at three groups: the first was treated with radical mastectomy, the second with simple mastectomy with radiation therapy, and the third with simple mastectomy alone. The 5-year relapse-free survival rate was 68 percent in the radical mastectomy group, 71 percent in the simple mastectomy with radiation therapy group, and 63 percent in the simple mastectomy group. Obviously, there is no significant difference in these numbers. At 10 years, there also is no significant difference in disease-free survival, distant disease-free survival, or survival.[11,12]

Robbins and colleagues[13] reported 735 patients undergoing radical mastectomy. Similar to Fisher, the groups were divided into those patients receiving postoperative x-ray therapy and those receiving no therapy to the remaining regional lymph nodes. Their conclusions also were similar. Local and regional disease were lower with postoperative radiation to the remaining nodes, but survival was identical in both groups.

Hermann and associates[14] conducted a study of 1,593 patients. The 5- to 15-year survival was equal with simple mastectomy versus local lumpectomy versus modified radical mastectomy. No radiation therapy was used. The number of positive axillary lymph nodes was prognostic and indicative of disseminated disease; however, the 5- to 15-year survival in each of the groups was equal. Papaioannou[15] concluded that regional lymph nodes should be preserved since they stimulate systemic immunity.

From this literature review, one can conclude that *survival* is unaffected by regional lymphadenectomy or radiation ablation in breast cancer.

Colorectal Cancer. Some recent data concerning colorectal cancer also have been published supporting the view that regional lymphadenectomy has no value for cure in cancer therapy. In a study by Gunderson and Sosin,[16] survival was related directly to local tissue invasion but not to lymph node status. Recurrence rate was 72 percent in those patients with negative nodes and 71 percent in those patients with positive nodes with local tissue invasion.

In a study by Wood and colleagues,[17] it was found that local tumor invasion was a prognostic factor in colorectal cancer. The 5-year survival in patients with Dukes C lesions with positive nodes but no local invasion was approximately 79 percent; in those patients with C1 lesions and local invasion, survival was 20 percent; in those patients with Dukes B lesions and no local invasion, survival was 80 percent. In those patients with Dukes B lesions and local invasion, survival was 45 percent. They concluded that survival was related to local tissue invasion but not lymph node status.

Head/Neck Cancer. Snyderman and colleagues[18] reported on the extracapsular spread of carcinoma in cervical lymph nodes. They also found that survival in head and neck carcinoma was related to extracapsular spread of tumor but not to local lymph node status. The 3-year survival in those patients with negative nodes was 71 percent; in those patients with positive nodes, survival was 79 percent. The 3-year survival was 45 percent in those patients with extracapsular spread of tumor.

LYMPH NODE METASTASES ARE DISSOCIATED FROM SURVIVAL

Thyroid Cancer. Franssila[19] reported his results for prognosis in thyroid carcinoma. The 10-year survival for papillary thyroid carcinoma with positive nodes was

79 percent; with negative nodes, survival was 81 percent. When all types of thyroid carcinoma (papillary, follicular, mixed) were analyzed together, the overall survival rate was 57 percent. Survival was not related to the presence of local lymph node metastases. The 10-year survival, however, was affected by the presence of *distant* metastases. The 10-year survival for all types with distant positive nodes was 11 percent; with distant negative nodes, survival was 67 percent.

Carcinoid. Similar results can be found with carcinoid. Moertel and colleagues[20] reported on the life history of carcinoid tumor of the small intestine. The 5-year survival with nodal metastases was 71 percent. The 5-year survival with no nodal metastases was 64 percent. Again, local nodal metastases had no influence on long-term survival.

Gastric Carcinoma. For gastric carcinoma, many have advocated an extended gastrectomy, which usually requires total gastrectomy, distal pancreatectomy, splenectomy, and removal of the greater and lesser omentum. The proximity of the stomach to the spleen, pancreas, and greater and lesser omentum requires this type of therapy if regional lymph nodes are to be removed. Also of note is that the lymphatics follow the arterial supply to the stomach.

Prognosis in gastric carcinoma also is dependent on whether the primary tumor lies in the proximal, middle, or distal one-third of the stomach. Midstomach lesions have a better prognosis than the distal lesions, which have a better prognosis than the proximal lesions. The level of invasion of the primary tumor also correlates with nodal involvement. When the serosa of the stomach is involved, invariably there are multiple positive regional nodes.

No prospective, randomized trials have been performed on gastric carcinoma. The largest United States series was done by Gilbertson.[21] He studied 1,983 patients and used retrospective controls. The overall 5-year survival was a dismal 10.2 percent. The operative mortality with partial gastrectomy was 25.6 pecent; yet with total gastrectomy, the operative mortality jumped to 33.3 percent. The 5-year survival rate for patients operated on for cure dropped from 28 percent to 17 percent when extended gastrectomy was used. The 5-year survival for patients operated on for cure with positive lymph nodes dropped from 18 percent to 9 percent when extended gastrectomy was employed. The overall 5-year survival decreased from 12.2 percent to 8.8 percent.

OCCULT QUIESCENT LYMPH NODE METASTASES

There appears to be a group of tumors in which occult quiescent lymph node metastases are present for many years with no deleterious effects on the host.

Medullary Thyroid Carcinoma. Block and colleagues[22] conducted a study on the management of a medullary thyroid carcinoma. Medullary thyroid carcinoma is unique in that its presence can be indicated by high serum calcitonin levels. It was found that calcitonin levels were elevated postoperatively in over one-third of patients and that this indicated presence of residual disease in the local-regional nodes. These micrometastases appeared to remain dormant during the entire seven-year follow-up period of the study.

Similarly, Jackson and colleagues[23] published the clinical course after definitive operation for medullary carcinoma of the thyroid. Calcitonin levels were normal postoperatively in only one-third of the patients; survival averaged 68.5 years in those patients presenting without pheochromocytoma.

REGIONAL LYMPH NODE DISSECTION—COMPLICATIONS

Regional lymphadenectomy is not without complication. Urist and colleagues[24] reported on the surgical morbidity after regional lymphadenectomy in 204 melanoma patients. Forty-eight of these patients had cervical lymphadenectomy, 98 patients had axillary lymphadenectomy, and 58 patients had groin lymphadenectomy. One-fourth of the 204 patients showed short-term wound-related problems. Serona developed in 22 percent of these, nerve dysfunction or significant pain developed in 14 percent, and wound infection requiring wound revision occurred in 6 percent. Wound complications increased the hospital stay to between 0.6 to 4.8 days. Lymphedema was present in 26 percent of the groin dissection patients at greater than six-month or longer follow-up. Eight percent had significant functional deficit secondary to this lymphedema.

SUMMARY

From the review of the literature, it is apparent that the concepts of tumor biology are evolving slowly. Cancer cells seem to disseminate relatively early in the course of the disease. However, the presence of circulating cancer cells does not predict outcome. Tumor-host factors appear to govern the absence or presence of local and distant metastases. Patients do not survive if the interaction of host factors and neoplastic cells results in progressive growth.

From the literature, we can conclude the following:

1. Lymph nodes function poorly as barriers to tumor cells.
2. Prophylactic lymphadenectomy does not improve survival in many tumors.
3. Lymph node metastases can be dissociated from survival in many tumors.
4. Occult quiescent metastases are present for many years in some tumors.
5. Regional lymph node dissection is not without complication.

The timing of lymph node metastases (early vs. late) may indicate tumor aggressiveness. Lymph node metastases, therefore, are indicators for but not governors of survival. Regional lymphadenectomy has no impact upon *survival* and will, of necessity, increase complications.

The issue of the therapeutic value of regional lymphadenectomy has been summarized by Weiss: "Local therapy aimed at lymph nodes themselves will no more effectively control distant metastases than removal of the speedometer from a car will reduce its speed."[25]

REFERENCES

1. Fisher, B. and Fisher, E.R.: Barrier function of lymph node to tumor cells and erythrocytes. Cancer, 20:1907–1913, 1967.
2. Pressman, J.J., Simon, M.B., Hand, K., and Miller, J.: Passage of fluids, cells, and bacteria via direct communications between lymph nodes and veins. Surg. Gynecol. Obstet., 115:204–214, 1962.
3. Veronesi, U. Adamus, J., Bandiera, D.C., et al.: Inefficacy of immediate node dissection in stage I melanoma of the limbs. N. Engl. J. Med., 297:627–630, 1977.
4. Sim, F.H., Taylor, W.F., Ivins, J.C., Pritchard, D.J., and Soule, E.H.: A prospective, randomized study of the efficacy of routine elective lymphadenectomy in management of malignant melanoma. Cancer, 41:948–956, 1978.
5. Day, C.L., Sober, A.J., Lew, R.A., et al.: Malignant melanoma patients with positive nodes and relatively good prognoses. Cancer, 47:955–962, 1981.
6. Eldh, J., Boeryd, B., and Peterson, L-E: Prognostic factors in cutaneous melanoma in stage I. Scand. J. Plas. Reconstr. Surg., 12:243–255, 1978.
7. Cady, B., Legg, M.A., and Redfern, A.B.: Contemporary treatment of malignant melanoma. Am. J. Surg., 129:472–482, 1975.
8. Fisher, B., Montague, E., Remond, C., et al.: Comparison of radical mastectomy with alternative treatments for primary breast cancer: Prospective, randomized clinical trial. Cancer, 39:2827–2839, 1977.
9. Crile, G., Jr.: Results of simple mastectomy without irradiation in the treatment of operative stage I cancer of the breast. Ann. Surg., 168:330–336, 1968.
10. Cancer Research Trial. Management of early cancer of the breast: International Multicenter Trial. Br. Med. J., 1:1035–1038, 1976.
11. Fisher, B., Bauer, M., Margolese, R., et al.: Five-year results of a randomized clinical trial comparing total mastectomy and segmental mastectomy with or without radiation in the treatment of breast cancer. N. Engl. J. Med., 312(11):665–673, 1985.
12. Fisher, B., Redman, C., Fisher, E.R., et al.: Ten-year results of a randomized clinical trial comparing radical mastectomy with or without radiation. N. Engl. J. Med., 312(11):674–681, 1985.
13. Robbins, G.F., Lucas, J.C., Fraclhia, A.A., et al.: An evaluation of postoperative prophylactic radiotherapy in breast cancer. Surg. Gynecol. Obstet., 122:979–982, 1966.
14. Hermann, R.E., Esselstyn, C.B., Crile, G., Jr., et al.: Results of conservative operations for breast cancer. Arch. Surg., 120:746–751, 1985.
15. Papaioannou, A.: The contribution of regional lymph nodes in the resistance against breast cancer: Practical applications. J. Surg. Onc., 25:232–239, 1984.
16. Gunderson, L.I. and Sosin, H.: Areas of failure at reoperation following "curative surgery" for adenocarcinoma of the rectum. Cancer, 34:1278–1292, 1974.
17. Wood, C.B., Gillis, C.R., Hole, D., Malcom, A.J., and Blumgart, L.H.: Local tumor invasion as a prognostic factor in colorectal cancer. Br. J. Surg., 68:326–328. 1981.
18. Snyderman, N.L., Johnson, J.T., Schramm, V.L., et al.: Extracapsular spread of carcinoma in cervical lymph nodes. Cancer, 56:1597–1599, 1985.
19. Franssila, K.O.: Prognosis in thyroid carcinoma. Cancer, 36:1138–1146, 1975.
20. Moertel, C.G., Sauer, W.G., Dockerty, M.B., and Bagenstoss, A.H.: Life history of the carcinoid tumor of the small intestine. Cancer, 14:901–912, 1961.
21. Gilbertson, V.A.: Results of treatment of stomach cancer. An appraisal of efforts for more extensive surgery and a report of 1,983 cases. Cancer, 23(6):1305–1308, 1969.
22. Block, M.A., Jackson, C.E., and Tashjian, A.H.: Management of occult medullary thyroid carcinoma. Arch. Surg., 113:368–372, 1978.
23. Jackson, C.E., Talpos, G.B., and Kambours, A.: The clinical course after definitive operation for medullary thyroid carcinoma. Surgery, 94:995–1001, 1983.
24. Urist, M.M., Maddox, W.A., Kennedy, J.E., and Balch, C.M.: Patient risk factors and surgical morbidity after regional lymphadenectomy in 204 melanoma patients. Cancer, 51:2152–2156, 1983.
25. Weiss, S.: The significance of the circulating cancer cell. Can. Treat. Rev., 2:55–72, 1975.

V-B: REGIONAL LYMPH NODE DISSECTION IS BOTH THERAPEUTIC *AND* DIAGNOSTIC

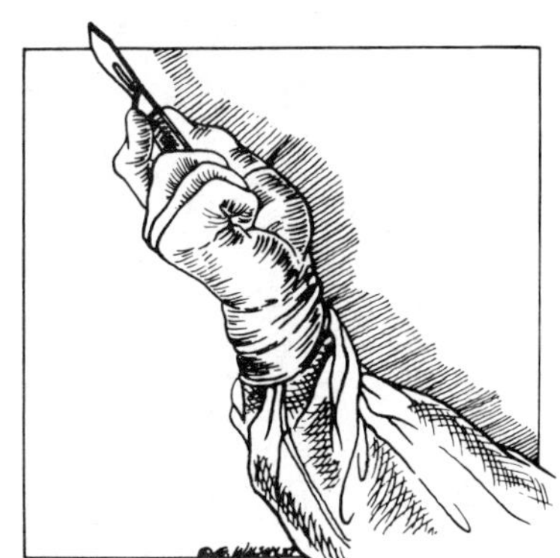

JOHN A. RIDGE, M.D., Ph.D.

The question of whether lymph node dissections are therapeutic really considers the nature of cancer. Is cancer a "Halstedian" disease that spreads to lymph nodes and then sequentially to distant sites, or does the tumor spread in no orderly way? The issue is important to surgeons because operations have limitations. An operation can remove tumor to prevent advanced local disease, obtain tumor-free margins around a cancer, and remove regional nodes that are likely to be involved.

This discussion will demonstrate that lymph node dissection is both diagnostic and therapeutic. Cure may be defined as survival for a given period of time, as interruption of the disease's "force of mortality," or as freedom from cancer for the remainder of life.[1] The cancers under consideration here are melanoma (where there is no responsible dissenting opinion), gastric cancer (a classic "Halstedian cancer"), and breast cancer (where removal of involved regional lymph nodes is curative).

Lymph node dissection is so widely accepted as therapy for melanoma that it is impossible to find a series of melanoma patients with involved lymph nodes who were not treated by removal of the regional nodes. The only available information comes from a group of untreated patients, two-thirds of whom probably had Stage I disease. The 5-year survival of these untreated patients was only 10 percent,[2] much less than the 26 to 40 percent survival of patients whose involved lymph nodes were removed.[3-5] As shown in Table I, this difference is significant.

If patients without palpable lymphadenopathy were submitted to lymph node dissection, the 5-year survival was even longer, rising to 46 to 53 percent.[3-6] As shown in Table II, it also is notable that the 5-year survival falls with increasing numbers of involved lymph nodes.[4] Patients with only one tumor-bearing lymph node had a 5-year survival of 58 percent, while those with more than four lymph nodes involved had a 5-year survival of 10 percent. As shown in Table III, this is a significant difference.

This brief review of the melanoma literature demonstrates important features of lymph node involvement:

TABLE I.   LYMPH NODE DISSECTION CAN CURE MELANOMAS

CLASS	NUMBER	5-YEAR SURVIVAL (%)
Untreated (all)	3/ 29[2]	10
Palpable nodes	8/ 31[2]	26
	41/106[3]	39
	23/ 82[4]	28
	26/ 64[5]	40

[2]Block and Hartwell: Ann. Surg., 154:74, 1961.
[3]Goldsmith, et al.: Cancer, 26:606, 1970.
[4]Balch, et al.: Ann. Surg., 193:377, 1977.
[5]Veronesi, et al.: Cancer, 49:2420, 1982.

TABLE II. DEGREE OF NODE INVOLVEMENT AFFECTS SURVICAL

Microscopic Compared with Gross Disease	
TYPE OF INVOLVEMENT	5-YEAR SURVIVAL (%)
Palpable	26[2]
	39[3]
	28[4]
	40[5]
Microscopic	48[3]
	48[4]
	46[5]
	53[6]

[2]Block and Hartwell: Ann. Surg., 154(S):74, 1961.
[3]Goldsmith, et al.: Cancer, 26:606, 1970.
[4]Balch, et al.: Ann. Surg., 193:377, 1981.
[5]Veronesi, et al.: Cancer, 49, 2420, 1982.
[6]Roses, et al.: Ann. Surg., 198:65, 1983.

TABLE III.   NUMBER OF NODES INVOLVED AFFECTS SURVIVAL*

SURVIVAL WITH TUMOR-BEARING NODES	
NODES INVOLVED	5-YEAR SURVIVAL (%)
1	58
2, 3, 4	27
4+	10

This difference is significant (p < 0.001)

*From Balch, C.M., Soong, S.J., Murad, T.M., et al.: A multifactorial analysis of melanoma. III. Prognostic factors in melanoma patients with lymph node metastases (stage II). Ann. Surg., 193:377–388, 1981.

1. Lymph node dissections enhance the 5-year survival.
2. Bulk disease of the nodes is worse than microscopic tumor spread.
3. Involvement of increasing numbers of lymph nodes worsens the prognosis.

What about gastric cancer? The conventional therapy available in the United States is woefully inadequate. Five-year survival with the (treated) disease ranges from 5 to 17 percent in 11 series; and in 7 of those 11 reports, the 5-year survival is less than 10 percent.[7] Such dismal results, essentially regardless of the operation employed, have led many surgeons to the erroneous conclusion that lymph node dissections will not benefit patients with gastric cancer. This impression is due to the advanced state at which most gastric cancers are detected in America. Seventy percent of gastric cancers have involved nodes more than 3 cm from the primary neoplasm or on the opposite side of the stomach (termed Stage III in the following discussion).

Such tumors cannot be cured by any operation, regardless of its extent, because patients with lymph nodes on both sides of the stomach already have distant disease.[8] As shown in Table IV, fully 70 percent of Stage III patients who came to necropsy within one month of a "curative" operation that ostensibly extirpated their tumor were found to have residual disease—usually a liver or lung metastasis. In contrast, no patient with Stage I or Stage II gastric cancer had residual tumor found at autopsy. Since surgical therapy cannot hope to cure disease outside of the margins of resection, it is not surprising that no benefit is found from lymph node dissection in most cases of gastric cancer.

Thus, the true value of extended surgery is seen only when survival with Stage I or Stage II gastric cancer is considered.[9-11] Table V indicates that the usual procedure performed in the United States is the subtotal gastrectomy, which involves resection of the appropriate portion of the stomach, contiguous viscus, and both omenta. The extended total gastrectomy entails resection of the entire stomach, the distal esophagus, the first part of the duodenum, the spleen, both omenta, the distal pancreas, and the celiac nodes. This is a big operation, but it shows a real benefit. In all parts of the stomach, the extended total gastrectomy offers a 2.5- to 5-fold higher survival than does the subtotal gastrectomy. In most cases the differences are significant. The results for antral lesions (only 11 extended total gastrectomies were performed for antral gastric cancer) are particularly impressive.

A single surgeon reported his personal series of more than 400 operations for gastric cancer.[12] Traditional subtotal gastrectomy was performed until 1963 when he changed therapy to extended subtotal gastrectomy involving meticulous lymph node

**TABLE IV.   NODES AND DISTANT DISEASE IN
GASTRIC CANCER***

EARLY AUTOPSY AFTER CURATIVE RESECTION

Stage I-II	0/8 residual disease
Stage III	10/13 residual disease

This difference is significant (p < 0.01)

*From Papachristou, D.N. and Fortner, J.G.: Is gastric cancer generalized at the time of surgery? J. Surg. Oncol., 18:27–29, 1981.

TABLE V.   EXTENDED RESECTIONS CAN CURE
GASTRIC CANCER*

5-YEAR SURVIVAL FOR STAGES I AND II (PERCENT)		
Fundus	68	13	<0.01
Cardia	83	16	<0.03
Midstomach	42	17	NS
Antrum	100	37	<0.02
	n = 100	n = 114	

*From Shiu, M.H., Papachristou, D.N., Kosloff, C., and Eliopoulos, G.: Selection of operative procedure for adenocarcinoma of the midstomach. Twenty years' experience with implications for future treatment strategy. Ann. Surg., 192:730–737, 1980; Papachristou, D.N. and Fortner, J.G.: Adenocarcinoma of the gastric cardia. The choice of gastrectomy. Ann. Surg., 192:58–64, 1980; Papachristou, D.N. and Fortner, J.G.: Selection of gastrectomy for adenocarcinoma arising in the gastric fundus. J. Surg. Oncol., 21:165–169, 1982.

TABLE VI.   A BIGGER OPERATION CURES MORE
GASTRIC CANCER*

5-YEAR SURVIVAL AFTER RESECTION			
SITE	EXTENDED	SUBTOTAL	p
Serosa	45% (113/251)	18% (33/179)	< 0.001
Nodes	39% (95/245)**	18% (32/181)	< 0.001

*From Kodama, Y., Sugimachi, K., Soejima, K., et al.: Evaluation of extensive lymph node dissection for carcinoma of the stomach. World J. Surg., 5:243, 1981.
**EGC n = 23

dissections. Table VI shows that, in patients whose primary lesion extended to the serosa, the 5-year survival for extended dissection was 45 percent, in contrast to 18 percent after traditional subtotal gastrectomy. In patients with involved lymph nodes, the 5-year survival of extended subtotal gastrectomy was 39 percent, while that for subtotal gastrectomy was 18 percent. Again, this is a significant difference. It is noteworthy that only 23 patients with involved nodes (less than 10 percent) had early gastric cancer. In fact, some of the 5-year survivors actually had nodes involved on the opposite side of the stomach from the primary neoplasm (Stage III). The extended resection cured some patients with Stage III gastric cancers.

Thus, in the case of gastric cancer, the evidence shows that:

1. Lymph node dissections may cure patients with positive nodes.
2. Extended resections increase the frequency of 5-year survival 200 to 300 percent if the disease is regional.

Even cancer of the breast, perhaps the paradigm for the "alternative," non-Halstedian view of cancer, responds well to lymph node dissection.

TABLE VII. PATIENTS WITH UNTREATED BREAST CANCER DIE*

CASES	SURVIVAL RATE (%) YEARS		
	5	10	15
651	16		
100	18	5	0
250	18	4	1

*Adapted from Bloom, H.J.G., Richardson, W.W., and Harries, E.J.: Natural history of untreated breast cancer (1805–1933): Comparison of untreated and treated cases according to histological grade of malignancy. Br. Med. J., 2:216, 1962.

Breast cancer is a fatal disease. Studies of the untreated tumor show that the 10-year survival is only about 5 percent[13] as shown in Table VII. In contrast, locoregional therapy by mastectomy offers cure, even to patients with involved nodes. Two studies have been published that offer 30-year follow-up of patients treated by radical mastectomy.[14,15] Though one reports the data in terms of actuarial survival while the other reports "crude survival," their results are comparable when corrected for aging and other causes of death. Both studies include many patients with advanced breast cancers. No woman died of breast cancer after 23 years in either series.

Following 1,259 patients from a single institution[14] who were treated by radical mastectomy, the 30-year actuarial survival for patients with Stage II breast cancer was 35 percent. The survival for patients with Stage III breast cancer was 17 percent! (Table VIII).

Similarly, as shown in Table IX, when 1,458 patients from a single private practice were followed for 30 years,[15] 24 percent had died without evidence of disease (NED); and 13 percent were still alive without evidence of cancer. Only 7 percent of the patients were lost to follow-up!

Examination of the survivors is instructive. Table X shows that 67 percent of the 184 30-year survivors had no involved lymph nodes in their specimens. However, 60 of the 30-year survivors had involved lymph nodes behind or medial to the pectoralis minor muscle (Levels II and III nodes).

TABLE VIII. RADICAL MASTECTOMY CAN CURE BREAST CANCER*

STAGE	NED SURVIVAL RATE (%) YEARS			
	5	10	20	30
I (487)	84	76	66	66
II (473)	52	44	35	35
III (299)	39	20	17	17

*From Ferguson, D.J., Meier, P., Karrison, I., et al.: Staging of breast cancer and survival rates: An assessment based on 50 years of experience with radical mastectomy. J.A.M.A., 248:1337–1341, 1982.

**TABLE IX.　1,458 RADICAL MASTECTOMIES—
30-YEAR FOLLOW-UP***

OUTCOME	PERCENT
Died of breast cancer	57
Lost to follow-up	7
Died NED	24
Alive NED	13

*From Adair, F., Berg, J., Joubert, L., and Robbins, G.F.: Long-term follow-up of breast cancer patients: The 30-year report. Cancer, 33:1145–1150, 1974.

A fundamental tenet of the "non-Halstedian" alternative theory of cancer spread, that lymph nodes represent only an indicator of tumor behavior, would suggest that women with tumor in Level II or Level III nodes have aggressive, widely disseminated disease. Nonetheless, many women survived 30 years after radical mastectomy—a "locoregional" therapy. Admittedly, some received hormonal therapy.

Hence:

1. Lymph node dissections alone can cure women with breast cancer in lymph nodes, and
2. Many patients with advanced lymph node involvement may not die of their cancer if those lymph nodes are removed.

Surgical therapy for melanoma, gastric cancer, and breast cancer offers striking results. Some 40 percent of melanoma patients with limited tumor burden in their lymph nodes may be cured by node dissection. A similar fraction of appropriately staged patients with gastric cancer is cured by radical operations. Fifteen to 35 percent of breast cancer patients are cured by radical mastectomy, even with high axillary nodes involved.

These results support a "modified Halstedian" view of cancer. Table X shows that cancer begins as a local process (Stage I). It spreads by local invasion and begins to involve regional nodes. Perhaps there is even "systemic" spread that may be survived if the tumor burden is reduced (Stage II). Eventually, the tumor only *appears* to be a

**TABLE X.　30-YEAR SURVIVORS OF RADICAL
MASTECTOMY***

CLASS	NUMBERS	PERCENT
Nodes negative	124/184	67
Nodes positive	60/184	33
Level I	26/184	14
Levels II-III	34/184	18

*From Adair, F., Berg, J., Joubert, L., and Robbins, G.F.: Long-term follow-up of breast cancer patients: The 30-year report. Cancer, 33:1145–1150, 1974.

regional problem, and insurmountable systemic dissemination has occurred (Stage III). This is followed by the gross appearance of distant metastases (Stage IV). A surgeon should not be disheartened if his operations cannot cure Stage III and Stage IV cancers.

An operation can remove tumor to prevent advanced local disease. It can obtain local tumor-free margins and remove involved nodes. Operations should not be abandoned because they cannot cure patients with substantial distant tumor burden.

The challenge for the surgeon is to submit only the proper patients to lymph node dissections. Under these circumstances, lymph node dissection is therapeutic!

REFERENCES

1. Harris, J.R. and Hellman, S.: Observations on survival curve analysis with particular reference to breast cancer treatment. Cancer, 57:925–928, 1986.
2. Block, G.E. and Hartwell, S.W., Jr.: Malignant melanoma: A study of 217 cases. Part I: Epidemiology. Ann. Surg., 154(suppl):74–87, 1961.
3. Goldsmith, H.S., Shah, J.P., and Kim, D.H.: Prognostic significance of lymph node dissection in the treatment of malignant melanoma. Cancer, 26:606–609, 1970.
4. Balch, C.M., Soong, S.J., Murad, T.M., et al.: A multifactorial analysis of melanoma. III. Prognostic factors in melanoma patients with lymph node metastases (stage II). Ann. Surg., 193:377–388, 1981.
5. Veronesi, U., Adamus, J., Bandiera, D.C., et al.: Delayed regional lymph node dissection in stage I melanoma of the skin of the lower extremities. Cancer, 49:2420–2430, 1982.
6. Roses, D.F., Harris, M.N., Rigel, D., et al.: Local and in-transit metastases following definitive excision for primary cutaneous malignant melanoma. Ann. Surg., 198:65–69, 1983.
7. Dupont, J.B., Jr., Lee, J.R., Burton, G.R., and Cohn, I., Jr.: Adenocarcinoma of the stomach: Review of 1,497 cases. Cancer, 41:941–947, 1978.
8. Papachristou, D.N. and Fortner, J.G.: Is gastric cancer generalized at the time of surgery? J. Surg. Oncol., 18:27–29, 1981.
9. Shiu, M.H., Papachristou, D.N., Kosloff, C., and Eliopoulos, G.: Selection of operative procedure for adenocarcinoma of the midstomach. Twenty years' experience with implications for future treatment strategy. Ann. Surg., 192:730–737, 1980.
10. Papachristou, D.N. and Fortner, J.G.: Adenocarcinoma of the gastric cardia. The choice of gastrectomy. Ann. Surg., 192:58–64, 1980.
11. Papachristou, D.N. and Fortner, J.G.: Selection of gastrectomy for adenocarcinoma arising in the gastric fundus. J. Surg. Oncol., 21:165–169, 1982.
12. Kodama, Y., Sugimachi, K., Soejima, K., et al.: Evaluation of extensive lymph node dissection for carcinoma of the stomach. World J. Surg., 5:241–246, 1981.
13. Bloom, H.J.G., Richardson, W.W., and Harries, E.J.: Natural history of untreated breast cancer (1805–1933): Comparison of untreated and treated cases according to histological grade of malignancy. Br. Med. J., 2:213–221, 1962.
14. Ferguson, D.J., Meier, P., Karrison, I., et al.: Staging of breast cancer and survival rates: An assessment based on 50 years of experience with radical mastectomy. J.A.M.A., 248:1337–1341, 1982.
15. Adair, F., Berg, J., Joubert, L., and Robbins, G.F.: Long-term follow-up of breast cancer patients: The 30-year report. Cancer, 33:1145–1150, 1974.

DEBATE VI

Hepatic Resections

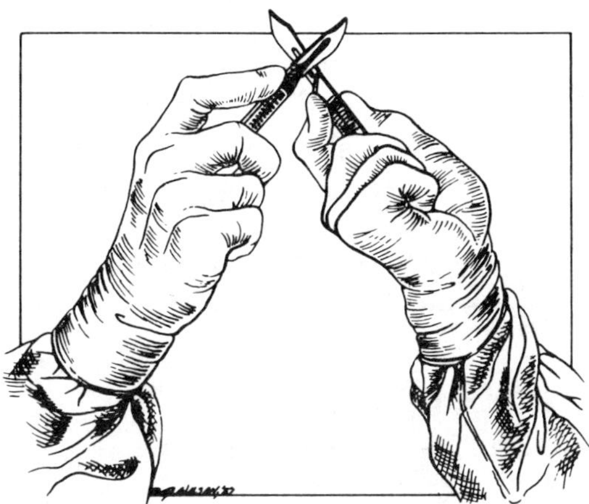

Should we debunk debulking? When neoplastic disease spreads beyond the confines of the locoregional site, is it not then systemic? Surgery is uniquely capable of eliminating local neoplastic disease. Intuitively, surgery is uniquely incapable of definitively dealing with a systemic process. Can there be any value in decreasing (but not eliminating) systemic tumor burden?

In the following pages, Dr. Teter builds a formidable argument against offering a patient with metastatic hepatic disease the opportunity for distant resective therapy. He reasons that, until effective concomitant adjuvant therapy is available, the risks of a major surgical procedure (hepatic resection) do not warrant the unlikely possibility that surgeons can influence the inexorable course of Stage IV colorectal cancer—we are simply rearranging the deck chairs on the Titanic.

Conversely, Dr. Davis remains enthusiastically optimistic concerning our ability to redirect by surgery the course of patients with metastatic colorectal cancer. She does not want to abandon patients with Stage IV disease. Dr. Davis does not rely on pessimistic intuition or therapy, she relies solely on facts.

Approximately 10,000 patients with colorectal cancer and liver metastasis who can be considered candidates for hepatic resection present each year. Their prognosis without therapy or with chemotherapy alone is dismal. As with all surgical procedures, the complications diminish with increasing experience. The morbidity of hepatic lobectomy and even trisegmentectomy in experienced hands is now startlingly low.

In a matched control series from Memorial, the 4-year survival in patients undergoing hepatic resection of metastatic disease was approximately 40 percent, while the survival in the control group was zero! Ultimately, we must all determine whether these results may be translated to the patient population we see in our own hospitals. We still need better adjuvant therapy for this systemic disease and more precise methods of selecting candidates for major hepatic resective surgery.

VI-A: RESECTION OF COLORECTAL HEPATIC METASTASIS: NO

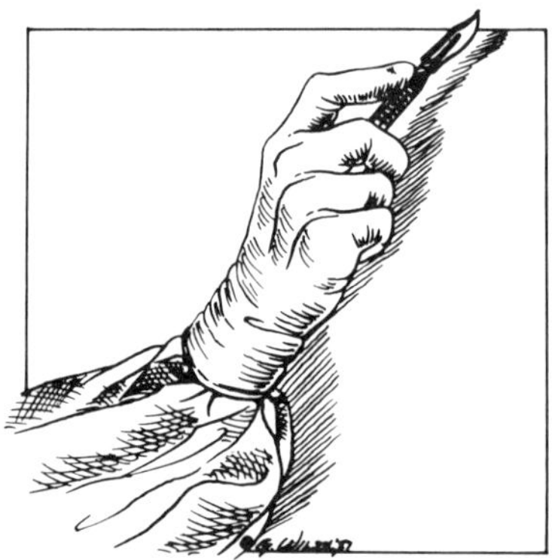

ALLEN L. TETER, M.D.

Over the past three decades of modern oncological therapy for colorectal carcinoma, nothing has proven more dismal in terms of success or cure than treatment of colorectal metastasis to the liver. At present, with regard to radiation and chemotherapy, no significant improvement in 5-year survival has been seen. Even with newer and more potent intravenously administered chemotherapeutic agents, single or in combination, median survivals still are disheartening, being only a few months more than the usual six to nine months in nontreated patients.

When resection of hepatic metastasis was proposed in the early 1970s with 5-year survival rates varying from 25 to 30 percent,[1,2] it is understandable why many oncological surgeons as well as oncologists jumped on the bandwagon. Even more influential in following the course of resection are the current survival data that have been recorded by Starzl and colleagues[3] and Fortner and colleagues.[4] Actuarial survival rates as high as 57 percent at five years have to be viewed with interest and not something at which to shrug our shoulders.[3]

However, we must keep in mind several points that are not immediately apparent. Firstly, all the patients that are included in these studies were highly selected with either single or multiple hepatic metastasis confined to one lobe; secondly, these patients generally were younger and healthier; and, thirdly, the tumors were slower growing with better cellular differentiation. Additionally, these studies do not demonstrate what percentage of the patients who were alive at five years were actually disease free.

It is one thing to say that a patient's survival rate is higher with hepatic resection. However, to say that the cure rate is improved forces me to raise a question.

Indeed, the validity of our reservations is borne out by looking at Foster's series, where 20 of 61 5-year survivors, after resection of hepatic metastasis, died of recurrent disease 7.5 years from the time of initial operation.[1] For these patients, all that has been done is to extend the time of the inevitable. I ask then, "Are we really doing these patients a favor?" At three years, 60 to 70 percent of patients still die of their disease. Many of these patients were treated initially for a solitary colorectal metastasis to the liver, and it is these patients whom we have considered to be favorable for resective therapy.

So, what does this say to us? It says two things. Firstly, it tells us that we do not have an accurate and sensitive means of staging these carcinomas. Obviously, those patients who were thought to be favorable candidates for hepatic resection with a single metastasis were actually at a more advanced stage of metastatic spread.

Secondly, we do not have a good understanding of the biologic behavior or nature of this kind of metastatic cancer. It is interesting that, if we were to select the very same patients who underwent hepatic resection and just follow them for three years,[3] survival rates would range from 10 to 20 percent.

Let's elaborate on this issue. Assume we were to say to a patient with colorectal hepatic metastasis that he has a choice of either:

A. *surgery,* which has an operative mortality of 10 to 20 percent, a 5-year survival rate of 25 to 30 percent, and still he would have a 30 percent chance of dying of cancer at 7.5 years, or
B. *no surgery,* with a likelihood of living three years.

We then comment that we cannot guarantee that after surgery his lifestyle would be better than it would be at three years after diagnosis without treatment. Could we honestly expect him to consent to such a surgery? I don't think so.

To recapitulate then, in order for hepatic resection to be beneficial to a patient with colorectal metastasis to the liver, several things need to be provided. Firstly, a more accurate and sensitive diagnostic tool is necessary to determine the actual state of the tumor.

Secondly, a better understanding of the natural history of the disease is necessary in order to permit selection of the more favorable patients who might have a higher chance for cure.

Thirdly, we must acknowledge that hepatic metastatic disease bespeaks a systemic, Stage IV process.[5] In order for hepatic resection to become acceptable therapy for colorectal hepatic metastasis, therefore, effective adjuvant therapy must be developed.

The patients who undergo hepatic resection represent only 5 to 10 percent of the population who develop hepatic metastasis. Thus, the high selectivity of patients in these studies must be acknowledged.

As surgeons, we can only admit that resection of hepatic metastasis alone is not the answer for treatment of colorectal metastasis. For the majority of patients with the disease, by the time it is diagnosed it must be considered a systemic disease. Hence, we must approach the systemic neoplastic process with that in mind; and hepatic resection, if it is to be utilized, must be combined with adjuvant therapy.

Recently, encouraging results have been reported by Niederhuber and colleagues[6] by infusing mitomycin C and 5-fluoro-deoxyuridine into the hepatic artery. This group noted an 83 percent response rate in 50 patients with tumor confined to the liver over a period of 13 months, with a median survival that extended to 25 months. These tumors were not considered to be resectable. One can imagine, then, that the rates of cure might be much higher if intrahepatic arterial infusion with these two chemotherapeutic agents were to be combined with hepatic resection in selected patients.

Should a patient not be considered a candidate for hepatic resection because of the extent of metastatic involvement? Didolkar and colleagues[7] have shown an improvement in survivability with hepatic dearterialization and intra-arterial chemotherapy. Of 30 patients studied, this group had a 3-year survival rate of 40 percent, which compares favorably to that of highly selected resected patients. So, there does appear to be an improvement with systemic chemotherapy for a systemic disease.

In summary, then, hepatic resection for colorectal metastasis cannot be recommended to all patients—this is obvious. Only 5 to 10 percent of patients are considered candidates for resection. Of those 5 to 10 percent, at least 60 to 70 percent still will die of recurrent disease at three years. Of those who survive to five years, roughly 30 percent of them still will be harboring disease and ultimately will die at 7.5 years following surgery.[8] This bears witness to the fact that colorectal carcinoma is a systemic disease by the time metastasis appears in the liver. Hence, it needs to be treated as a systemic disease; and resection of colorectal metastasis cannot be advocated without the concomitant use of adjuvant therapy.[9]

It is better not to agonize over trying to define the favorable candidate for resection. We must find the patient who has lesions in the liver that can be resected anatomically.

Then, let us acknowledge that hepatic metastatic disease bespeaks a systemic neoplastic process. Unless we can develop and provide concurrent systemic therapy for a systemic process, we are simply rearranging the deck chairs on the Titanic.

REFERENCES

1. Foster, J.H.: Survival after liver resection for secondary tumors. Am. J. Surg., 135:389–394, 1978.
2. Wagner, J.S., Adson, M.A., vanHeerden, J.A., et al.: The natural history of hepatic metastases from colorectal cancer. A comparison with resective treatment. Ann. Surg., 199(5):502–508, 1984.
3. Iwatsuki, S., Shaw, B.W., and Starzl, T.E.: Experience with 150 liver resections. Ann. Surg., 197(3):247–253, 1983.
4. Fortner, J.G., Silva, J.S., Golbey, R.B., et al.: Multivariate analysis for a personal series of 247 consecutive patients with liver metastases from colorectal cancer. I. Treatment by hepatic resection. Ann. Surg., 199(3):306–316, 1984.
5. Steele, G., Jr., Osteen, R.T., Wilson, R.E., et al.: Patterns of failure after surgical cure of large liver tumors. A change in the proximate cause of death and a need for effective systemic adjuvant therapy. Am. J. Surg., 147:554–559, 1984.
6. Niederhuber, J.E., Ensminger, W., Gyves, J., et al.: Regional chemotherapy of colorectal cancer metastatic to the liver. Cancer, 53:1336–1343, 1984.
7. Didolkar, M.S., Elias, E.G., Whitley, N.O., et al.: Unresectable hepatic metastases from carcinoma of the colon and rectum. Surg. Gynecol. Obstet., 160:429–436, 1985.
8. Thompson, H.H., Thompkins, R.K., and Longmire, W.P., Jr.: Major hepatic resection—A 25-year experience. Ann. Surg., 197(4):375–388, 1983.
9. Adson, M.A., VanHeerden, J.A., Adson, M.H., Wagner, J.S., and Ilstrup, D.M.: Resection of hepatic metastases from colorectal cancer. Arch. Surg., 119:647–651, 1984.

VI-B: RESECTION OF COLORECTAL HEPATIC METASTASIS: YES

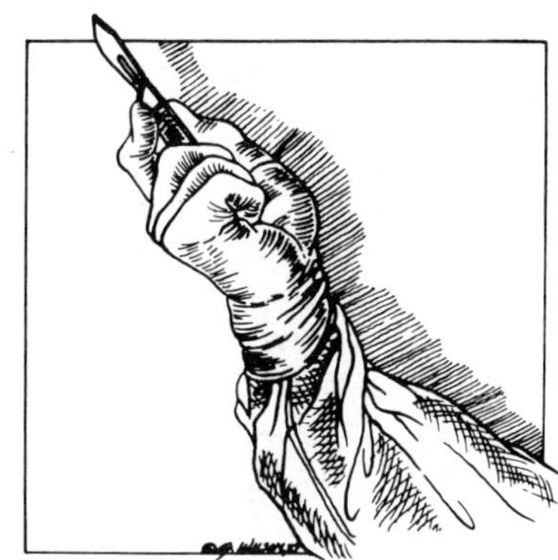

DEBORAH K. DAVIS, M.D.

Hepatic resection of metastatic disease is emphatically an effective therapeutic option. I will support this position with three statements:

1. Resection is effective in that survival is improved over the natural course of the disease.
2. The morbidity and mortality of resection are acceptable.
3. Hepatic resection is superior to any kind of systemic or regional chemotherapy.

This discussion will be limited to resection for colorectal metastases as this is the most common setting in which debate regarding resection versus chemotherapy will arise.

One hundred twenty thousand (120,000) cases of colorectal cancer occur each year. Forty to 70 percent of these have hepatic metastases. "Twenty percent are considered candidates for resection." This is an oft repeated statement, but what are the criteria for resectable disease? Most will accept single nodule or multiple nodules within a single lobe as resectable disease. But what of the patient with disease requiring trisegmentectomy? Is the risk-benefit ratio of major resection acceptable? I propose that it is.

To support treatment of any kind, one must show that treatment is superior to results without treatment. In other words, therapy must influence the natural history of the disease. The survival for untreated colorectal metastasis is categorically dismal.

Table I is a summary of studies showing the survival after diagnosis and no further treatment for hepatic metastases.[1] Three points to note: the median survival is 1.4 to 21.5 months; the 5-year survival is essentially zero; survival correlates with the degree of hepatic involvement. Keep these numbers in mind as we review the results of chemotherapy.

What are the results of chemotherapy? The studies of systemic 5-fluorouracil (5-FU) as a single agent in chemotherapy for large bowel cancer are:

TABLE I. SURVIVAL AFTER DIAGNOSIS OF LIVER METASTASIS—NATURAL HISTORY WITHOUT THERAPY*

REFERENCES	PATIENTS	DEGREE OF LIVER INVOLVEMENT	MEAN (mo)	PATIENT SURVIVED			
				1 YEAR	2 YEARS	3 YEARS	5 YEARS
Colorectal Cancer							
Pestana, et al. (1964)	353	All degrees	9.0				
Jaffe, et al. (1968)	177	All degrees	5 (med.)	21%			
Bengmark and Hafstrom (1969)	38	All degrees	7.8	21%	0%		
Cady, et al. (1970)	269	All degrees	13	33%	14%	7%	1%
Wood, et al. (1976)	15	Solitary	16.7	60%		13%	
	11	Localized	10.6	27%		10%	
	87	Widespread	3.1	6%			
Pettavel and Morgenthaler (1978)	12	Minimal	21.5	100%			0%
	41	Moderate	6.9		0%		
	30	Widespread	1.4	0%			
Blumgart and Allison (1982)	15	Solitary		38%			
	13	Localized		45%			
	76	Widespread		14%			

*Modified from Foster, J.H.: Treatment of metastatic disease of the liver: A skeptic's view. Sem Liver Dis, 4(2):171, 1984.

1. The SWOG study in 1976 included 42 patients in whom the response rate was 9.5 percent.
2. The COG study in 1977 included 198 patients in whom the response rate varied from 13 to 33 percent. The median survival was only 58 weeks, and four different regimens were included.
3. The ECOG study in 1980 included 67 patients and showed a response rate of 16 percent, and the median survival was only 31 weeks.[1]

Is systemic chemotherapy really better than no treatment at all? The patient with untreated colorectal metastasis has a median survival of 3 to 24 months. Systemic chemotherapy with 5-FU does not improve survival, and the response rate is only 20 percent. Polychemotherapy has a higher response rate although survival is only slightly improved. Cady and Oberfield[2] showed that the effectiveness of systemic chemotherapy decreases with increasing liver involvement. In those patients with less than 25 percent liver replacement, median survival was 16 months. For patients with 24 to 50 percent liver replacement, median survial was 13 months. For patients with 75 percent liver replacement, median survival was 8 months. Again, the patients with more disease have the most dismal natural history and the worst survival without treatment; and chemotherapy is even less effective in these patients. But—what if all their tumors could be removed by lobectomy, extended lobectomy, or even tri-segmentectomy?

The oncologic community thought there was new hope after Ensminger and colleagues[3] compared systemic versus regional chemotherapy and showed an 83 percent response rate with intrahepatic chemotherapy and a median survival of 21 months. However, subsequent studies have not achieved this response rate. Again, median survival is only 21 months. Is this really any better than the natural history of the disease without treatment?

Table II is a summary of the studies of hepatic artery infusion therapy for metastatic cancer. Note the response rate of 35 to 83 percent and a median survival of only 5 to 13.5 months. This treatment is not without morbidity. Is this truly better than no treatment at all?

What are the problems with the chemotherapy studies?

1. There are few randomized trials comparing systemic versus intra-arterial versus no treatment versus resection.
2. The studies fail to distinguish between the stages of disease. Are they single nodules, multiple nodules, unilobular, or multilobular?
3. The studies lack precise criteria of response to therapy. Many studies look at diminution of palpable liver size, CEA, and the liver function tests rather than an objective decrease in tumor volume. If 83 percent of patients respond to chemotherapy by decreasing the carcinoembryonic antigen or liver function test, have you treated their tumor or simply poisoned the rest of their functioning liver?
4. The studies do not account for the natural course. The studies have shown no increase in survival with chemotherapy. Has the treatment been of any value in palliation if not in survival? Most patients are asymptomatic from their hepatic metastases. How do you palliate an asymptomatic patient?

TABLE II.　HEPATIC ARTERY INFUSION THERAPY FOR METASTATIC CANCER*

YEAR	NO. PATIENTS	DISEASE	AGENT	RESPONSE RATE	TOXICITY	SURVIVAL AND/ OR COMMENT
1979	31	Colorectal	5-FU	34%	Moderate	Median, 10 months; mean, 13.5 months
1982	18 (91 P)	Colorectal	5-FU, 5-FUDR, radiation	—	2 deaths	Median, 8 months
1982	60 (IP)	Colorectal	5-FUDR	83%	Moderate	Too early to calculate mean or median
1982	20	Colorectal	5-FU + mitomycin	55%	Moderate	Median, 8 months
1983	50 (IP)	Colorectal	5-FUDR	83%	Moderate	Too early to assess
1983	23	Colorectal	5-FUDR	39%	Severe	No figures given
1983	27	Colorectal	5-FU	41%	Severe	No difference when compared with systemic therapy
1983	17 (IP)	Colorectal	5-FUDR	35%	—	—
1983	29	Colorectal	5-FUDR	35%	—	Median, 5 months

*Modified from Foster, J.H.: Treatment of metastatic disease of the liver: A skeptic's view. Sem. Liver Dis., 4(2):174, 1984.

5. The studies do not identify patients with resectable disease. Were these patients receiving chemotherapy because they were thought to be unresectable? By whom were they thought to be unresectable, the medical oncologist or the general surgeon?

The history of hepatic resection for neoplasia probably began with Langenbuch in 1888 when he performed the first wedge resection of the liver. In 1899 Keene performed the first left lobectomy, and Wendel is credited with performing the first right lobectomy in 1901. Then came a period of time in which wedge resections for small nodules were deemed appropriate; however, the thought persisted that more extensive disease was to be turned over to the oncologist. Only in recent years, with improved techniques of anesthesia and hepatic resection, has partial hepatectomy been considered a viable option.

Table III shows reports of hepatic resection for colorectal metastases. The numbers speak for themselves. Clearly, resection is superior to the survival results with no treatment alone or with chemotherapy. Two observations:

1. The morbidity and mortality of major resection diminish with the experience of the operator as witnessed by Dr. Starzl and colleagues[4] in a study in which 24 patients had a 0 percent operative mortality, a 1-year survival of 91 percent, and a 2- to 3-year survival of 73 percent.
2. In time, with the improvement of surgical and anesthetic techniques, future series will exhibit similarly superb surgical results.

What about the complications of removing part of the patient's liver? The most common complication postoperatively is subphrenic abscess. The biggest immediate problem with extensive resection is control of dead space. This is improved with resection techniques and the use of better drainage systems. In the majority of patients who presented with subphrenic abscess, the abscess could be drained adequately by CT-guided needle aspiration.[4]

Is the morbidity of a lobectomy greater than that of a trisegmentectomy? Intuitively, one would expect this to be so; however, many of the studies do not categorize complications with respect to the extent of resection. Therefore, this sup-

TABLE III.   HEPATIC RESECTION FOR COLORECTAL METASTASES

			SURVIVAL		
STUDY	NO. PATIENTS	OPERATIVE MORTALITY	1 YR	2 YR	3 YR
Foster	192	11%	—	44%	—
Bengmark	32	6.3%	—	—	25%
Fortner	68	8%	88%	48%	48%
Wilson, Adson	60	1.7%	—	—	28%
Adson, van Heerden	34	5.9%	82%	58%	41%
Starzl 1983	24	0%	91%	73%	73%

*Adapted from Iwatsuki, S., Shaw, B.W., and Starzl, t.C., et al.: Experience with 150 liver resections. Ann. Surg., 197(3):252, 1983.

position cannot be supported statistically. This is an important point, however, for it is those patients with extensive disease who have the worst prognosis without treatment and the poorest response to chemotherapy. If, however, they can be resected by extended lobectomy or even trisegmentectomy, the risk-benefit ratio, despite a slightly increased morbidity, is acceptable.

A study by Attiyeh and colleagues[5] included 25 patients collected over a 26-year period and showed that, in those patients with wedge resections, the 3-year survival was 56 percent; and those patients with major resection had a 3-year survival of 58 percent. There was no difference between these groups. Their conclusions were that obligatory lobectomy is not necessary, that resection with a rim of normal tissue is sufficient, and that large metastases do not preclude resection or cure.

A study by Adson and vanHeerden[6] included 34 patients, 12 of whom had segmentectomy, 19 had lobectomy, and 3 had trisegmentectomy. The operative mortality was from 5 to 9 percent. The 1-year survival was 82 percent, the 2-year survival was 58 percent, and the 3-year survival was 41 percent. They found that the significant factors in survival postresection were residual or recurrent hepatic disease. Factors that were not significant included the age and sex of the patient, whether the patient had multiple or single metastases, and the interval between diagnosis and hepatic disease.

In a study by Fortner and colleagues,[7] of 60 patients with an operative mortality of 7 percent—27 having right lobectomy, 14 trisegmentectomy, 10 left lobectomy, and 9 left lateral segmentectomy—the 3-year survival was 66 percent for those patients with Stage I, which was tumor confined to the region of resection, and 58 percent for Stage II, regional spread to bile ducts and intrahepatic vessels. Wilson and Adson[8] included in their retrospective study matched controls (patients with resectable liver disease) who, for whatever reason, received no treatment beyond removal of the primary tumor (Figure 1). This is the only direct comparison that exists of patients with similar disease who undergo surgery or no treatment. The number of patients undergoing liver resection was 40 and survival at four years was approx-

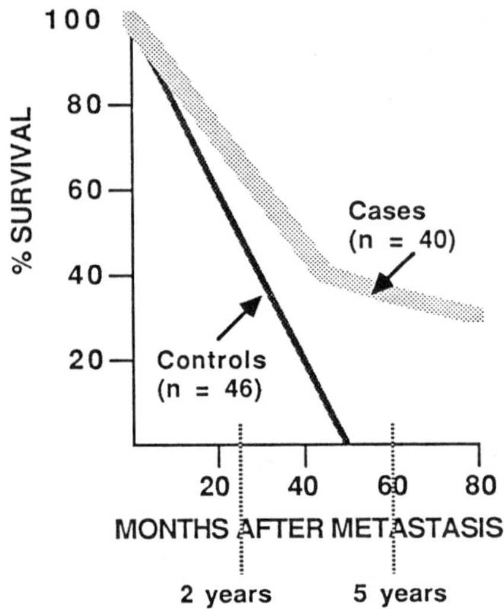

FIGURE 1. From Wilson, S.M., Adson, M.A.: Surgical treatment of hepatic metastases from colorectal cancers. Arch. Surg., 111:330–333, 1976.

imately 40 percent. However, in the matched controls of 46 patients, the 4-year survival was zero! Any comparison of matched patients who received only chemotherapy does not exist.

The oncologists say, of course, that the statistics for chemotherapy are bad in that patients with bad disease do poorly; i.e., patients whose tumors are unresectable. However, I propose that many of the patients included in their poor survival data are not truly unresectable. It is in these patients with extensive disease in which the disparity between the results of surgery and chemotherapy is so impressive. The burden of proof is on the oncologist to show that for identical disease chemotherapy can provide better survival with less morbidity than resection.

In conclusion, hepatic resection for metastatic disease is effective. The morbidity and mortality for resection are acceptable. The resection for extensive disease is more effective than chemotherapy alone.

REFERENCES

1. Foster, J.H.: Treatment of metastatic disease of the liver: A skeptic's view. Semin. Liver Dis., 4(2):170–179, 1984.
2. Cady, B. and Oberfield, R.A.: Chemotherapy of hepatic metastases from carcinoma of the colon. Am. J. Surg., 127:220–227, 1974.
3. Ensminger, W.D., Rosowsky, A., Raso, V., et al.: A clinical-pharmacological evaluation of hepatic arterial infusions of 5-fluoro-2-deoxyuridine and 5-fluorouracil. Cancer Res., 38:3784–3792, 1978.
4. Iwatsuki, S., Shaw, B.W., and Starzl, T.E.: Experience with 150 liver resections. Ann. Surg., 197(3):247–253, 1983.
5. Attiyeh, F.F., Wanebo, H.J., and Stearns, M.W.: Hepatic resection for metastasis from colorectal cancer. Dis. Colon Rectum, 21:160–162, 1978.
6. Adson, M.A. and vanHeerden, J.A.: Major hepatic resections for metastatic colorectal cancer. Ann. Surg., 191:576–583, 1980.
7. Fortner, J.G., Silva, J.S., Golbey, R.B., et al.: Multivariate analysis of a personal series of 247 consecutive patients with liver metastasis from colorectal cancer. Ann. Surg., 199(3):306–316, 1984.
8. Wilson, S.M., and Adson, M.A.: Surgical treatment of hepatic metastases from colorectal cancers. Arch. Surg., 111:330–333, 1976.

DEBATE VII

Anesthesia

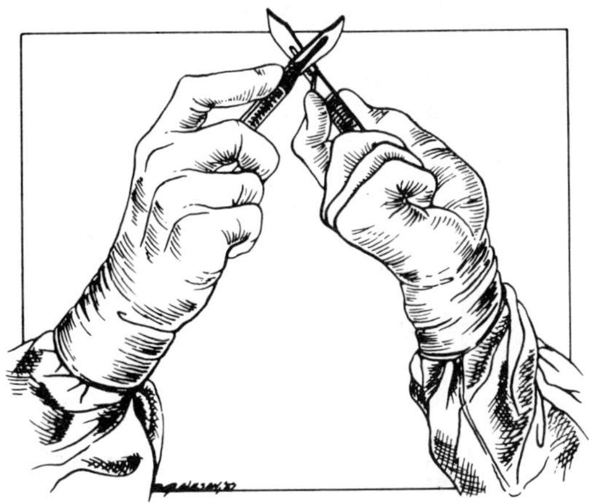

In the conduct of one task, I have always been completely satisfied with my own performance—that task is breathing. Yet, as surgeons, how often have we listened to our patients say, "I would rather be asleep."? During my standard preoperative visit, I always caution that "There is no course of no risk."

Anesthesia and surgery are inherently risky. The responsible anesthesiologist and surgeon constantly search for methods of decreasing that risk. Is regional anesthesia such a method?

Clearly, regional anesthesia is a realistic alternative for many, if not most, surgical procedures. Cardiopulmonary complications account for the majority of anesthetic-related morbidity/mortality. During a regional anesthetic, the patient himself (what greater incentive) can monitor, signal, and correct any imbalance in cardiopulmonary function.

In the subsequent discussions, Dr. Horesh develops strong safety, pathophysiologic, and financial arguments in favor of regional anesthesia. She presents huge series of patients operated on with both techniques in which the morbidity of regional anesthesia is strikingly lower. She awes us with the many, many potential complications associated with general anesthesia; and she points out specific advantages of regional anesthesia relative to fibrinolysis, pulmonary embolism, and DVT.

Perhaps the regional vs. general anesthesia controversy is as good as any controversy in medicine to demonstrate the formidable power of a *selective* literature search. Dr. Ebeling presents studies indicating absolutely no difference in the safety of the anesthetic techniques. He exposes professional football as substantially riskier than a general anesthetic (Eat your heart out, Walter Mitty!), and he quotes a study disparaging the use of upper extremity blocks in " . . . anyone whose fingers and hands are needed for fine work." Is regional anesthesia permissible, then, only for philosophers and foundry workers?

Clearly, the space program has created an explosion in biomedical technology, permitting second-to-second monitoring of blood pressure, EKG, EEG, end-tidal carbon dioxide, and oximetric tissue perfusion in the anesthetized patient. While general anesthesia does increase the responsibility of the anesthesiologist, it similarly augments his control. Maintenance and monitoring of hemodynamic/pulmonary/neurologic functions are transferred to a trained specialist rather than relegating these vital concerns to the frightened, premedicated patient.

VII-A: REGIONAL ANESTHESIA IS BETTER THAN GENERAL ANESTHESIA

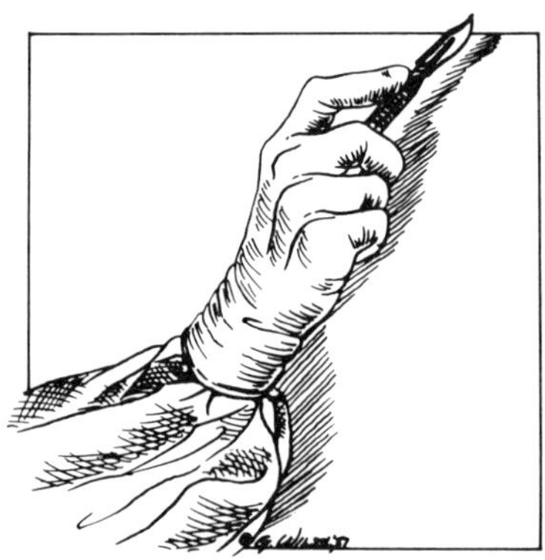

IRENE R. HORESH, M.D.

Soon after Morton's first general anesthetic, it became obvious that general anesthesia was not the means by which the pain associated with surgery should be alleviated; and the search began for a better technique. It was less than 40 years later that Carl Kohler established regional anesthesia with a topical application of cocaine. It was William Halsted who went further and applied cocaine to the area around the nerve trunk to further refine the art of regional anesthesia.

Harvey Cushing once administered a general anesthetic, experiencing complications that would substantively influence his career. This is what he wrote to his father in a letter several years later: "As the operation started, there was a sudden great gush of fluid from the patient's mouth, most of which was inhaled." This, no doubt, was an early account of aspiration of gastric contents associated with general anesthesia. This complication subsequently resulted in the patient's death. This event, no doubt, affected Cushing's interest in anesthesia and in improving the art and science of anesthesiology. He was the first to use anesthesia charts and one of the first to advocate routine measurement of blood pressure intraoperatively. In addition, he coined the term "regional anesthesia." This 1920 quotation of Cushing's says:

> Please put this [collection of Ether charts] in a corner of the Treadwell Library, where someday some young fellow may brush the dust from it and say, "Who were these fellows anyhow, and what is this 'ether' they are talking about? Do you mean that people used to be put to sleep by the inhalation of drugs in the 19th century?"[1]

I think this adequately illustrates Cushing's pessimism about the future of general anesthesia and predicts the widespread use of regional anesthesia.

The definition of regional anesthesia is "the use of local anesthetic to provide analgesia in various parts of the body by topical application, by injection in the vicinity of a peripheral nerve ending or major nerve trunk, or by the instillation within the epidural or subarachnoid spaces"[2] (Figure 1[3]). As one can imagine, there are books and books written on the techniques of providing regional anesthetic and the selection of the type of regional anesthetic for the patient and the procedure. Upper and

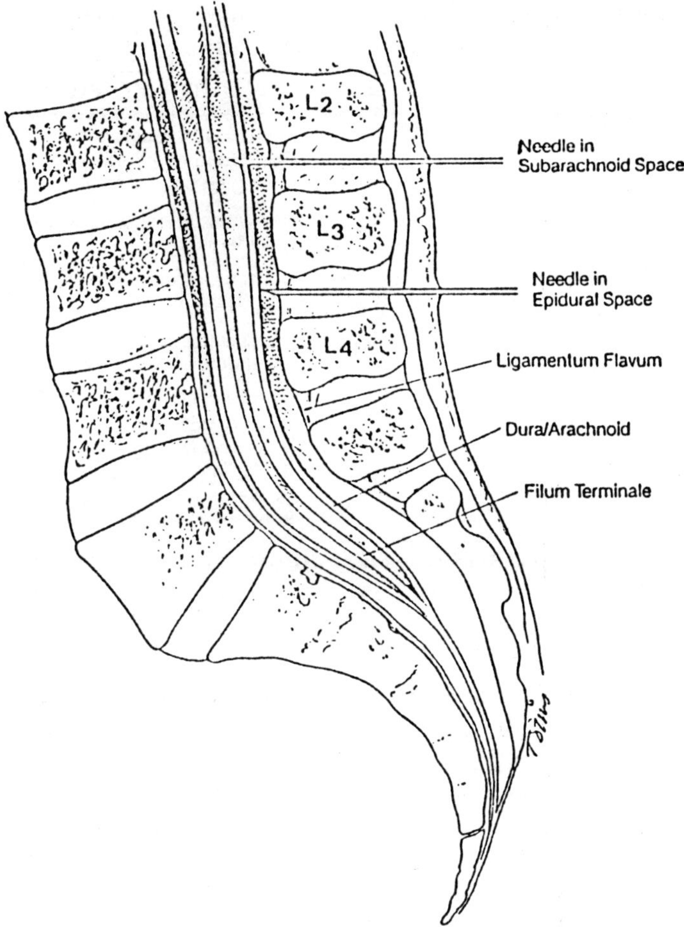

FIGURE 1. From Raj, P. Prithvi ed.: Handbook of Regional Anaesthesia. New York, Churchill Livingstone, 1985, p. 231.

lower abdominal surgery, urologic surgery, pelvic surgery, obstetrical surgery, and lower extremity surgery, particularly in the hip area, can be achieved using epidural, subdural, and regional anesthesia (Table I).[3] In addition, continued postoperative pain relief may be provided with an in-dwelling catheter for regional anesthesia.

Surgery of the upper extremity can be achieved with either cervical, brachial, axilliary, or other distal extremity maneuvers for achieving local analgesia. Regional blocks of the face and neck can allow pain relief on a variety of facial and neck procedures.

In summary, please acknowledge that analgesia may be provided in almost all anatomic areas by regional anesthesia. The majority of this discussion will be focused on the specific benefits of regional anesthesia.

The benefits of regional anesthesia can be categorized into three areas:

TABLE I. SUGGESTED TECHNIQUES OF REGIONAL ANESTHESIA ACCORDING TO SURGICAL PROCEDURE*

SURGERY	LEVEL	BLOCK
Splenectomy	T_4–T_6	Continuous subarachnoid block Continuous epidural 1.5–2 ml/dermatome or single-shot epidural
Nephrectomy	T_6–T_4	Continuous epidural (single-shot), epidural or subarachnoid block
Retroperitoneal iliac renal implant	T_8	Continuous epidural (single-shot) epidural or subarachnoid block
Parathyroid	C_1–C_4	Deep cervical plexus, superficial branches of cervical plexus, or local infiltration
Vascular access Scribner shunt Cimino brescia Arteriovenous Fistula	C_5–T_1	1. Interscalene 2. Supraclavicular 3. Infraclavicular 4. Axillary 5. Nerve block at the elbow 6. Local infiltration

*From Raj, P. Prithvi, ed.: Handbook of Regional Anaesthesia. New York, Churchill Livingstone, 1985, p. 40.

1. The complications of general anesthesia are avoided. If that were the only benefit, it would still be a strong argument in favor of pursuing regional anesthesia in lieu of general anesthesia.
2. There are specific pathophysiological considerations.
3. The last benefit is cost. Flanagan and Bascom[4] reported Winkler's unpublished comparison of the cost savings of doing hernia repair under regional anesthesia versus hernia repair under general anesthesia in which Winkler found $900 per patient savings.

Dr. Orkin wrote a wonderful book on the *Complications in Anesthesiology*. It is a large book, and these are just a few of the high points of the complications. In my research I found no similar text for the complications of regional anesthesia.

In thinking about general anesthesia, I ask you to bear in mind that there is a total and absolute dependence on the anesthesiologist for even the most fundamental of processes, such as airway maintenance, ventilation, and even positioning. We all have horror stories of problems that have occurred—pressure, trauma—because the anesthesiologist was not attentive in moving the patient. This is a rather mundane responsibility but one that can create incredibly significant problems if inadequately conducted. In addition to those things, the anesthesiologist also is administering a systemically toxic agent. Lastly, there is no communication between patient and surgeon, and patient and anesthesiologist. We are relying purely on instrumentation, our monitoring systems, and our own technical skills.

The complications of regional anesthesia may be related to one or more of the following factors:

1. Poor preparation of patient and materials.

2. Poor technique.
3. Inattention to pharmacological constraints, such as overdosing of medication and wrong solution.
4. Interaction of regional anesthetic blockade with pre-existing medications or the patient's pathophysiologic status.
5. Associated but unrelated misadventures.[5]

Grouping the first three together, I think you can realize that those really are not complications of regional anesthesia at all. If you do not have the technical skills to do the procedure, if you do not have time to discuss the procedure with your patient, and if you do not know how to mix solutions or know the doses of medication, it probably is best not to administer anesthesia.

Item 4 is the one that represents a true complication of regional anesthetics, of which there certainly are some. An example of this might be the arachnoid penetration associated with epidural blocks; and pre-existing pathophysiology might be hypoxemia, resulting in hypotension.

Item 5 might be the administration of a regional anesthetic during an electrical power failure. This might result in a complication but not a complication of regional anesthesia—a truly associated but unrelated series of events.

Let's look at some specific areas in which regional anesthesia is of particular benefit. This is by no means a comprehensive list. Cunningham and colleagues[6] have reported on 100 consecutive cases involving abdominal vascular surgery with epidural anesthesia. I chose this report because there is quite a bit of concern about using epidural anesthesia in cases in which there will be systemic heparinization. This group of investigators had been using epidural anesthesia routinely and doing abdominal vascular surgery since the 1960s. Nevertheless, they set about to look at 100 consecutive patients in the mid-1970s.

These patients underwent mostly resection of aortic abdominal aneurysms, although there were also a variety of intra-abdominal procedures for vascular problems. Low-dose systemic anti-coagulation was used. There were absolutely no complications related to the epidural anesthetic with the exception of 10 cases of mild hypotension that responded to fluid. So, of 100 patients and 100 epidurals, there were no problems.

A group of anesthesiologists and radiologists have found an added benefit in using epidural anesthesia during arteriography. They reported 59 patients undergoing arteriography.[7] All 59 patients had epidural anesthesia. Fifty-one of them had absolutely no signs of either subjective or objective pain. Eight of the patients complained of mild burning when the contrast material was injected. This is clearly an effective method of alleviating pain associated with arteriography. They additionally realized a marked improvement in the quality of their radiographs, presumably due to the dilatation in the peripheral vessels that occurs during administration of epidural anesthesia. There was dilatation of both the distal small arteries and the collateral vessels. This group of investigators have become very strong advocates of the use of epidural anesthesia for arteriography, and they have continued to use this technique. A footnote to this article was that, subsequent to the submission of the article, 200 additional patients were treated in this manner without complications.

The next thing I want to discuss with you is a topic of interest to all of us regardless of our specific area of interest. It will be within the framework of an orthopedic procedure—total hip replacement. Now, let's look at the relationship between regional anesthesia and deep venous thrombosis (DVT). This is a problem with which we all deal and have had tragedies.

Deep venous thrombosis occurs in 20 to 80 percent of patients who undergo a total hip replacement. This is the most common cause of postoperative death in the group undergoing total hip replacement. Modig and colleagues[8] studied 60 patients who were to undergo total hip replacement. Thirty patients had epidural anesthesia with postoperative pain relief by this method, and 30 had general anesthesia with routine parenteral narcotics postoperatively. There were no antiplatelet drugs or antithrombotic agents used, and both patient groups received the same postoperative physical therapy. The patients underwent bilateral phlebography and chest radiographs combined with perfusion lung scanning at 14 days preoperatively and 11 days postoperatively. The results were quite striking.

The two groups varied to no significant degree in terms of age, height, weight, sex, duration of operation, or postoperative hematocrit, although there were marked differences between intraoperative blood loss, with the epidural group losing less blood, therefore requiring less intraoperative transfusion. There was DVT of the popliteal and/or femoral veins in 13 percent of those undergoing epidural as compared with 67 percent of those undergoing general anesthesia; DVT involving calf and thighs, 40 percent epidural and 77 percent general; pulmonary emboli (PE) diagnosed in 10 percent versus 33 percent. This is quite a bit of difference. Bear in mind that this was a group that was extremely well monitored for PE. Not all of the patients who had documentation of pulmonary emboli had symptoms of PE.

Along the same line, epidural and general anesthesia seem to impact on fibrinolysis and coagulation after total hip replacement. Thirty patients were offered the opportunity to choose their anesthetic.[9] Fourteen chose epidural and 16 chose general anesthesia for total hip replacement. On each hospitalized day preoperatively and postoperatively for one week, venous blood samples were drawn for evaluation of fibrinolysis inhibition and capacity to activate Factor VIII. Again, the two groups did not vary in terms of height, weight, age, sex, or postoperative hematocrit. However, there was the same difference in intraoperative blood loss, and, therefore, in rate of transfusion.

Figure 2 relates fibrinolysis inhibition as compared to aminocaproic acid in both the general anesthesia patient and the extradural patient.[10] The stars at the top above the general anesthesia data show level of significance. Clearly, patients following regional anesthesia clot better and hold that clot better.

Another area of potential concern has been regional anesthesia in patients with a neurological deficit or with abnormal spinal anatomy. Reynolds and colleagues[11] have done quite a bit of work to dispel these fears. They evaluated 24 patients with a variety of spinal and neurological diseases and subjected them to surgery under epidural anesthesia. They reported absolutely no complications after using epidural anesthesia with the exception of two patients who did not get an adequate block and had to undergo general anesthesia. They concluded that they have had no problems using epidural anesthesia in the face of a neurological deficit or abnormal spinal anatomy.

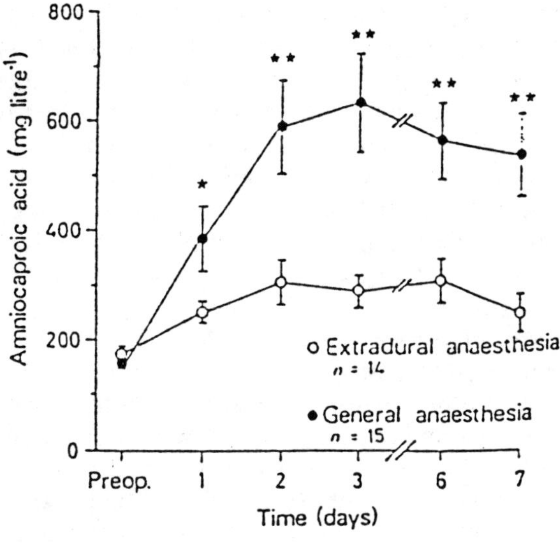

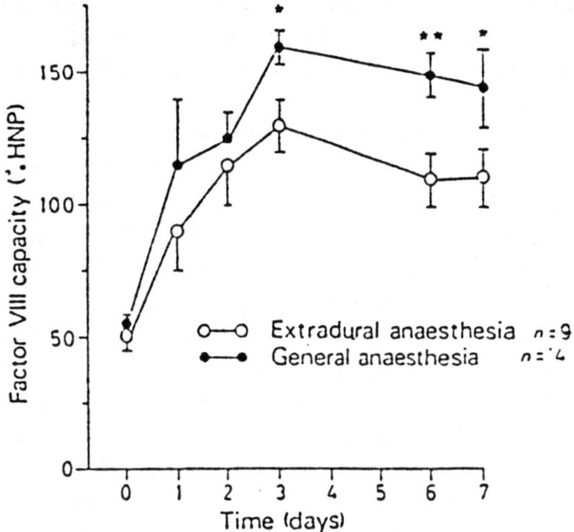

FIGURE 2. Role of extradural and of general anesthesia in fibrinolysis and coagulation after total hip replacement. From Modig, J., Borg, T., Bagge, L., and Saldeen, T.: Role of extradural and of general anaesthesia in fibrinolysis and coagulation after total hip replacement. Br. J. Anaesth., 55:627, 1983.

The biggest risk of doing carotid endarterectomy is intraoperative cerebral ischemia resulting in patients who have a permanent deficit. Why not leave the patient awake and ask, "Do you have a neurological deficit?" If he or she says "Yes," stop, back off, and rethink what you are doing. Jopling and colleagues[12] looked at over 300 patients in a retrospective manner. Sixty-two patients got general anesthesia with electroencephalographic monitoring, and over 250 got regional anesthesia.

Regional anesthesia for this procedure consisted of both superficial and deep cervical blocks with local infiltration of agent if needed. The patients subsequently were observed for deficits upon clamping of the carotid artery. If changes occurred, if the patient was not able to speak or not able to count or had loss of consciousness, a shunt was placed and the endarterectomy was performed.

This group found that they were able to reduce the use of shunts as well as save their patients from the non-neurological complications associated with general anesthesia. Their rate of non-neurological complications associated with general anesthesia was 13 percent. They concluded that regional anesthesia spares their patient population the substantial risks of general anesthesia.

One group of vascular surgeons and anesthesiologists[13] wanted to resolve the question of whether to monitor patients during carotid endarterectomy using EEG, jugular venous oxygen tension, or stump pressures. Another group[9] compared EEG monitoring, stump pressure, and neurological status during regional anesthesia. They took a prospective look at 134 patients undergoing carotid endarterectomy. A shunt was placed based on the development of a deficit; not on the basis of EEG or on the basis of stump pressure, only on the basis of neurological examination. They found that 10 percent of patients developed deficits, one was permanent and the other nine resolved with placement of the shunt. Four patients had unchanged EEGs but had deficits. None of the patients had EEG changes but no deficits, and stump pressure was not helpful in any way. Thus, EEG and stump pressure actually may be misleading during carotid surgery.

Lastly, I have chosen a paper to exhibit the advantages of regional anesthesia because the numbers are so impressive. Second trimester dilatation and evacuation of the uterus is a procedure that is done very frequently in this country. MacKay and colleagues[14] looked retrospectively at 9,500 patients. Over 4,000 of these underwent general anesthesia and 5,000 benefitted by regional anesthesia—a paracervical or ultracervical block. Serious complications were defined as a temperature over 38 degrees for greater than three days, hemorrhage requiring transfusion, or complications requiring unintended abdominal surgery such as laparotomy, hysterotomy, or hysterectomy. The rate of serious complications under local anesthesia was 0.3 per 100 abortions, while there was an incidence of 0.72 complications per 100 abortions during general anesthesia. Thus, there was a 2.5 times greater risk of serious complications under general anesthesia. If, in addition, you factor in the savings in cost, the group receiving regional anesthesia calculated a savings of over $3 million. If the more than 50 percent of women undergoing regional anesthesia could have been increased to 90 percent, there would have been a significant improvement not only in the health of the group with fewer complications but also in realizing an additional saving of almost $3 million.

The benefits of regional anesthesia have been appreciated since antiquity. The inherent benefits of a regional anesthetic coupled with the risks and complications of general anesthesia make regional anesthesia the technique of choice in a myriad of surgical procedures.

REFERENCES

1. Kirsch, N.: Harvey Cushing: His contribution to anesthesia. Anesth. Analg., 65:288–293, 1986.
2. Savarese, J.: Basic and clinical pharmacology of local anesthetic drugs. In Anesthesia , 2nd Ed. Miller, R.D. (ed.). New York, Churchill Livingstone, 1986.
3. Raj, P. Prithvi, ed.: Handbook of Regional Anaesthesia. New York, Churchill Livingstone, 1985.
4. Flanagan, L., Jr., and Bascom, J.U.: Herniorrhaphies performed upon out-patients under local anesthesia. Surg. Gynecol. Obstet., 153:557–560, 1981.
5. Bromage, Philip: Complications of regional anesthesia. Thirty-fifth annual refresher course lectures and clinical update program. American Society of Anesthesiologists, Inc., 1984.
6. Cunningham, F.O., Egan, J.M., and Inahara, T.: Continuous epidural anesthesia in abdominal vascular surgery: A review of 100 consecutive cases. Am. J. Surg., 139:624–627, 1980.
7. Miller, P.A., Lennart, F., Johnsrude, I.S., et al.: Epidural anesthesia in aortofemoral arteriography. Ann. Surg., 192:227–231, 1980.
8. Modig, J., Borg, T., Karlstrom, G., et al.: Thromboembolism after total hip replacement: Role of epidural and general anesthesia. Anesth. Analg., 62:174–180, 1983.
9. MacKenzie, P.J.: Local anesthesia for orthopedic surgery. J. Anesth., 58:779–789, 1986.
10. Modig, J., Borg, T., Bagge, L., and Saldeen, T.: Role of extradural and of general anesthesia in fibrinolysis and coagulation after total hip replacement. Br. J. Anaesth., 55:625–629, 1983.
11. Reynolds, A.F., Dautenhahn, D.L., Fagraeus, L., and Pollay, M.: Safety and efficacy of epidural analgesia in spine surgery. Ann. Surg., 303:225–227, 1985.
12. Jopling, M.W.: Anesthesia for carotid endarterectomy: A comparison of regional and general techniques. Anesthesiology, 59:A217, 1983.
13. Evans, W.E., Hayes, J.P., Waltke, E.A., and Vermilion, B.D.: Optimal cerebral monitoring during carotid endarterectomy: Neurologic response under local anesthesia. J. Vasc. Surg., 2:775–777, 1985.
14. MacKay, H.T., Schulz, K.F., and Grimes, D.A.: Safety of local vs. general anesthesia for second-trimester dilatation and evacuation abortion. Obstet. and Gynecol., 66:661–665, 1985.

VII-B: GENERAL ANESTHESIA IS BETTER THAN REGIONAL ANESTHESIA

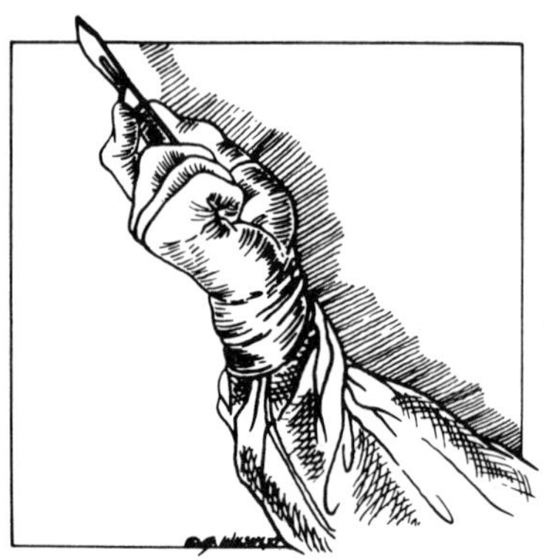

JOHN D. EBELING, M.D.

To discuss the relative advantages and disadvantages of general anesthesia and regional anesthesia, baseline risk first must be established. Lunn and colleagues[1] reported on anesthesia-related mortality in 108,878 cases. The overall 6-day mortality after surgery was 0.6 percent. Using a system similar to the ASA system of risk, the inhospital mortality ranged from 0.3 percent for good-risk patients to 57.8 percent for moribund patients. The higher overall mortality rates by operative region were: intracranial, 9.7 percent; intrathoracic, 8.6 percent; and upper abdominal, 6.6 percent. The most commonly associated risk factors were concomitant coronary artery disease and chronic pulmonary disease. Anesthesia was believed to be causative of death in 0.8–0.9 per 10,000 cases and involved in death 1–2 per 10,000 cases.[1,2]

Thirty-two deaths from a total of 197 patients were deemed entirely due to anesthesia. Three deaths were due to inadequate preoperative preparation. Fifteen deaths were due to faulty technique. Eleven deaths were due to accidents such as aspiration, failure to intubate, malignant hyperthermia, and bronchospasm. Five of the anesthetic deaths were judged totally unavoidable.[1]

A similar retrospective study by Hovi-Viander[3] detailed 626 deaths from 338,-934 procedures. An "anesthetic mortality" was found to be 10.7 percent, or 67, of the 626 total deaths, which compares with the English study.[1] Twelve patients died during the procedure—four during induction, four during maintenance anesthesia, three while awakening, and one in the recovery room. Of the anesthetic deaths, 48 percent were caused by fluid mismanagement or respiratory insufficiency. Twelve patients died of cardiac complications. Five deaths were from technical complications and eight were from unknown causes.[3]

The mortality risk of anesthesia of 0.02 percent compares favorably to the risk of being involved in a fatal automobile accident, which is 0.028 percent yearly, and is one-half the yearly mortality associated with playing professional football.[4]

Steen and colleagues[5] looked at the incidence of myocardial reinfarction in 587 patients with documented previous myocardial infarcts. Of the 587 patients, 96 patients underwent transurethral resection of the prostate. There was no difference found in the reinfarction rate when spinal anesthesia was compared to general anesthesia for transurethral resection of the prostate. Two reinfarctions occurred in the spinal group of 44 patients compared to one reinfarction in the general anesthetic group of 52 patients.

McKenzie and colleagues[6] compared spinal anesthesia to general anesthesia in a randomized, prospective study of 180 operations for femoral neck fracture. There was no statistical difference in the two groups with respect to preoperative and operative therapy. Mean age was 75. There were no differences statistically in mortality or pulmonary complications, although there was a trend toward higher mortality in the general anesthetic group.

These two studies[5,6] examined the mortality rates of spinal anesthesia and general anesthesia in a population at high anesthetic risk and did not find a statistical difference in mortality between the two groups. The next two studies compared complications between general and spinal anesthesia in ambulatory surgery patients. This group is at less anesthetic risk; but, due to the nature of ambulatory surgery, lesser complications may assume larger significance.

Meridy and colleagues[7] reviewed 1,553 ambulatory surgery cases. All patients were ASA Classes I and II. Surgeries were grouped into seven categories: 34.2 percent gynecologic, 16.2 percent general, 15 percent dental, 14.6 percent orthopedic, 9 percent ENT, 7.6 percent urologic, and 3.4 percent ophthalmologic. Seventy-six percent of the patients received general anesthesia. There was a 2.4 percent transfer rate; 1.8 percent of transfers were due to surgical complications and 0.64 percent were due to anesthesic complications. Ten patients were transferred for anesthetic complications consisting of nausea and vomiting. All of these patients had general anesthesia. No deaths were reported in this series.

Dawson and Wallace[8] reviewed 10 years of experience with greater than 60,000 ambulatory surgery patients. The patients were primarily ASA Classes I and II, although Class IIIs were not excluded. Approximately 85 percent of the cases had general anesthesia. A wide variety of regional anesthetic techniques were used also. Dissatisfaction was reported with epidural anesthesia due to an 8 percent failure rate. Overall there were no reported deaths, cardiac arrests, or cases of malignant hyperthermia. Common complications were nausea, 30 percent; emesis, 20 percent; and postoperative hypotension, 10 percent. The hospital transfer rate was 0.2 percent overall but increased to 0.59 percent in patients greater than 64 years of age. This increased to 1.41 percent in ASA Class III patients.

These two outpatient studies show that general anesthesia remains the anesthesia of choice in an ambulatory setting without prohibitive hospital transfer rates or morbidity. Although recovery time with regional anesthesia is often less compared to general anesthesia, this may be prolonged with the addition of IV sedation. Regional anesthesia carries its own set of complications. With today's medical/legal climate, complications can be disastrous, especially when general anesthesia is a safe alternative.

Regional anesthesia usually takes more time to effect than general anesthesia. In one series,[8] 8 percent of epidurals were inadequate; and in another series,[9] 9.5 percent of brachial plexus blocks were inadequate anesthesia. In cases of inadequate regional anesthesia, the patient is then exposed to the risk of two anesthetics. With today's operating room costs and time constraints, an inadequate block may be a significant consideration.

The incidence of spinal headaches also can be a troublesome problem. The incidence in a series of 10,098 spinal anesthetics was 11 percent, or 1,111, with most resolving in the first week,[10] while in another study nausea and vomiting with spinal anesthesia occurred in 13 to 42 percent of cases.[11]

Meningitis and epidural abscess are rare but important complications of spinal and epidural anesthesia. There are 15 reported cases in which epidural anesthesia precipitated epidural abscess. Infections of any type are probably a contraindication to spinal and epidural anesthesia.[11-14]

Epidural anesthesia in vascular patients who are anticoagulated has resulted in epidural hematoma and neurological deficit, although selected large series of epidurals in anticoagulated patients have shown no hematomas.[11,15-17]

Adhesive arachnoiditis resulting in cauda equina syndrome is a rare but devastating complication of spinal anesthesia.[11,18]

Accidental total spinal anesthesia is reported with both epidural and paravertebral blocks.[11] Dawkins[19] reported an incidence of 0.2 percent of this complication with epidural anesthesia. Total spine anesthesia requiring intubation and resuscitation also has been reported with local anesthesia of the nasal passages and in trigeminal V2–V3 blocks.[21,22]

Brachial plexus blocks in one series had a 9 percent incidence of inadequate surgical anesthesia.[9] There is a 1 percent rate of pneumothorax which can rise to 4 percent with the supraclavicular approach associated with brachial plexus blocks.[21,23]

The incidence of postblock neurologic sequelae, as in spinal and epidural anesthesia, exists but is difficult to define. The frequency is not rare. One series cites six out of 432 cases and another 17 out of 300 cases of postblock neurologic sequelae after brachial plexus blocks. Woolley and Kandam[9] recommend avoidance of brachial plexus blocks in patients whose fingers and hands are needed for fine work.

Using fluoroscopic examination, Knoblanche[24] found a 67 percent incidence of phrenic nerve block following brachial plexus block. There were no cases of respiratory insufficiency, but he postulates respiratory embarrassment in marginal patients. In any event, bilateral blocks are contraindicated.

General anesthesia remains the standard of care in anesthesia. Regional anesthesia undoubtedly has advantages when applied to individual patients, but in large studies it is not proven to decrease overall mortality when compared to general anesthesia. The complications of regional anesthesia can be as disastrous as those of general anesthesia. While general anesthetic does increase the responsibility of the anesthesiologist, it similarly augments his control. Maintenance and monitoring of hemodynamic/pulmonary/neurologic functions are transferred to a trained specialist rather than relegating them to the frightened, premedicated patient.

REFERENCES

1. Lunn, J.N., Hunter, A.R., and Scott, D.B.: Anesthesia related surgical mortality. Anaesthesia, 38:1090–1096, 1983.

2. Tinker, J. H. and Roberts, S.L.: Anesthesia risk. In Anesthesia, 2nd Ed. Miller, R.D. (ed.). New York: Churchill Livingstone, 1986, pp. 359–381.
3. Hovi-Viander, M.: Death associated with anesthesia in Finland. Br. J. Anaesth., 52:483–489, 1980.
4. Eiseman, B.: What Are My Chances? Philadelphia: W.B. Saunders Company, 1980, p. 16.
5. Steen, P.A., Tinker, J.H., Sait, T., et al.: Myocardial reinfarction after anesthesia and surgery. J.A.M.A., 239:2566–2570, 1978.
6. McKenzie, P.J., Wishart, H.Y., Demar, M.S., et al.: Comparison of the effects of spinal anaesthesia and general anaesthesia on postoperative oxygenation and perioperative mortality. Br. J. Anaesth., 52:49–53, 1980.
7. Meridy, H.W.: Criteria for selection of ambulatory surgical patients and guidelines for anesthetic management: A retrospective study of 1,553 cases. Anesth. Analg., 61:921–926, 1982.
8. Dawson, B. and Wallace, A.R.: Anaesthesia for adult surgical outpatients. Can. Anaesth. Soc. J., 27:409–416, 1980.
9. Woolley, J.E. and Vandam, L.D.: Neurological sequelae of brachial plexus nerve block. Ann. Surg., 149:53–60, 1959.
10. Vandam, L.D. and Dripps, R.D.: Long-term follow-up of patients who received 10,098 spinal anesthetics. J.A.M.A., 161:586–591, 1956.
11. Vandam, L.D.: Complications of spinal and epidural anesthesia. In Anesthesiology. Yao, F-S.S. and Artusio, J.F., Jr. (eds.). Philadelphia: J.B. Lippincott Company, 1983, pp. 75–105.
12. Kilpatrick, M.E. and Girgis, N.I.: Meningitis—a complication of spinal anesthesia. Anesth. Analg., 62:513–515, 1983.
13. Loarie, D.J. and Fairley, H.B.: Epidural abscess following spinal anesthesia. Anesth. Analg., 57:351–363, 1978.
14. Berman, R.S. and Eisele, J.H.: Bacteremia, spinal anesthesia, and development of meningitis. Anesthesiology, 48:376–377, 1978.
15. Odoom, J.A. and Sih, I.L.: Epidural analgesia and anticoagulant therapy. Anaesthesia, 38:254–259, 1983.
16. Janis, K.M.: Epidural hematoma following postoperative epidural analgesia: A care report. Anesth. Analg., 51:689–692, 1972.
17. Tadikordo, L.K. Rao and El-Etr, A.A.: Anticoagulation following placement of epidural and subarachnoid catheters. Anesthesiology, 55:618–620, 1981.
18. Reisher, L.S., Hochman, B.N., and Plumer, M.H.: Persistent neurologic deficit and adhesive arachnoiditis following intrathecal 2-chloroprocaine injection. Anesth. Analg., 59:452–454, 1980.
19. Dawkins, C.J.M.: An analysis of the complications of extradural and caudal block. Anaesthesia, 24:554–563, 1969.
20. Gay, G.R. and Evans, J.A.: Total spinal anesthesia following lumbar paravertebral block. Anesth. Analg., 50:344–348, 1971.
21. Murphy, T.M.: Complications of diagnostic and therapeutic nerve blocks. In Complications in Anesthesiology. Orkin, F.K. and Cooperman, L.H. (eds.). Philadelphia: J.B. Lippincott Company, 1983, pp. 106–116.
22. Hill, J.N., Gershon, N.I., and Gargiulo, P.O.: Total spinal blockade during local anesthesia of the nasal passages. Anesthesiology, 59:144–146, 1983.
23. DeJong, R.H.: Axillary block of the brachial plexus. Anesthesiology, 22:215–225, 1961.
24. Knoblanche, G.E.: The incidence and aetiology of phrenic nerve blockade associated with supraclavicular brachial plexus block. Anaesth. Intens. Care, 7:346–349, 1979.

DEBATE VIII

Should All Postoperative Vascular Surgical Patients Receive Aspirin?

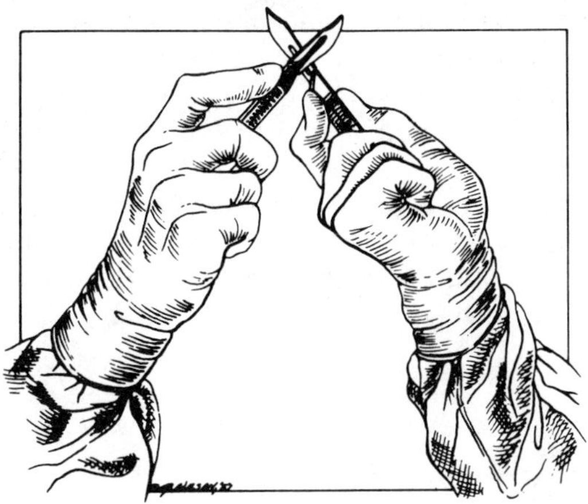

The definition of a miracle drug is "any drug that will do what the label says it will do."

Vascular surgeons can successfully attach both large and small conduits in a multitude of positions for the replacement of diseased blood vessels. None of these conduits, however, successfully mimics endothelial cell lining function. Endothelial cell physiologists have determined that these cells provide a potent anatomic and humoral deterrent to platelet adherence/activation and thrombus formation.

Conversely, all currently available prosthetic and biologic conduits promote thrombosis to variable degrees. When platelets contact the foreign surface of a prosthetic graft or the subendothelial collagen of a biologic graft, they undergo the release reaction.

Platelet cyclooxygenase converts arachidonic acid to cyclic endoperoxides, which are metabolized either to thromboxanes (potent vasoconstrictors and platelet activators) or prostacyclins (potent vasodilators and platelet pacifiers). Therefore, thromboxanes are bad and prostacyclins are good. But, aspirin irreversibly inhibits cyclooxygenase, which blocks production of both.

Dr. Berguer presents data to suggest that low-, middle-, or high-dose aspirin does not prevent platelet activation *in vitro* or *in vivo*. Presumably this is because aspirin prevents production of both good (prostacyclin) and bad (thromboxane) hormones. In addition, in all three major prospective, randomized clinical studies evaluating aspirin following femoropopliteal bypass grafting, the influence of the drug on graft patency (what the patient really cares about) was unimpressive. Dr. Berguer concludes that more doctors should prescribe less aspirin. Very low-dose aspirin may have theoretic (if not clinical) appeal. Perhaps surgeons should extend this principle to its logical limits by prescribing the very lowest dose—none.

Conversely, Dr. Whitehill has found a differential sensitivity of endothelial cell cyclooxygenase to aspirin. Thus, it should be possible to preferentially block thromboxane cyclooxygenase and achieve a net balance that favors endothelial cell prostacyclin production. Ultimately, it is the prostacyclin to thromboxane ratio that is important, not the absolute level of either.

Indeed, experimentally aspirin *unequivocally* reduces thrombosis of vascular grafts in animals. Is this of veterinary significance only? Dr. Whitehill presents a prospective, randomized group of over 700 patients following coronary artery bypass grafting in whom graft patency was significantly higher at 10 days and one year in the aspirin-treated group. In addition, he indicates that Dacron grafts continue to activate and accumulate platelets in man for many years. Aspirin should prevent this. If low-dose aspirin is started *very early* following vascular surgery, it should be logical, effective, and cheap.

Both advocates construct a rational case from basic physiologic tenets. Both advocates refer to well-designed and relevant animal studies. Both advocates present conscientious prospective, randomized clinical studies. Based on these data, both advocates disagree conclusively.

VIII-A: ALL POSTOPERATIVE VASCULAR SURGICAL PATIENTS SHOULD RECEIVE ASPIRIN

THOMAS A. WHITEHILL, M.D.

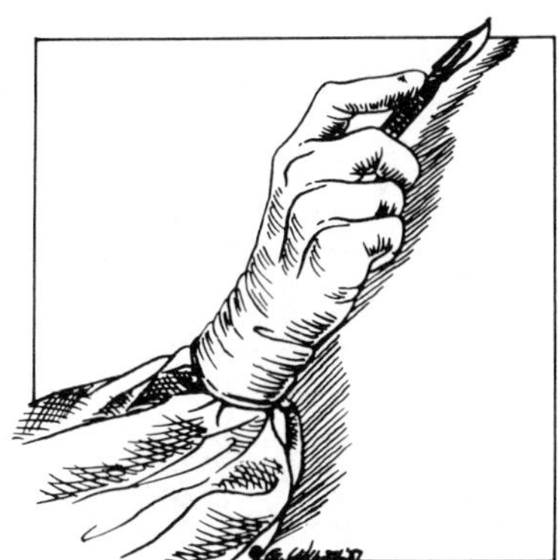

Paralleling the proliferation of various prosthetic materials for arterial replacement, the field of vascular surgery has developed rapidly. As a result, symptoms of tissue ischemia often can be alleviated through the use of artificial conduits to divert blood flow beyond known occlusive disease. Advances in biomaterial science have granted greater strength and durability to these prosthetics, such that they can be implanted to replace aneuysms or to relieve occlusions of large arteries. In the high-flow, low-resistance aortic position, these materials perform well with a low incidence of thrombotic complications. However, postoperative graft thrombosis becomes prevalent when these same prosthetic materials are used to bypass medium- or small-sized arteries.

It is because of the increased thrombotic tendency in this low-flow, high-resistance setting that vascular surgeons prefer to use autogenous saphenous vein graft (ASVG) rather than an equivalent prosthetic conduit. However, the ASVG is often inadequate or unavailable for bypass purposes and a prosthetic alternative needs to be employed. It is in these instances that some adjuvant means of improving prosthetic graft patency needs to be used to reduce the inherent rate of graft thrombosis.[1]

It is well known that platelets play a major role in the formation of thrombi, especially in the arterial system. Their involvement in initiating thrombus formation on artificial surfaces also is well recognized. Platelets do not adhere to normal endothelial-lined surfaces. Intact endothelium presents a physical and humoral barrier between the flowing blood and the thrombogenic subendothelial collagen and smooth muscle. But, when a prosthetic graft is placed either in an artifical *in vitro* flow loop or in an *in vivo* position and is exposed to circulating blood, platelets rapidly adhere to the luminal surface at a rate that varies with the physical properties of the graft material. This same adherence also readily occurs on the damaged endothelium of tramatized vein grafts. Platelets also may be involved in the formation of progressive late-term lesions of the arterial system such as recurrent stenoses, anastomotic neoinitimal fibrous hyperplasia (ANFH), and arteriosclerotic plaque. As a result, the use of adjuvant antithrombotic drug therapy (e.g., aspirin) has evolved in an attempt to prevent or modify these thrombotic and stenotic events.

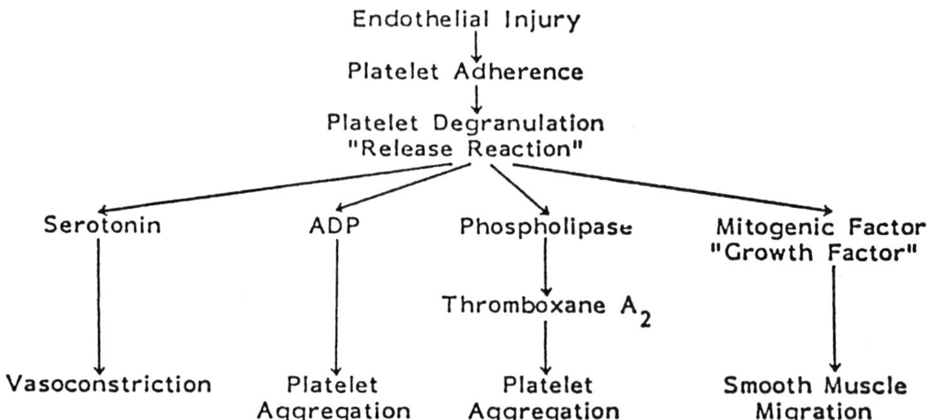

FIGURE 1.   Platelet Function: Platelets' response to endothelial injury. From DeWeese, J.A.: Antiplatelet agents. In Vascular Surgery: Principles and Practice. S.E. Wilson, F.J. Veith, R.W. Hobson, and R.A. Williams (eds.). New York: McGraw-Hill, 1987, p. 253.

PLATELET FUNCTION, ENDOTHELIUM, AND ASPIRIN

Platelets respond quickly to endothelial injury—they do this by adhering to the exposed subendothelial structures. They also adhere readily to the artificial luminal surfaces of vascular grafts (Figure 1[2]). Following initial adherence, the platelets undergo a "release reaction" with resultant degranulation of their cytoplasmic contents. This propagates further adherence with resultant platelet aggregation or clumping, all of which is under the continued direction of various chemical mediators of the degranulation response. ADP, serotonin, and phospholipase are among the products of the release reaction. ADP is a potent platelet aggregator whereas serotonin has prominent vasoconstrictive activity. Liberated phospholipase releases arachidonic acid from membrane phospholipids. Cyclooxygenase readily converts this to cyclic endoperoxides that are, in the presence of thromboxane synthetase, converted to thromboxane A_2 (TxA_2), a potent platelet aggregator and strong vasoconstrictor. Platelet activation begets further release of platelet-derived TxA_{22} as well as release of a smooth muscle and fibroblast mitogen. This mitogenic factor, or platelet-derived growth factor (PDGF), is responsible for migration and proliferation of smooth muscle cells and fibroblasts at sites of injury or platelet deposition.[3]

Aspirin inhibits platelet aggregation by blocking cyclooxygenase and therefore the generation of TxA_2 from arachidonic acid (Figure 2). This effect is achieved by acetylation of a serine residue in the active site of the enzyme. The aspirin effect is unique to nonsteroidal antiinflammatory drugs due to its irreversible acetylation of the membrane-cyclooxygenase complex. Lack of cyclooxygenase activity lasts the lifespan of platelets (7 to 10 days) because of their low protein synthetic capability. Inhibition of cyclooxygenase also decreases aggregation and release that are dependent on thromboxane A_2.

Cyclooxygenase also is found in endothelial cells and is responsible for the synthesis by these cells of the prostaglandin inhibitor of platelet aggregation, prostacyclin

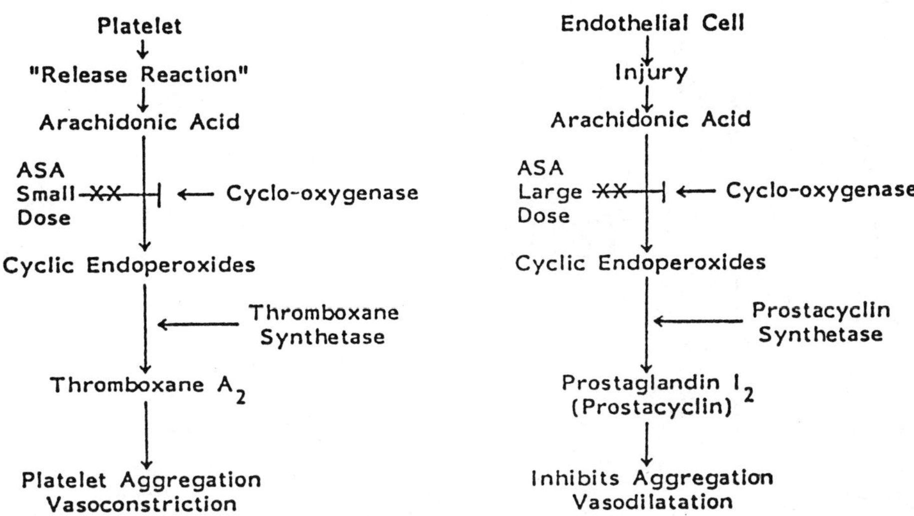

FIGURE 2. Platelet and vessel wall arachidonic acid pathways: antagonistic results of varying doses of ASA on platelet aggregation and vasoconstriction. From DeWeese, J.A.: Antiplatelet agents. In Vascular Surgery: Principles and Practice. S.E. Wilson, F.J. Veith, R.W. Hobson, and R.A. Williams (eds.). New York: McGraw-Hill, 1987, p. 254.

(prostaglandin I_2, PGI_2). PGI_2, which originates from the same precursor as TxA_2, inhibits platelet aggregation and releases and causes vasodilatation and thus is believed to render the vessel lining inert to platelet interactions.

Endothelial cyclooxygenase also can be inactivated by aspirin; however, it is less sensitive than the platelet enzyme and can be regenerated rapidly. Work done by Jaffe and colleagues[4] showed that, when endothelial cells were exposed to 5uM aspirin for varying periods of time, PGI_2 production declined (Figure 3). After five minutes of aspirin exposure, PGI_2 production fell to 36 percent of control values; after one hour, endothelial cell PGI_2 production was <3 percent of control. This inhibition was found to be a nonlinear function of aspirin dosage. Resumption of endothelial cell PGI_2 production after inhibition by aspirin was linear and found to be related to net protein synthesis as determined by cycloheximide inhibition (Figure 4).[4] Because PGI_2 and TxA_2 exert opposite effects on stimulated platelets, much effort has been directed toward exploiting the differential sensitivity of platelet and endothelial cell cyclooxygenase to aspirin to achieve a net balance that favors endothelial cell PGI_2 production and inhibition of platelet TxA_2 synthesis.

In many of the studies on the effect of pharmacologic interventions on graft patency, aspirin has been used together with dipyridamole. In animals and in man, dipyridamole appears to potentiate the antiaggregating effect of aspirin in a synergistic fashion. It is thought that this potentiation is due to inhibition of platelet phosphodiesterase, causing an increase in platelet cAMP levels. An increase in cAMP levels inhibits cyclooxygenase activity and blocks the ADP activation of aggregation. This diminishes platelet adherence to damaged vessel walls as well as decreases platelet aggregation and release induced by all stimuli.

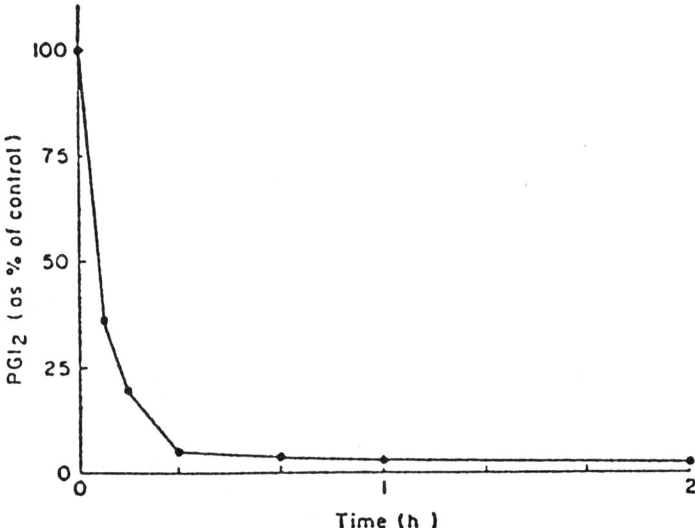

FIGURE 3. Time-course of inhibition by aspirin of endothelial PGI$_2$ production. From Jaffe, E.A. and Weksler, B.B.: Recovery of endothelial cell prostacyclin production after inhibition by low doses of aspirin. J. Clin. Invest., 63:533, 1979.

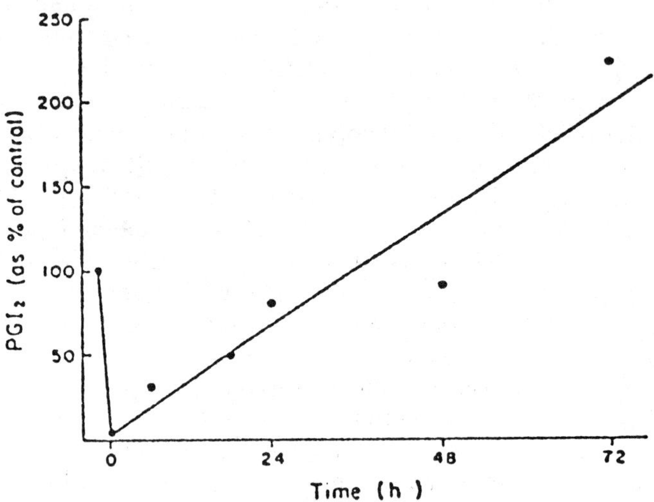

FIGURE 4. Time-course of recovery of endothelial cell PGI$_2$ after inhibition by aspirin. From Jaffe, E.A. and Weksler, B.B.: Recovery of endothelial cell prostacyclin production after inhibition by low doses of aspirin. J. Clin. Invest., 63:534, 1979.

ASPIRIN AND ANIMAL STUDIES

Prevention of Thrombus Deposition at the Operative Site.   The role of aspirin in preventing early graft thrombosis in the animal model has been evaluated extensively. Early graft closure is often a result of diffuse thrombus formation on the luminal flow surface. Pharmacologic inhibition of platelet function may reduce prosthesis-related thrombus formation sufficiently to prevent thrombotic occlusion of small caliber grafts. Aspirin given with or without dipyridamole to nonhuman primates and canines reduced initial and ongoing platelet consumption after placement of Dacron grafts and reduced time-related intimal thickening in autologous vein and PTFE grafts.

Harker and colleagues[5] have has shown in baboons that aspirin treatment interrupts platelet consumption by prosthetic grafts as determined by ^{51}Cr-labeled platelet consumption.[5] An increase in platelet consumption accompanies the exposure of subendothelial tissues that follows desquamation of arterial endothelial cells. This reduction in platelet survival may, therefore, be a useful *in vivo* indicator of the amount of nonendothelialized thrombogenic surface exposed to circulating blood. Platelet survival in baboons progressively returned to control values within six weeks following surgery (Figure 5). Changing platelet survival measurements correlated directly with histologic studies of the graft luminal surface in these animals, showing that complete endothelialization of the graft surface gradually occurred. In contrast, normalization of platelet survival took place in humans at nine months. This species-dependent difference is well supported and will be discussed later.

Allen and colleagues[6] have reported the effects of aspirin and its withdrawal on platelet deposition on control and endothelial cell-seeded grafts in the dog model. Their studies, using radiolabeled platelets, indicated that 325 mg of aspirin daily, beginning 24 hours preoperatively, was effective in reducing platelet deposition and improving early graft patency. Abrupt withdrawal of aspirin at two weeks post-implantation resulted in a dramatic increase in platelet deposition on control grafts accompanied by a concomitant rise in the rate of graft thrombosis.

Although a number of questions regarding the role of PGI_2 and TxA_2 in the development of thrombus formation have not been answered completely, it is known

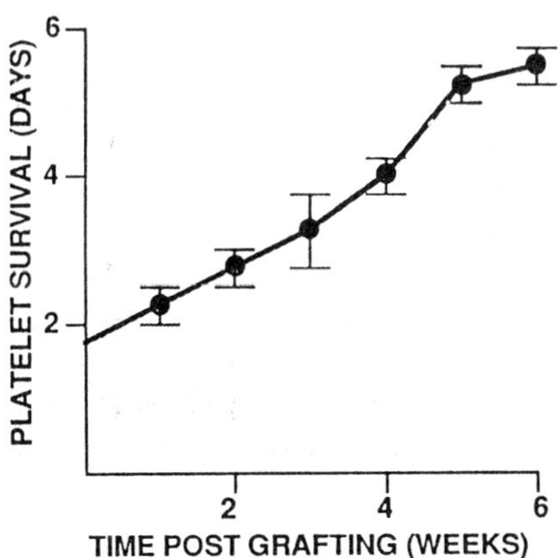

FIGURE 5. Serial platelet survival times in baboons with aortic grafts. From Harker, L.A., Slichter, S.J., and Sauvage, L.R.: Platelet consumption by arterial prostheses: The effects of endothelialization and pharmacologic inhibition of platelet function. Ann. Surg., 186:598, 1977.

that the degree of their physiologic effect in the cardiovascular system is determined mainly by their quantitative alignment.

Zammit and colleagues[7] placed Dacron carotid interposition grafts in mongrel dogs. Grafted animals (control) received no antiplatelet agents while an equal number of grafted animals (treatment) received aspirin intraoperatively. Both groups were followed serially with angiography to determine graft patency rates. Perioperative TxA_2 and PGI_2 were monitored to determine if the ratio of the two mediators was indicative of the antithrombotic nature of the host toward implanted prosthetic graft and whether this was affected by aspirin. Low TxB_2/PGI_2 ratio animals maintained patency without aspirin therapy. High TxB_2/PGI_2 ratio animals occluded uniformly, despite aspirin therapy. However, the intermediate ratio dogs treated with aspirin were less prone to graft thrombosis—a similar ratio in the untreated group resulted in graft closure. Animals in both the control and treatment groups that occluded grafts in this study had a higher *in vitro* platelet aggregation response to ADP.

However, enhancement of ADP-induced aggregation during the postoperative period seen in all of the control groups was partially reduced in the aspirin-treated group. Collagen-induced platelet aggregation also was partially inhibited in the medicated group during the perioperative period and remained uniformly higher in the controls throughout the same period. This study demonstrated a protective effect on the early patency of small-caliber prostheses in the canine model with daily oral aspirin administration. The degree and duration of this effect depended upon the preoperative baseline ratio of TxA_2 to PGI_2 in each subject.

Prevention of Anastomotic Neointimal Fibrous Hyperplasia (ANFH). ANFH eventually occurs to some degree in all vein grafts and at the anastomotic junctions in all prosthetic grafts. This hyperplasia is responsible for up to 50 percent of late graft failures in both the coronary and peripheral circulation. It is apparent from the aforementioned studies that aspirin reduces platelet aggregability and may decrease eventual intimal thickening in prosthetic grafts. Clinical data indicate that antithrombotic therapy may be expected to offer more protection against acute graft failure caused by thrombosis than against late failure caused by intimal thickening and smooth muscle cell proliferation as enhanced by platelet-derived growth factor (PDGF). This conclusion is evident from a comparison of rates of occlusion early (within the first month) and late after surgery.

However, the relationship between platelet deposition and subsequent intimal thickening has not been clearly defined. Thrombus accumulation at suture lines immediately after surgery may become further organized and thickened by the infiltration and proliferation of underlying smooth muscle cells and fibroblasts. This may be in response to an unknown mediator or repeatedly catalyzed by anastomotic trauma, by compliance mismatch, or by ongoing cyclical stress. However, there is accumulated data that suggest that ANFH may well be due to continual platelet deposition and stripping. Platelet-derived growth factor (PDGF) is a polypeptide found in the alpha granules of platelets. Upon thrombin stimulation, platelets release PDGF and the releasate stimulates smooth muscle cells to divide and migrate. ANFH requires this migration and proliferation of medial smooth muscle cells. Ongoing maturation and expansion of the lesion then continues with hyperplasia of myofibroblasts and deposition of collagen.[3]

Following observations by Ross and colleagues[3] that platelet factors were required for smooth muscle cell growth, studies were undertaken to determine if antibody-induced thrombocytopenia could interfere with the intimal hyperplastic response induced by arterial de-endothelialization.

Friedman and colleagues[8] decreased and maintained mean platelet counts of 5.6×10^3 in rabbits using a highly specific sheep anti-rabbit platelet sera (APS). Control rabbits maintained mean platelet counts of 3.63×10^5 while receiving normal sheep sera for the same period of time. Selective aortic de-endothelialization was then carried out in both groups using a standard intraaortic balloon catheter technique. At a minimum of 28 days follow-up, intimal thickening in aortas from rabbits treated with APS was strikingly suppressed—the mean intimal thickness was 18 cell layers—this translates to less than 10 percent of the control thickness upon de-endothelialization. Re-endothelialization was not affected by APS treatment. Related work, using a continuous injury model (indwelling catheter), showed that the mean weight of raised lesions in the control group (Figure 6[9]) was six to seven times greater than in the experimentally treated APS group (P < 0.001) (Figure 7). Thus, a decreased number of functioning platelets with a concomitant decrease in available PDGF brought about less subintimal wall thickening upon short-term vessel healing.

In two different experiments, Oblath and colleagues[10] looked at the effect of ASA and dipyridamole (DPM) on the formation of ANFH. Dacron and PTFE grafts were used to bypass short segments of canine femoral arteries. Treated animals received aspirin and DPM. One hundred percent of the grafts in the treated animals remained patent at four months without evidence of ANFH, whereas only 60 percent of control

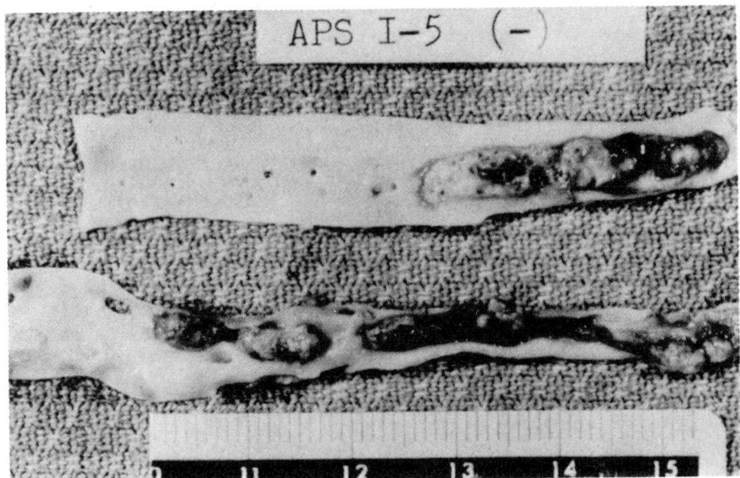

FIGURE 6.   Control aorta showing extensive raised thromboatherosclerotic lesions. From Moore, S., Friedman, R.J., Singal, D.P., et al.: Inhibition of injury induced thromboatherosclerotic lesions by anti-platelet serum in rabbits. Thrombos Haemostas (Stuttg.), 35:75, 1976.

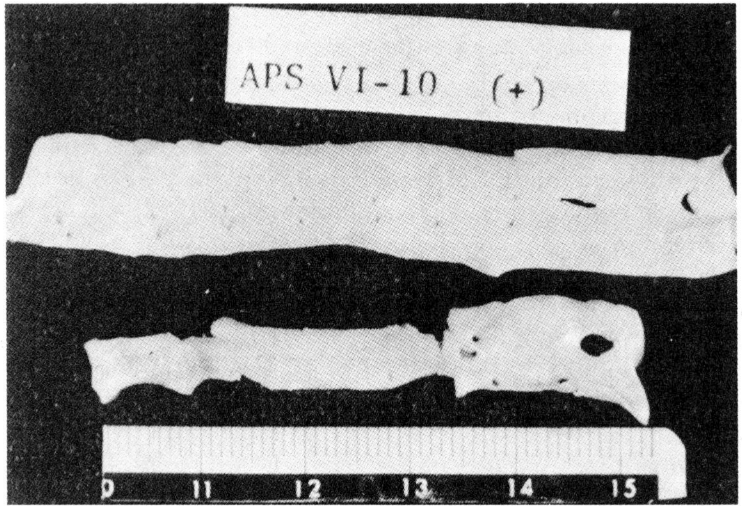

FIGURE 7. Rabbit aorta which received antiplatelet serum. From Moore, S., Friedman, R.J., Singal, D.P., et al.: Inhibition of injury induced thromboatherosclerotic lesions by anti-platelet serum in rabbits. Thrombos. Haemostas. (Stuttg.) 35:76, 1976.

grafts remained patent at that time. There was stenosis at the proximal anastomoses secondary to ANFH in seven of these 20 (35 percent) control grafts. This compares to a 0 percent incidence of stenosis in the treated cohorts. In a related experiment, grafts were also removed postoperatively from both groups at the time of predetermined maximal platelet adherence (two hours following operation) and placed in a scintillation counter. Radiolabeled platelet counts on the control grafts were significantly elevated above those of the aspirin-treated graft counts in all animals (261K vs 101K, $p < 0.005$) with Dacron grafts; counts were also significantly elevated in all control animals (158K vs 56K, $p < 0.05$) with PTFE grafts. In these experiments, antiplatelet therapy prevented the development of ANFH at the anastomoses of prosthetic vascular grafts, presumably secondary to reduced platelet adherence to the graft.

ASPIRIN AND CLINICAL STUDIES

From the presented experimental studies in animals, it has become apparent that aspirin, with or without dipyridamole, can protect against the formation of mural thrombus and to some degree limit neointimal thickening. Similar studies in man have confirmed these observations. Various investigators have demonstrated that synthetic aortofemoral or femoropopliteal grafts continue to accumulate platelets even as late as a decade after surgery and that this platelet accumulation can be reduced by the administration of antithrombotic drugs.

In a study by Goldman and colleagues,[11] the accumulation of [111]indium-labeled autologous platelets in Dacron aortofemoral grafts was measured one week following

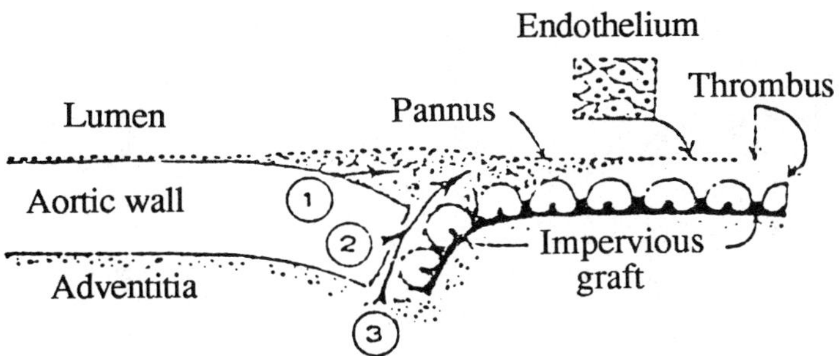

FIGURE 8. Pannus growth at an anastomosis between the aorta and an impervious graft. From Berger, K., Sauvage, L.R., Rao, A.M., and Wood, S.J.: Healing of arterial prostheses in man: Its incompleteness. Ann. Surg., 175:121, 1972.

surgery and at intervals of six months to one year. Gamma images taken three days after the early post-injection image demonstrated continued and widespread graft radioactivity and, therefore, platelet accumulation on the grafts. Similar images in a 12-month-old graft demonstrated that continued platelet accumulation became confined mainly to the anastomoses.

Platelet accumulation also continued to occur on the left limb of a 9-year-old bifurcation graft but not on the previously thrombosed right limb. It was concluded from this study that platelet accumulation on Dacron grafts does diminish with time but persists beyond the period of altered platelet survival and continues perhaps indefinitely.

Related work also describes absent or incomplete endothelial cell coverage of chronic graft flow surfaces; the treatise shows a decreased number of adherent platelets in response to aspirin therapy in PTFE and Dacron grafts.

Knowing that there is an incompleteness of vascular graft healing in man, Berger and colleagues[12] have dealt quite extensively with the conceptualization of vascular graft incorporation in man. With time, a certain migratory hyperplastic response takes place on the luminal surface of implanted grafts (Figure 8). Certain tracts of intraluminal pannus grow in from the divided ends of the native vessels so as to cover anastomoses and replace thrombus or the compacted fibrin layer overlying the adjacent portions of perianastomotic graft. In man, as contrasted to many animal models, this process is quite incomplete.

This incomplete intraluminal vascular healing or incorporation by adjacent arterial tissue in man reflects a deficit of total endothelialization over the new graft flow surface. The functional significance of this incomplete healing is shown by the work of Clagett and colleagues,[13] who demonstrated that platelet survival is continually decreased by a noncompleted endothelial lining. Even 32 months after implantation, canines with aortic grafts (whose biology of graft incorporation most closely parallels that of man) demonstrated decreased platelet survival. In Table I, compare the differences in 6-keto PGF_{1a} content and platelet anti-aggregatory activity of prosthetic pseudointima with that of native aorta. Knowing that man incompletely heals vascular grafts and most certainly continues to deposit platelets on even the most gently handled vein graft, it is easy to postulate that there is also continuous platelet aggregation and release going on in the associated prosthetic grafts.

TABLE I. PRODUCTION OF 6 KETO PGF$_{1a}$ AND PLATELET ANTIAGGREGATORY ACTIVITY BY PROSTHETIC PSEUDOINTIMA AND AORTA*

	TRIS BUFFER (CONTROL)	PSEUDOINTIMA NEAR ANASTOMOSES (n = 15)	PSEUDOINTIMA, MID-PROSTHESIS (n = 15)	PROSTHESIS LACKING PSEUDOINTIMA OR COVERED WITH THROMBUS (n = 14)	PSEUDOINTIMA SOAKED IN INDOMETHACIN (n = 14)	AORTA (n = 15)	AORTA SOAKED IN INDOMETHACIN (n = 10)
6 keto PFG$_{1\alpha}$ (ng/cm^2)	0	13.1 ± 3.8	12.7 ± 4.0	1.6 ± 0.2	0.2 ± 0.1	26.1 ± 2.1	2.4 ± 0.8
Collagen-induced aggregation of normal platelets (%)	100	6.4 ± 1.6	8.2 ± 1.9	74.2 ± 8.4	53.8 ± 14.7	3.5 ± 1.4	30.4 ± 6.3

NOTE: All results, mean ± SEM.
*From Clagett, G.P., Robinowitz, M., Maddox, Y., et al.: The antithrombotic nature of vascular prosthetic pseudointima. Surgery, 91:92, 1982.

TABLE II. EFFECT OF ANTITHROMBOTIC DRUGS ON VASCULAR GRAFT PATENCY

			PATENCY	
INVESTIGATORS	DRUG	ADMINISTRATION STARTED	TREATED	PLACEBO
Aortocoronary Grafts				
Mayer et al.	ASA/DPM	1, postop	92% at 3-6 months	77% (113 pts)
Chesebro et al.	ASA DPM	7 hr, postop 2, preop	89% at 12 months	75% (407 pts)
Brown et al.	ASA/DPM ASA	2-3, postop 2-3, postop	86% 88%	79% 79%
Femoropopliteal Grafts				
Green et al.	ASA/DPM or ASA	1-2, preop	Improved for above-knee bypasses at 12 months (49 patients)	

McDaniel and colleagues[14] have shown that the perioperative time provides for a windfall of abnormal coagulation. In their study of 24 patients, they found that platelet reactivity increased significantly during the early perioperative period and that Factor VIII-related antigen increased and antithrombin III decreased during that same period of time. All of these indices point to an increased risk of thrombosis during the period of surgical manipulation. After administration of 325 mg of aspirin, the abnormal platelet activity ceased and the involved patients were at a lessened risk with a decreased hypercoagulable state than their nontreated peers. These findings remain significant in that multiple studies have well documented that the operative patient is one at risk for hypercoagulability. Thus, it seems very prudent to protect the perioperative patient with aspirin.

A number of clinical trials examining the effectiveness of antithrombotic agents in preventing aortocoronary or femoropopliteal graft failures have now been reported (Table II). In the aortocoronary bypass studies, saphenous vein grafts were used, whereas in the femoropopliteal studies both saphenous vein and synthetic grafts were employed. The administered dosages of drugs in those studies varied but in most circumstances were 325 mg of aspirin and 75 mg of dipyridamole three times each day.

At the Mayo Clinic, patients were randomized between treatment (preoperative dipyridamole plus aspirin added immediately postoperatively) and placebo groups. Immediate postoperative occlusions occurred in 10 of 351 medicated patients (3 percent) versus 38 of 362 placebo patients (10 percent). At one year follow-up, individual graft patency determined arteriographically reflected a similar difference in that 11 of 478 treated grafts occluded versus 25 of 486 placebo-treated grafts.[15] A similar study by Brown and colleagues[16] found aspirin alone to be as effective as aspirin plus dipyridamole when started after surgery. These reports indicate that aspirin therapy can prevent at least some of the early postoperative thromboses associated with cornonary artery bypass grafting.

Green and colleagues[17] randomized 49 patients undergoing PTFE peripheral artery bypass into groups treated with aspirin and dipyridamole, aspirin alone, or placebo. There was a significant benefit at one year from aspirin or aspirin and dipyridamole treatment in patients undergoing above-knee bypass. Drug treatment was started before surgery. A similar study comparing aspirin and dipyridamole to placebo treatment was reported by Kohler and colleagues[18] for patients receiving either saphenous vein or PTFE grafts and could not demonstrate a benefit from drug therapy. In this trial, drug administration was initiated during the first postoperative day.

The reason for the differing outcomes of these trials is evident in that antithrombotic agents need to be given to patients at the time of greatest vulnerability, intraoperatively or preoperatively. Kohler's study suffered from having small numbers of patients in subgroups particularly prone to thrombosis, and the numbers were too small for a statistical comparison to be made.

CONCLUSIONS

Several overall conclusions emerge from a comparison of the data provided by these animal and clinical trials.

1. Aspirin is experimentally effective in preventing thrombotic material from accumulating on the raw surface of a suture line, patch, or graft. In all reports demonstrating improved patency in the aspirin-treated groups, the drug was administered either preoperatively or immediately after surgery. If the initiation of aspirin therapy was delayed beyond two days after surgery, no benefit could be demonstrated.
2. Aspirin experimentally can prevent the development of anastomotic neointimal fibrous hyperplasia (ANFH) leading to early restenosis after repair. It does this by inhibiting platelet adherence and aggregation.
3. In particular clinical trials, such as the one by Chesebro and colleagues,[15] drug therapy was of most benefit in preventing *early* graft failure. Less benefit could be demonstrated at later times. However, as it has been shown that Dacron grafts continue to accumulate platelets for many years in man, it also seems logical that, where platelet-inhibiting drug therapy is indicated, it should be continued indefinitely.

REFERENCES

1. Clowes, A.W.: The role of aspirin in enhancing arterial graft patency. J. Vasc. Surg., 3:381–388, 1986.
2. DeWeese, J.A.: Antiplatelet agents. In Vascular Surgery. Principles and Practice. S.E. Wilson, F.J. Veith, R.W. Hobson, and R.A. Williams (eds.). New York: McGraw-Hill, 1987, p. 253.
3. Ross, R., Glomset, J., Karija, B., et al.: A platelet-dependent serum factor that stimulates the proliferation of arterial smooth muscle cells in vitro. Proc. Natl. Acad. Sci. USA, 71:1207, 1974.

4. Jaffe, E.A. and Weksler, B.B.: Recovery of endothelial cell prostacyclin production after inhibition by low doses of aspirin. J. Clin. Invest., 63:532–535, 1979.
5. Harker, L.A., Slichter, S.J., and Sauvage, L.R.: Platelet consumption by arterial prostheses: The effects of endothelialization and pharacologic inhibition of platelet function. Ann. Surg., 186:594–601, 1977.
6. Allen, B.T., Long, J.A., Welch, M.J., et al.: Effect of aspirin therapy and its withdrawal on control and endothelial cell seeded grafts. Surg. Forum, 34:470–472, 1983.
7. Zammit, M., Kaplan, S., Sauvage, L.R., et al.: Aspirin therapy in small-caliber arterial prostheses: Long-term experimental observations. J. Vasc. Surg., 1:839–851, 1984.
8. Friedman, R.J., Stemerman, M.B., Wenz, B., et al.: The effect of thrombocytopenia on experimental atherosclerotic lesion formation in rabbits. Smooth muscle proliferation and re-endothelialization. J. Clin. Invest., 60:1191–1201, 1977.
9. Moore, S., Friedman, R.J., Singal, D.P., et al.: Inhibition of injury induced thromboatherosclerotic lesions by anti-platelet serum in rabbits. Thrombos Haemostas (Stuttg.), 35:70–81, 1976.
10. Oblath, R.W., Buckley, F.D., Green, R.M., et al.: Prevention of platelet aggregation and adherence to prosthetic vascular grafts by aspirin and dipyridamole. Surgery, 84:37–44, 1978.
11. Goldman, M.D., Norcott, H.C., Hawker, R.J., et al.: Platelet accumulation on mature Dacron grafts in man. Br. J. Surg., 69(Suppl):38–40, 1982.
12. Berger, K., Sauvage, L.R., Rao, A.M., and Wood, S.J.: Healing of arterial prostheses in man: Its incompleteness. Ann. Surg., 175:118–127, 1972.
13. Clagett, G.P., Robinowitz, M., Maddox, Y., et al.: The antithrombotic nature of vascular prosthetic pseudointima. Surgery, 91:87–94, 1982.
14. McDaniel, M.D., Pearce, W.H., Yao, J.S.T., et al.: Sequential changes in coagulation and platelet function following femorotibial bypass. J. Vasc. Surg., 1:261–268, 1984.
15. Chesebro, J.H., Fuster, V., Elveback, L.R., et al.: Effect of dipyridamole and aspirin on late vein-graft patency after coronary bypass operations. N. Engl. J. Med., 310:209–214, 1984.
16. Brown, B.G., Cukingham, R.A., DeRouen, T., et al.: Improved graft patency in patients treated with platelet-inhibiting therapy after coronary bypass surgery. Circulation, 72:138–146, 1985.
17. Green, R.M., Roedersheimer, L.R., and DeWeese, J.A.: Effects of aspirin and dipyridamole on expanded polytetrafluoroethylene graft patency. Surgery, 92:1016–1026, 1982.
18. Kohler, T.R., Kaufman, J.L., Kacoyanis, G., et al.: Effect of aspirin and dipyridamole on the patency of lower extremity bypass grafts. Surgery, 96:462–466, 1984.

VIII-B: ALL POSTOPERATIVE VASCULAR SURGICAL PATIENTS SHOULD NOT RECEIVE ASPIRIN

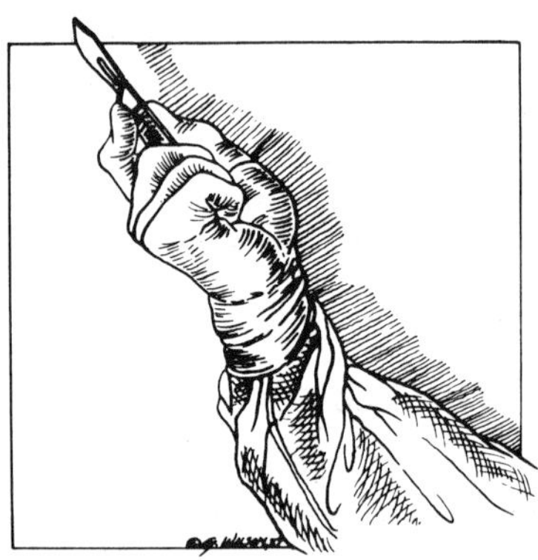

RAMON BERGUER, M.D.

Should all postoperative vascular patients receive aspirin? Probably not. The question then arises, "Why treat postoperative vascular patients at all?" With patency half-lives for femoropopliteal grafts at six to seven years and even lower for infrapopliteal grafts, a drug regimen that would increase long-term patency rates significantly would be welcome.[1,2]

Graft patency, then, is the key issue. I plan to demonstrate that clinical trials do not show conclusively that aspirin is of benefit in improving long-term patency for infrainguinal bypass grafts and that there is some experimental evidence to explain these negative observations.

Graft patency is affected by systemic factors such as the presence of diabetes and smoking. Regional factors exist such as severity of proximal and distal vascular disease, previous reconstructive surgery at the same site, graft material, and level of the distal anastomosis.[3,4]

Early graft occlusion usually is due to thrombosis, secondary to hemodynamic or technical problems in the perioperative period. On the other hand, late graft occlusion has been attributed to progression of vascular disease, degeneration of graft material, and, most recently, intimal hyperplasia leading to stenosis and eventual occlusion of the graft.[4-7]

Aspirin might be effective in preventing the stenosis and possible occlusion of vascular grafts by inhibiting the following:

1. *Platelet deposition at the site of endothelial damage* (Figure 1). Circulating platelets are activated by exposure to subendothelial collagen fibers and adhere to the damaged surface.[8] By blocking the platelet cyclooxygenase, aspirin may inhibit platelet activation and subsequent deposition.
2. *Thrombus formation* (Figure 2). As a result of the previous subendothelial collagen exposure, the platelets undergo release of intragranular thromboxane that acts as a potent stimulus to further platelet aggregation and thrombus formation.[8] By blocking the production of thromboxane, aspirin may inhibit this step.

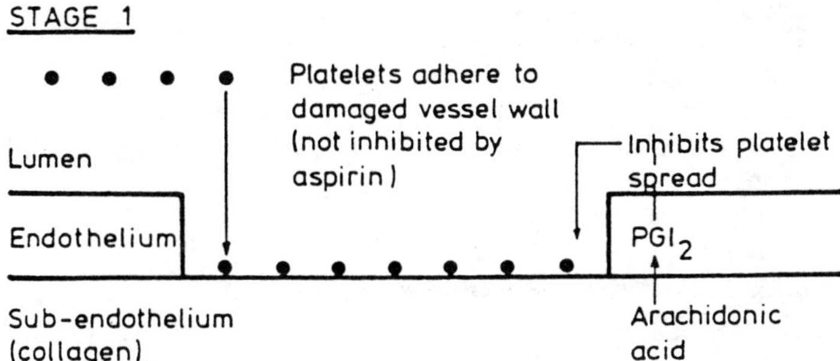

FIGURE 1. From Gershlick, A.H., Syndercombe-Court, Y.D.S., Murday, A.J., et al.: Adverse effects of high-dose aspirin on platelet adhesion to experimental autogenous vein grafts. Cardiovasc. Res., 19:775, 1985.

3. *Development of intimal hyperplasia* (Figure 3). It is postulated that during degranulation platelets release a platelet-derived growth factor that stimulates smooth muscle cells and fibroblast migration into the subendothelial space,[9] causing a fibrous neointimal hyperplasia and stenosis of the lumen of the vessel. Again, aspirin, by possibly inhibiting the previous two steps, may stop this longer term process and reduce the incidence of late graft stenosis and occlusion.[5]

Gershlick and colleagues[8] developed an animal model for studying these early and late changes in vein grafts. They used a reversed internal jugular vein interposition graft in the rabbit-common carotid artery. These authors demonstrated persistent and continued platelet activation by the interposed vein grafts lasting up to, but not longer than, four months following implantation (Figure 4). Many of these longer implanted grafts later developed intimal hyperplasia.[8]

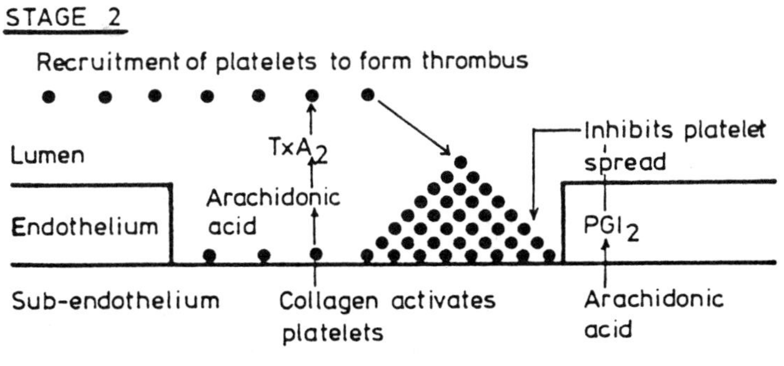

FIGURE 2. Thrombus formation. From Gershlick, A.H., Syndercombe-Court, Y.D.S., Murday, A.J., et al.: Adverse effects of high-dose aspirin on platelet adhesion to experimental autogenous vein grafts. Cardiovasc. Res., 19:775, 1985.

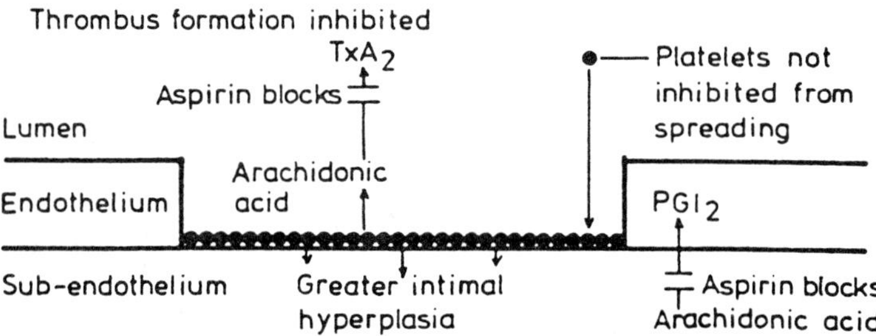

FIGURE 3. From Gershlick, A.H., Syndercombe-Court, Y.D.S., Murday, A.J., et al.: Adverse effects of high-dose aspirin on platelet adhesion to experimental autogenous vein grafts. Cardiovasc. Res., 19:775, 1985.

The same authors[10] found that platelet activation by the vein grafts was not prevented by low-, middle-, or high-dose aspirin plus dipyridamole and that this activation still lasted up to four months as before (Figure 5). Since platelet aggregation in response to arachidonic acid was suppressed completely in the high-dose group, they concluded that graft activation of platelets occurs via arachidonic *independent* pathways and probably is the result of exposure to subendothelial collagen. Aspirin, then, would be of no benefit in preventing initial platelet activation by the graft.

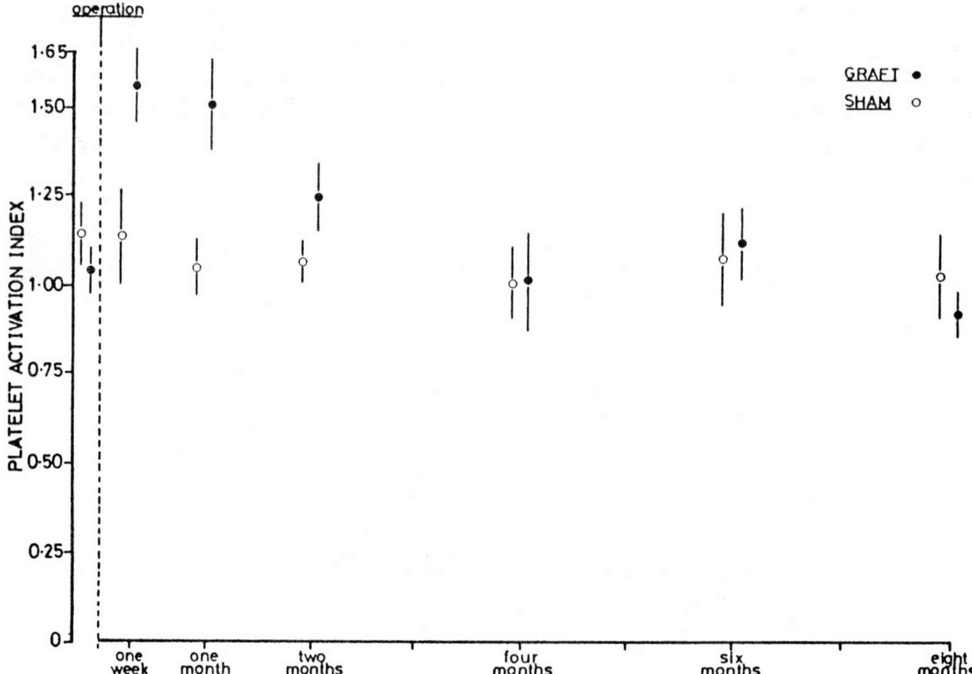

FIGURE 4. Platelet activation index (mean ± SEM) at set postoperative times in live animals. From Gershlick, A.H., Syndercombe-Court, Y.D.S., Murday, A.J., et al.: Platelet function is altered by autogenous vein grafts in the early postoperative months. Cardiovasc. Res., 18:122, 1984.

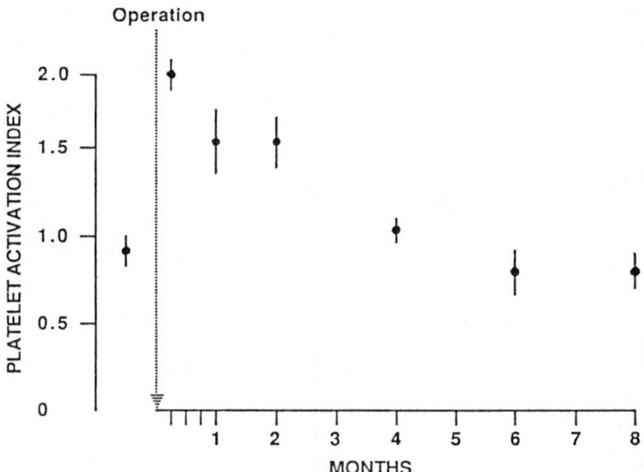

FIGURE 5.   Effect of aspirin plus dipyridamole on platelet activation. Platelet activation index (mean $\pm$ 1 SEM) at set post-operative times: Group A animals. Treatment: 10 mg·kg^{-1}·24h^{-1} ASA + 2 mg·kg^{-1}·6h^{-1} dipyridamole. Modified from Gershlick, A.H., Syndercombe-Court, Y.D.S., Murday, A.J., et al.: Activation of platelets by autogenous vein grafts is not prevented by acetylsalicyclic acid and dipyridamole. Cardiovasc. Res., 18:393, 1984.

In a similar study, Gershlick and colleagues[5] found that the thickness of intimal hyperplasia was increased in all three treatment groups relative to control, although only in the high-dose group did this reach statistical significance (Figure 6).

Others[11,12] have found no effect of aspirin on intimal hyperplasia and even have found a retarding effect of aspirin on endothelial regrowth after injury. These results cast a shadow of doubt on the effectiveness of aspirin in preventing intimal hyperplasia.

Finally, Gershlick and colleagues[13] studied prostacyclin levels and platelet deposition in the same model and found that high-dose aspirin significantly reduced prostacyclin levels and resulted in statistically greater platelet deposition on the vein grafts compared to controls (Figure 7).

The importance of prostacyclin in inhibiting platelet deposition and aggregation is well recognized and is supported by the following studies.[14-17] Weiss and Turitto[16] found that prostacyclin inhibits platelet spreading and thrombus formation on de-endothelialized rabbit aorta. Bush and colleagues[15] demonstrated significantly better patency rates of *in situ* versus reversed vein femoral-popliteal grafts and correlated this with finding a much higher blood prostacyclin/thromboxane ratio in the former group of patients. Dyerberg and colleagues[14] correlated the low incidence of atherosclerosis in Greenland Eskimos with their increased levels of eicosapentanoic acid in the blood. They then demonstrated that in rats this fatty acid is converted to prostacyclin by the vessel wall.

Up to now, we have seen that:

1. high-dose aspirin does not prevent platelet activation by vein grafts,
2. it may have no effect on or may increase intimal hyperplasia,
3. it inhibits prostacyclin production, and, thus,
4. it probably is harmful or of no effect in vascular patients.

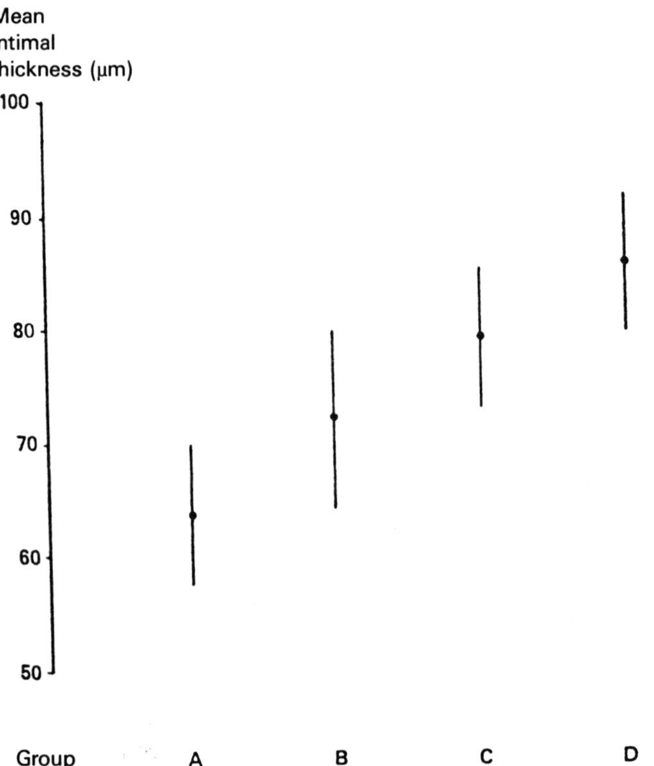

FIGURE 6. Intimal thicknesses (means with SEM) for the four groups of animals. From Murday, A.J., Gershlick, A.H., Syndercombe-Court, Y.D., et al.: Intimal thickening in autogenous vein grafts in rabbits: Influence of aspirin and dipyridamole. Thorax, 39:459, 1984.

However, the optimal "low dose" of aspirin that might selectively inhibit platelet cyclooxygenase and yet permit vessel wall prostacyclin production has not been established. Large inter-individual variations in aspirin blood levels with an identical aspirin dose have been observed, and the possible cumulative effect of every eight hours' dosing makes the definition of "low-dose" aspirin difficult.[18,19]

Until this potentially therapeutic "low dose" of aspirin is well established, the possibility of inhibiting prostacyclin synthesis in patients already at high risk for cardiovascular disease[20,21] may increase long-term platelet deposition and the possibility of stenosis and occlusion of native vessels and grafts.

There are three major prospective, randomized, and controlled clinical studies of the effectiveness of aspirin and dipyridamole on the long-term patency rates of femoropopliteal grafts.[7,22,23]

Green and colleagues[7] randomized 49 patients undergoing femoropopliteal grafts with expanded PTFE to three groups:

aspirin 325 mg + dipyridamole 75 mg. T.I.D.
aspirin 325 mg T.I.D.
placebo T.I.D.

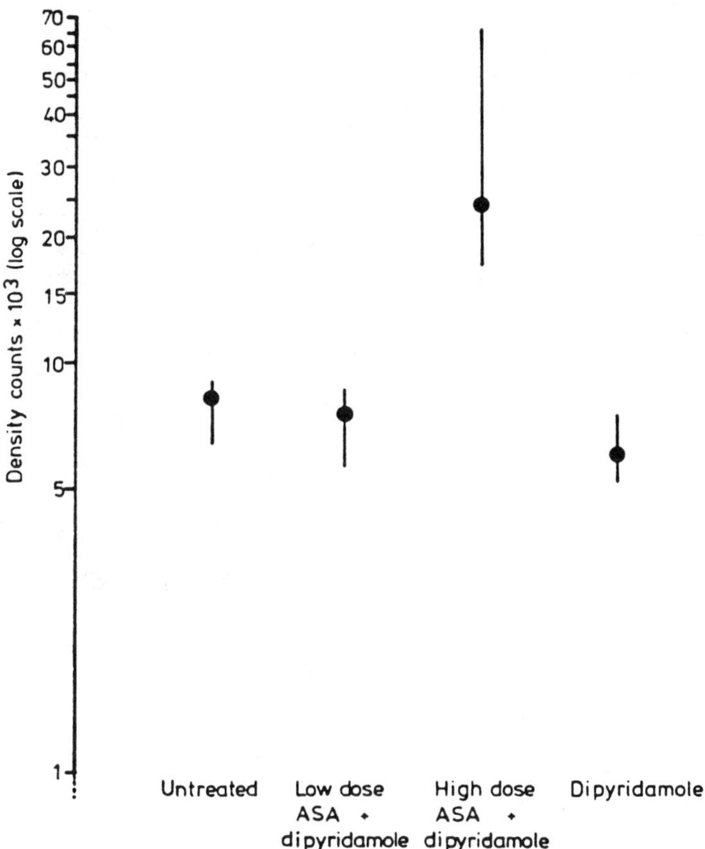

FIGURE 7.   Density counts from autoradiographs of vein grafts (median ± interquartile range). From Gershlick, A.H., Syndercombe-Court, Y.D.S., Murday, A.J., et al.: Adverse effects of high-dose aspirin on platelet adhesion to experimental autogenous vein grafts. Cardiovasc. Res., 19:773, 1985.

starting on the first postoperative day. Patients were seen at one-month intervals for one year. Treatment failure was defined as the first graft occlusion. Study groups were well matched in the indications for surgery and the presence of diabetes and smoking. However, there was a significantly larger number of patients with previous femoro-popliteal grafting in the placebo group, imparting a favorable bias to the treatment group (Table I). A statistically higher patency rate at one year was found in above-knee grafts only (Figures 8 and 9). They concluded that the one-year patency rates of PTFE femoropopliteal grafts can be improved significantly in above-knee bypasses by aspirin therapy alone or in combination with dipyridamole.

Kohler and colleagues[22] randomized 100 patients with 102 grafts undergoing either autologous vein or PTFE femoropopliteal bypasses to receive either

**TABLE I.   FACTORS (%) THAT COULD AFFECT
GRAFT PATENCY***

TREATMENT	SALVAGE	PRIOR FEM.-POP.	SMOKING	DIABETES
Placebo	88	41	53	48
ASA	75	6	56	37
ASA/DIP	87	19	56	50

*From Green, R.M., Roedersheimer, L.R., and DeWeese, J.A.: Effects of aspirin and dipyridamole on expanded PTFE graft patency. Surgery, 92: 1017, 1982.

aspirin 325 mg + dipyridamole 75 mg T.I.D. or
placebo T.I.D.

starting on the first postoperative day. Graft patency was assessed at three and six weeks and after that at three- to six-month intervals to 24 months. Failure was defined as the first graft occlusion. The study groups were well matched in this study (Table II). Cumulative patency rates were calculated up to 48 months (Figures 10, 11, and 12).

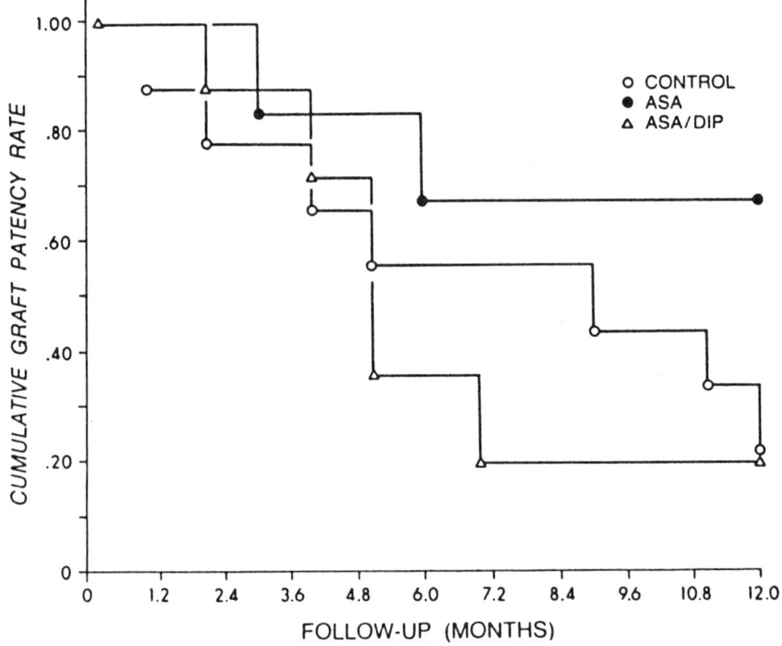

FIGURE 8.   Patients with below-knee PTFE grafts had higher 1-year cumulative patency rates when treated with ASA (65% versus 21% for placebo and 19% for ASA/DIP), but there were no statistically significant differences among the three groups. From Green, R.M., Roedersheimer, L.R., and DeWeese, J.A.: Effects of aspirin and dipyridamole on expanded PTFE graft patency. Surgery, 92:1020, 1982.

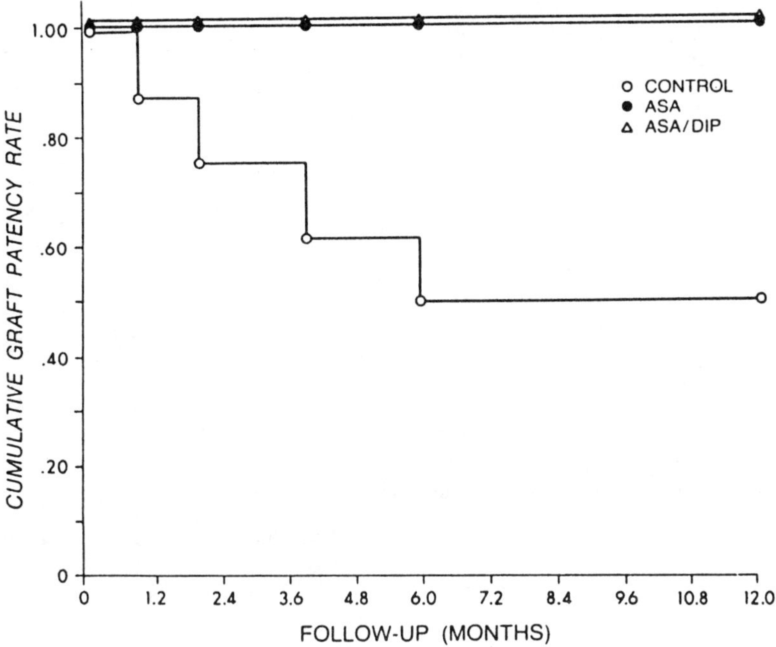

FIGURE 9.   Patients with above-knee PTFE grafts had statistically higher 1-year cumulative graft patency rates when treated with ASA alone (100%) or in combination with DIP (100%) as compared to placebo (50%) ($P = 0.05$). From Green, R.M., Roedersheimer, L.R., and DeWeese, J.A.: Effects of aspirin and dipyridamole on expanded PTFE graft patency. Surgery, 92:1020, 1982.

TABLE II.   STUDY GROUP PROFILE*

	TREATMENT	PLACEBO	TOTAL
No. of patients	44	44	88
Male	34	34	68
Female	10	10	20
Age (mean ± SD)	66 ± 12	66 ± 10	66 ± 11
Diabetic	15	15	30
History of smoking	32	33	65
Number of grafts	51	51	102
Indication for operation			
Claudication	16	19	35
Threatened limb	35	32	67
PTFE grafts	15	16	31
Vein grafts	36	35	71
Tibial grafts	8	10	18
Proximal popliteal grafts	21	22	43
Distal popliteal grafts	22	24	46
Previous femoropopliteal bypasses	5	6	11

*From Kohler, T.R., Kaufman, J.L., Kacoyanis, G., et al.: Effect of aspirin and dipyridamole on the patency of lower extremity bypass grafts. Surgery, 96:463, 1984.

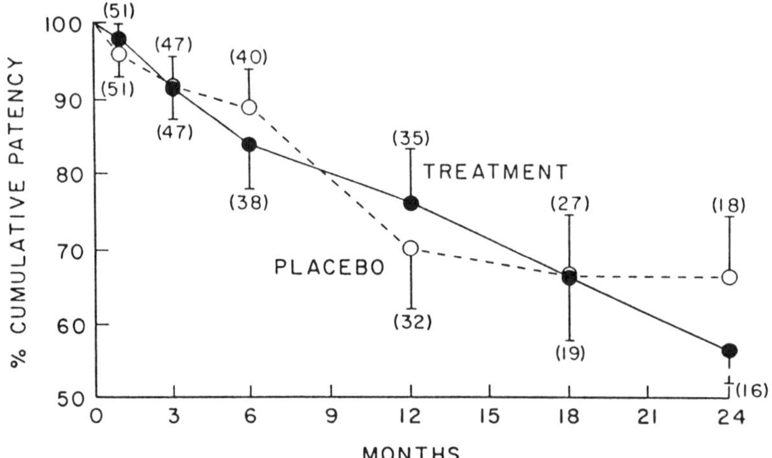

FIGURE 10.   Life table—all treatment group versus all placebo group. Bars indicate SE; the number of patients in each group is in parentheses. From Kohler, T.R., Kaufman, J.F., Kacoyanis, G., et al.: Effect of aspirin and dipyridamole on the patency of lower extremity bypass grafts. Surgery, 96:464, 1984.

The authors concluded that no benefit from drug therapy was obtained in this study.

Satiani[23] randomized 93 patients and 100 limbs to undergo PTFE, autologous vein, or composite femoropopliteal bypass grafting to receive either

aspirin 625 mg a day or
placebo a day

starting one to three days postoperatively. Failure was defined as the first graft occlusion. Follow-up was done at one week and then three- to six-month intervals. Length of follow-up was one to 51 months with the average being 12.9 months. Cumulative patency rates were calculated up to 24 months (Figure 13). The author concluded that no significant difference in patency rates was obtained in the treatment group and that further studies are needed before prescribing aspirin to postoperative vascular patients.

In summary, aspirin inhibition of thromboxane-induced platelet aggregation may prevent early graft thrombus formation. However, long-standing decreases in prostacyclin synthesis as a consequence of aspirin therapy, even at low doses, may allow chronic platelet deposition and increased intimal hyperplasia, especially in patients at high risk for cardiovascular disease. Finally, only one of three prospective, randomized, and controlled studies shows any benefit of aspirin and dipyridamole therapy in improving the patency rates of infrainguinal vascular grafts. More doctors should prescribe less aspirin. In fact, most doctors should prescribe none.

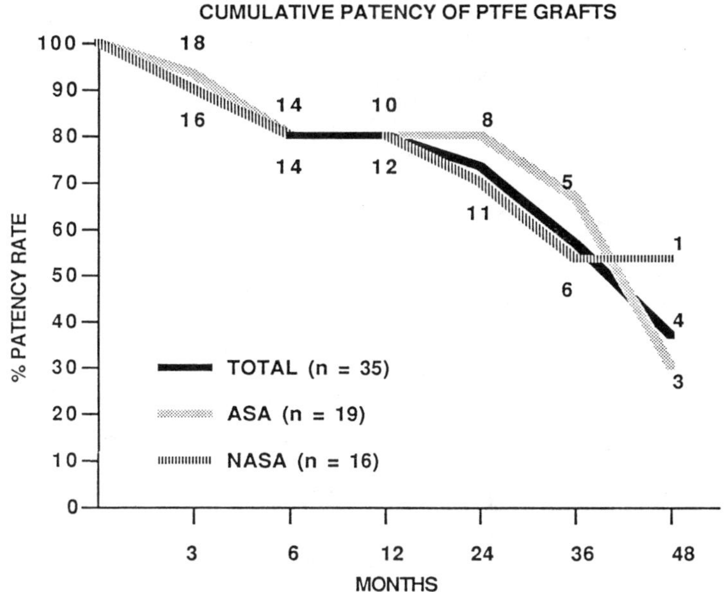

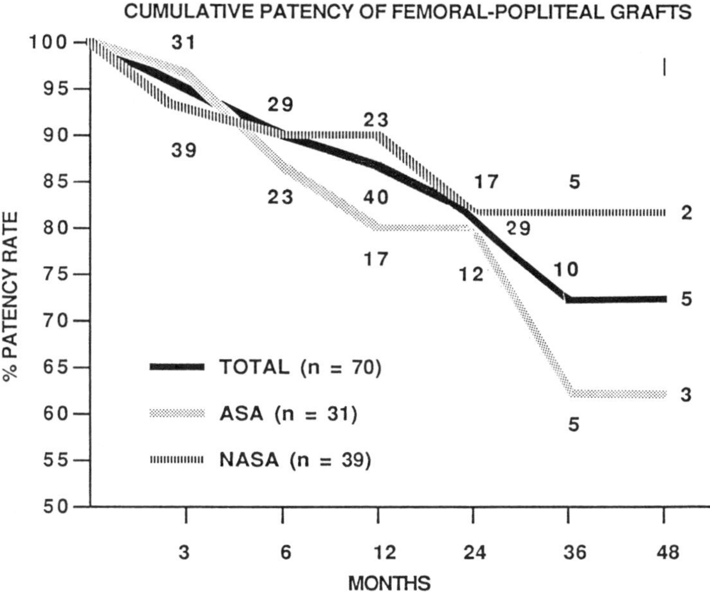

FIGURE 11. *(Top)* Cumulative patency rate of PTFE grafts treated with (ASA) and without (NASA) aspirin (p > .05). *(Bottom)* Cumulative patency rate by life table analysis of ASA (aspirin) and NASA (no aspirin) treated femoral popliteal bypass grafts (p > .05). Modified from Satiani, B.: A prospective, randomized trial of aspirin in femoral popliteal and tibial bypass grafts. Angiology, 36:611, 1985.

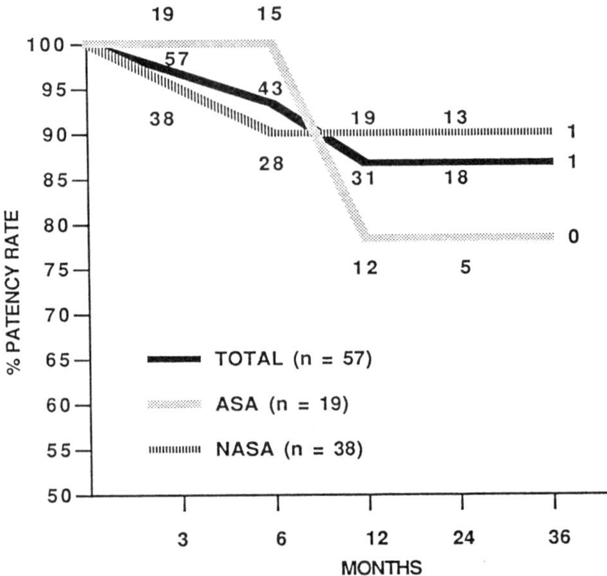

FIGURE 12. Cumulative patency rate of autogenous vein (AV) grafts treated with aspirin (ASA) and not treated with aspirin (NASA). No significant difference was noted between the two groups (p > .05). From Satiani, B.: A prospective, randomized trial of aspirin in femoral popliteal and tibial bypass grafts. Angiology, 36:610, 1985.

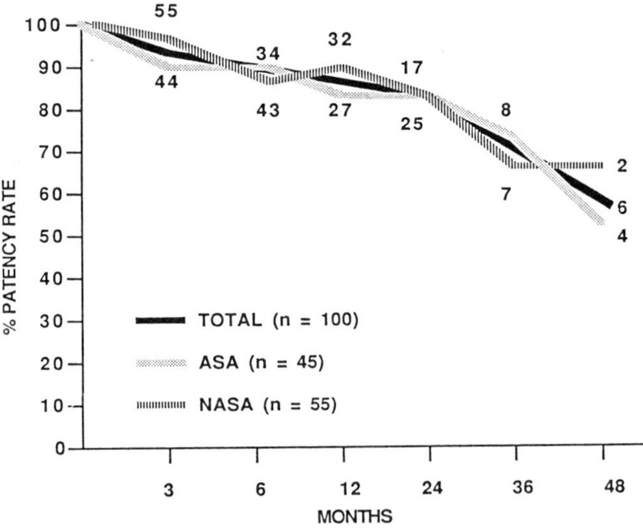

FIGURE 13. Cumulative patency rate by life table analysis of all grafts, those treated with aspirin (ASA) and grafts not treated with aspirin (NASA). No significant difference exists between ASA and NASA (p > .05). From Satiani, B.: A prospective, randomized trial of aspirin in femoral popliteal and tibial bypass grafts. Angiology, 36:610, 1985.

REFERENCES

1. Szilagyi, D.E., Hageman, J.H., Smith, R.F., et al.: Autogenous vein grafting in femoropopliteal atherosclerosis: The limits of its effectiveness. Surgery, 86:836–851, 1979.
2. Veith, F.J., Gupta, S.K., Ascer, E., et al.: Six-year prospective multicenter randomized comparison of autologous saphenous vein and expanded PTFE grafts in infra-inguinal arterial reconstructions. J. Vasc. Surg., 3:104–124, 1986.
3. Rutherford, R.B.: Vascular Surgery, 2nd ed. Philadelphia: W.B. Saunders, 1984.
4. Moore, W.S.: Vascular Surgery: A Comprehensive Review. New York: Grune & Stratton, 1983.
5. Murday, A.J., Gershlick, A.H., Syndercombe-Court, Y.D., et al.: Intimal thickening in autogenous vein grafts in rabbits: Influence of aspirin and dipyridamole. Thorax, 39:457–461, 1984.
6. Clowes, A.W.: The role of aspirin in enhancing arterial graft patency. J. Vasc. Surg., 3:381–388, 1986.
7. Green, R.M., Roedersheimer, L.R., and DeWeese, J.A.: Effects of aspirin and dipyridamole on expanded PTFE graft patency. Surgery, 92:1016–1026, 1982.
8. Gershlick, A.H., Syndercombe-Court, Y.D.S., Murday, A.J., et al.: Platelet function is altered by autogenous vein grafts in the early postoperative months. Cardiovasc. Res., 18:119–125, 1984.
9. Moncada, S. and Vane, J.R.: Arachidonic acid metabolites and the interactions between platelets and blood vessel walls. N. Engl. J. Med., 300:1142–1147, 1979.
10. Gershlick, A.H., Syndercombe-Court, Y.D.S., Murday, A.J., et al.: Activation of platelets by autogenous vein grafts is not prevented by acetylsalicyclic acid and dipyridamole. Cardiovasc. Res., 18:391–396, 1984.
11. Bomberger, R.A., DePalma, R.G., Ambrose, T.A., and Manalo, P.: Aspirin and dipyridamole inhibit endothelial healing. Arch. Surg., 117:1459–1464, 1982.
12. Clowes, A.W. and Karnovsky, M.J.: Failure of certain antiplatelet drugs to affect myointimal thickening following arterial endothelial injury in the rat. Lab. Inves., 36:452–464, 1977.
13. Gershlick, A.H., Syndercombe-Court, Y.D.S., Murday, A.J., et al.: Adverse effects of high-dose aspirin on platelet adhesion to experimental autogenous vein grafts. Cardiovasc. Res., 19:770–776, 1985.
14. Dyerberg, J., Bang, H.O., Stoffersen, E., et al.: Eicosapentanoic acid and prevention of thrombosis and atherosclerosis. Lancet, 2:117–119, 1978.
15. Bush, H.L., Graber, J.N., Jakubowski, J.A., et al.: Favorable balance of prostacyclin and thromboxane A2 improves early patency of human in situ vein grafts. J. Vasc. Surg., 1:149–159, 1984.
16. Weiss, H.J. and Turitto, V.T.: Prostacyclin inhibits platelet adhesion and thrombus formation on subendothelium. Blood, 53:244–250, 1979.
17. Echave, V., Koornick, A.R., Haimov, M., and Jacobson, J.H., II: Intimal hyperplasia as a complication of the use of the PTFE graft for femoral popliteal bypass. Surgery, 86:791–798, 1979.
18. Preston, F.E., Whipps, S., Jackson, C.A., et al.: Inhibition of prostacyclin and platelet thromboxane A2 after low-dose aspirin. N. Engl. J. Med., 304:76–79, 1981.
19. Pareti, F.I., D'Angelo, A., Mannucci, P.M., and Smith, J.B.: Platelets and the vessel wall: How much aspirin? Lancet, 1:371–373, 1980.
20. Carson, S.N., Demling, R.H., and Esquivel, C.O.: Aspirin failure in symptomatic atherosclerotic carotid artery disease. Surgery, 90:1084–1092, 1981.
21. Levine, P.H.: An acute effect of cigarette smoking on platelet function. A possible link between smoking and arterial thrombosis. Circulation, 48:619–623, 1973.
22. Kohler, T.R., Kaufman, J.L., Kacoyanis, G., et al.: Effect of aspirin and dipyridamole on the patency of lower extremity bypass grafts. Surgery, 96:462–466, 1984.
23. Satiani, B.: A prospective, randomized trial of aspirin in femoral popliteal and tibial bypass grafts. Angiology, 36:608–616, 1985.

DEBATE IX

In 1988 Is A Whipple Procedure Irrational And Imperfect?

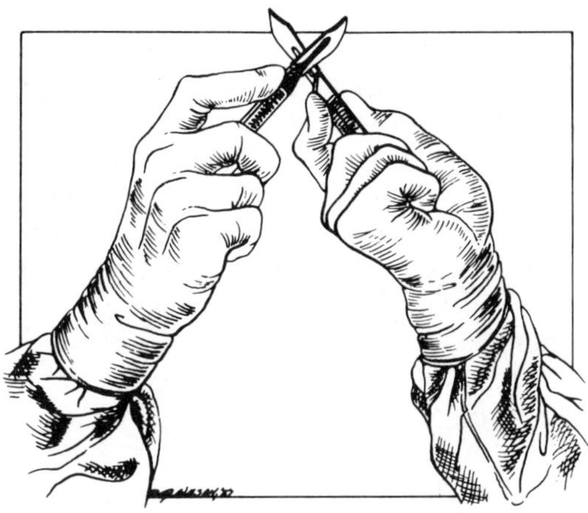

If the Congress of the United States were to pass a law making it illegal to perform a Whipple operation, would the plight of the patient with a pancreatic malignancy be improved or impaired? Clearly, periampullary/pancreatic cancer is a big problem requiring big therapy, a big surgeon, and a bold patient. Is a Whipple procedure too big?

Dr. Shannon argues that the surgical insult and physiologic price are too high and the curative potential is too low to warrant widespread application of Whipple's operation. The most favorable series now report an operative mortality that has just crept below 10 percent. In addition, when the Whipple procedure is performed for benign disease, the unique physiologic sequelae may be assessed. Postoperatively, there is a 12 percent incidence of new malabsorption, a 30 percent incidence of new diabetes mellitus, and a 6 percent incidence of cholangitis. Over the long term, 10 percent of patients will exhibit marginal ulceration, and 6 to 10 percent will suffer a pancreaticojejunal fistula (with an attendant 20 percent mortality). The cumulative complication rate may approach 60 percent, even in patients with benign disease.

In spite of this price, Dr. Shannon argues that the Whipple procedure is an inadequate cancer operation. Pancreatic cancer is multicentric in 30 percent of patients and metastasizes early to regional nodes. Experience with extended total pancreatectomy suggests that microscopic nodal metastasis will be found in up to 90 percent of patients. Presumably, these nodes might comfortably be left behind by the more limited Whipple procedure. Thus, patients deemed to have resectable pancreatic cancer should undergo a total pancreatectomy. Patients with demonstrable metastasis should avoid the physiologic ravages of pancreatic extirpation and receive a palliative bypass. The Whipple procedure (like most of the patients who have had one) is dead.

Conversely, Dr. Bell argues that the Whipple operation unequivocally provides a 40 to 50 percent 5-year survival in patients with carcinoma of the ampulla of Vater, common bile duct or duodenum, and islet cell carcinoma of the pancreas. Additional indications may be traumatic disruption of the pancreas/duodenum, incapacitating pancreatitis, or even hemorrhagic pancreatitis. Thus, a bypass procedure would deny up to 50 percent of patients with non-pancreatic periampullary tumors a real chance for cure.

Conversely, a total pancreatectomy is associated with an equal mortality when compared to the Whipple procedure and the morbidity is higher. Diabetes and steatorrhea are guaranteed. The spleen is not vestigial. No studies exist demonstrating superior survival following total pancreatectomy for equally staged pancreatic cancer.

Thus, in the patient who is less than 70 years old, is not alcoholic, and is a reasonable operative risk but who has a pancreatic cancer that is less than 2 cm in size and no demonstrable metastasis, the Whipple operation is not perfect; but no known therapy is better.

We must offer our patients hope and a chance for cure. No man is an average. Indeed, Joseph Stalin said, "A single death is a tragedy; one million deaths is a statistic."

IX-A: THE WHIPPLE OPERATION REMAINS VALUABLE SURGICAL THERAPY

REGINALD C. W. BELL, M.D.

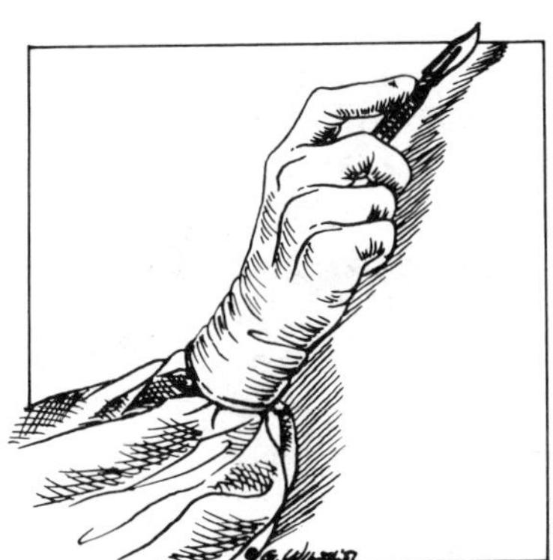

A Whipple operation is, indeed, a formidable operation to be undertaken by any surgeon. A Whipple procedure consists of division of the pancreas at the level of the superior mesenteric artery and involves resection of the stomach, duodenum, and the common bile duct. Reconstruction is performed by anastomosing the pancreas, the common hepatic duct, and the stomach to a Roux-en-Y limb of jejunum.

What are the indications for pancreatoduodenectomy? Carcinoma of the head of the pancreas is the most commonly cited indication. This is the most debatable indication and the one on which I will spend the most time. Carcinoma of the ampulla of Vater, common bile duct, or duodenum, and islet cell carcinoma of the head of the pancreas are well-accepted indications for a Whipple procedure. Other indications are traumatic disruption of the pancreatic head and duodenum, chronic pancreatitis with unremitting pain, or an undrainable pseudocyst. Pasquali and colleagues[1] have reported some cases of subtotal and total pancreatectomy for acute hemorrhagic pancreatic necrosis with operative mortalities that rank below the in-hospital mortality predicted with medical management by Ranson's criteria.

The majority of this discussion will be about cancer of the pancreas, specifically ductal adenocarcinoma. The question is whether a palliative operation, Whipple procedure, or total pancreatectomy should be performed. Those believing in palliation only would probably agree with the late Lord Cohen of Berkenhead who said, "The feasibility of an operation is not an indication for its performance."[2]

PALLIATIVE BYPASS VERSUS RESECTION

Crile[2] reported on 28 patients with a Whipple procedure for pancreatic ductal carcinoma with a median survival of five months and 28 patients with bypass without biopsy with a median survival of eight months. The cause of death in these bypass patients was not confirmed. At that time, he was dealing with a Whipple operative mortality of up to 40 percent. A major part of that operative mortality was related to the lethal nature of an open pancreatic biopsy.

The main objection to Crile's data is its high mortality. He admits that, with an operative mortality of less than 10 percent, one cannot argue strongly against the Whipple. The patients with better survival or equal survival with bypass patients are those who do *not* have biopsy-proven carcinoma of the head of the pancreas.

Gudjonsson and colleagues[3] analyzed 61 cases of resection for cure and 5-year survival in 15,000 patients. They concluded that radical surgery may benefit a small subgroup of patients with pancreatic cancer; but, as it has not improved the overall survival rate, it should be denied to patients as a curative procedure. This can be viewed as a ludicrous position. Just because we cannot influence *overall* survival of pancreatic cancer does not mean that we should not help whomever we can in whatever subgroup we can.

Approximately 15 percent of pancreatic ductal carcinoma indeed is resectable at the time of laparotomy. Shapiro[4] reviewed 16 series with 497 cases of radical surgery. Five-year survival was 4 percent, mean survival 14 months, and operative mortality 20 percent. He concluded, therefore, that 103 patients were denied immediately the 10 to 14 months of additional life in order for 20 patients to gain 60 months. If one calculates patient-months of survival, these numbers are indeed equal. However, this additional 10 to 14 months of life is misleading. In his series, bypass procedures had half the mortality of a Whipple procedure with a mean survival of seven months. So, by recalculating with his data, a Whipple procedure actually comes out *better* in terms of patient-months than does a bypass procedure. If bypass procedures are performed for all pancreatic head masses, then those patients with periampullary tumors will be denied a 90 percent chance of resection with an attendant 40 percent 5-year survival.

Gudjonsson and colleagues[3] demonstrated that 25 percent of intraoperatively diagnosed pancreatic cancers were not pancreatic in origin. Warren and colleagues,[5] in a study of 352 patients, showed that 10 percent of those intraoperatively diagnosed as pancreatic carcinomas were, in fact, periampullary carcinomas. They concluded that for this reason alone palliation should not be performed routinely when resectability seems possible. If the patient instead has an ampullary carcinoma, duodenal carcinoma, cystadenocarcinoma, islet cell carcinoma, or a common duct carcinoma, the 5-year survival is upwards of 35 to 50 percent.

Apart from curing those people with nonpancreatic periampullary tumors, is it also possible that in doing a Whipple procedure on a mass in the head of the pancreas one might cure a carcinoma of the head of the pancreas? Moossa and Levin[6] reported on 17 of 64 resected pancreatic ductal carcinomas that they termed early cancers. These met the following criteria: tumor diameter $\leq$ 2 cm, no histologic evidence of capsular invasion, absence of distant metastases at laparotomy, and absence of histologic lymph node involvement following careful examination of the resected specimen. Only one of these 17 patients died of metastatic pancreatic cancer after three years, presumably due to microscopic metastases undetected at the time of laparotomy.

It may be unfair to talk about *curative* resection because 5-year survival does not mean cure, and there are patients who die of metastatic disease following a Whipple operation at seven or eight years. However, there are no reported bypass patients who have lived five years except for one noted by Crile, and that patient was not biopsied. Tsuchiya and colleagues,[7] in Japan, have reported a 30 percent 5-year survival for resected small (≤ 2 cm) cancers. This increases to 37 percent for Stage I small cancers.

Pollard and colleagues[8] also found that there was a median survival of over 24 months and 71 percent 1-year survival in seven patients with T-1 neoplasms of 1 to 2 cm in size. Larger lesions had a significantly lower survival. This suggests that the patient with a small mass in the head of the pancreas that is a ductal adenocarcinoma may indeed be given a significantly prolonged symptom-free survival with a Whipple procedure, even if not completely cured.

Therefore, palliation should not be a routine procedure but should be limited to selected individuals. Patients over 70 years of age exhibit three times the mortality with a Whipple procedure than those under 70. A patient who has less than three years of life expectancy probably should not be resected. Distant metastases into the liver, omentum, peritoneum, and distant periaortic nodes preclude curative resection.

Local metastases and local spread do not preclude cure because there have been occasional reports of long-term survival with either local metastases or local spread. Most people do not recommend curative resection if one finds at least local nodal metastases. Longmire and Shafey[9] recommend looking for gross nodal involvement in three areas: the nodes along the hepatoduodenal ligament, the gastrohepatic artery and celiac access, and the inferior pancreaticoduodenal artery region. Nodes in these regions can be examined before the surgeon is committed to a Whipple procedure.

Moossa and colleagues[10] reported six patients with portal vein involvement. Four of these had actual invasion into the portal vein and died of metastases. Two had only inflammatory involvement of the portal vein. These were long-term survivors following a Whipple procedure. Likewise, if superior mesenteric vessels or the middle colic artery and transverse mesocolon are involved with local tumor, extensive resection has been performed with an occasional long-term survivor.

EXTENSIVE LOCAL DISEASE

What does one do in the resectable patient who has little hope for cure—the patient who has nodes involved grossly but who might still be resectable? Is it better to perform a Whipple operation anticipating a very rare long-term survivor, or should one perform a palliative bypass? Feduska and colleagues[11] reported 101 operations on patients with incurable but proportionately staged tumors. They defined palliation as the relief, even temporary, of any symptom or the return to work even on a part-time basis. Sixty patients treated with bypass had 53 percent palliation; 16 with Whipple procedure had 67 percent palliation. Four patients returned to work, two from each group. These numbers are too small to provide direction.

Significant considerations here are also the postoperative morbidity and the recuperation time. Although it is true that a Whipple procedure inflicts a higher morbidity than bypass, the number of postoperative hospital days quoted in most series is only two or three days apart. If one considers the chance for cure, albeit small, or prolonged survival, albeit small, offered to the patient with a Whipple procedure, I think one will agree that the larger operation at times may be worth the risks.

Open chemical splanchnicectomy at the time of a bypass has been reported by Sarr and Cameron to be 80 percent or more effective for long-term relief of pain.[12] This probably should be routinely added to any bypass procedure.

Regarding pancreatic cancer, a statement by Lord Smith of Marlow regarding resection versus palliation applies: "Although the average long-term results of pancreatoduodenectomy for cancer are very poor, no man is an average and resection does provide the *only* chance of cure. Individually, many patients might well opt for a considerable operative hazard with a small chance of cure rather than an inconsiderable hazard and no chance of cure."[13] We are talking more about a philosophical decision and the art of surgery than about hard scientific data.

WHIPPLE VERSUS TOTAL PANCREATECTOMY

If one is going to resect a mass in the head of the pancreas, should one do a total pancreatectomy or a Whipple procedure? The following must be considered in making this decision:

1. The curative intent is probably reserved for small, less than 2 cm, node-negative pancreatic cancers, although occasional 5-year survivors with positive nodes do exist.
2. The incidence of spreading or multicentric cancer is low enough that intraoperative sections should be used and can be used effectively.
3. True multicentric pancreatic carcinoma is probably systemic and, therefore, incurable upon presentation.
4. The actual lymphadenectomy of total pancreatectomy does not remove tissue in the drainage region of pancreatic head cancers. There is no evidence that the additional lymphadenectomy is curative.
5. Operative mortality is not lessened.
6. The postoperative morbidity and occasional mortality of a totally pancreatectomized patient with brittle diabetes are significant.
7. Steatorrhea should not be wished upon anyone.
8. The spleen is not an incidental organ.
9. No studies demonstrate a statistically better survival for equal stages of pancreatic cancer using total pancreatectomy.

The arguments in favor of a Whipple procedure are:

1.   There is preservation of endocrine function. Seventy percent of all patients of a Whipple procedure will remain free of diabetes; slightly less than this with pancreatic cancers. Seventeen percent already will have diabetes if they have pancreatic cancer upon presentation; 15 percent will develop diabetes postoperatively. Most often diabetes develops in a delayed fashion when the tumor recurs. Most importantly, glucagon levels will remain normal with only 10 to 15 percent of the pancreas left *in situ;* and, therefore, the Whipple diabetic is not the brittle diabetic as are total pancreatectomy patients. Brooks,[14] an advocate of total pancreatectomy, freely acknowledges this.

Thirty percent of patients following total pancreatectomy develop brittle diabetes. The mortality from this glucose intolerance is not insignificant. Three out of 65 patients died during hypoglycemic attacks;[15] two out of 51 died of uncontrolled diabetes in another study.[16]

2. There is preservation of exocrine function. Fifty percent of patients following a Whipple operation will maintain good exocrine function and be spared the steatorrhea that enzyme replacement cannot fully alleviate. DelPrato and colleagues[16] studied Type I diabetics, Whipple diabetics, and total pancreatectomy diabetics. Their data show that the high levels of gluconeogenic precursors, such as alanine, lactate, pyruvate, and glycerol, already reported in patients with diabetes due to total pancreatectomy after insulin withdrawal, do not become normal even in the presence of insulin. This finding shows that gluconeogenesis is primarily dependent upon pancreatic glucagon and confirms the role of glucagon in the development of diabetic hyperglycemia. Other studies also have demonstrated the failure of serum glucagon levels to rise in response to hyperglycemia.[17]

3. With a Whipple procedure, there is a decreased risk of marginal ulceration, a statistically significant three-fold decrease from 18 to 6 percent. These marginal ulcers are very aggressive. Death was caused at least partially by the ulcer in 22 percent of patients following total pancreatectomy, according to Grant and vanHeerden.[18]

Longmire[19] and Braasch and colleagues,[20] on opposite sides of the country, advocate a gastric and pylorus-sparing pancreatoduodenectomy, which almost totally eliminates the risk of marginal ulceration during the Whipple procedure. The addition of a vagotomy to a 50 percent gastrectomy in an attempt to alleviate marginal ulceration in the totally pancreatectomized patient was actually rejected by ReMine,[21] an early advocate of total pancreatectomy, because he reasoned that the combination of dumping syndrome and steatorrhea would relegate the patient to the bathroom itself.

4. The spleen is not an incidental organ. Total pancreatectomy involves removal of the spleen and splenic nodes; a Whipple procedure does not.

ARGUMENTS IN FAVOR OF TOTAL PANCREATECTOMY

The arguments in favor of total pancreatectomy include tumor multicentricity, wider lymphadenectomy, eradication of the pancreaticojejunal anastomosis, technical facility, elimination of postoperative pancreatitis, and improved survival.

What about tumor multicentricity? In the Mayo Clinic experience,[22] 31 percent of resected pancreatic carcinomas were multicentric; however, the original report includes carcinoma *in situ*. Ihse and colleagues[15] noted that, in 16 percent of their specimens, tumor cells were found far from the main lesion. Tryka and Brooks[23] found that 37 percent of 25 specimens had histologic evidence of tumor that, in their estimation, a Whipple procedure would have missed. However, in three of these nine patients, the tumor had spread up along the common bile duct. In four of the nine, the tumor had spread in continuity from a primary mass to the left. These are patients in whom a frozen section of the margins and extension to a subtotal or total pancreatectomy if frozen section margins were positive could be done within the framework of the Whipple operation. Blind total pancreatectomy is not warranted here. In five of the nine having truly multifocal disease with many islands of carcinoma *in situ,* an invasive carcinoma was found.

Two issues arise here:

1. Longmire, an advocate of *selective* rather than mandated total pancreatectomy, believes that here, too, intraoperative frozen section analysis can spare many patients a total pancreatectomy while resecting when indicated for multicentric tumor.

2. Multicentric tumors have a decidedly worse prognosis. VanHeerden and colleagues[24] showed that multicentric tumors had twice the 1-year mortality of unifocal tumors even with total pancreatectomy.

How about wider lymphadenectomy? Fortner[25] advocates a resection of the peripancreatic portal vein, transverse mesocolon, and a periaortic node dissection from the IMA to the diaphragmatic crura. Fortner is also in favor of an operation which, in his own data, has twice the operative mortality of the Whipple procedure. Most studies indicate that nodal involvement dramatically worsens prognosis. As vanHeerden[24] says, positive nodes connote systemic disease. Fortner himself has been unable to demonstrate that patients with nodal involvement or Stage II patients in his series are benefitted by his surgery.

What about eradication of the pancreaticojejunal anastomosis? Brooks[14] said that leakage accounts for 40 percent of the 10 to 20 percent mortality for a Whipple procedure. Both vanHeerden and colleagues[24] and Braasch and colleagues[20] have reported that the mortality overall due to leaking anastomosis is 1.5 to 2 percent. Most of the patients who leak can be treated conservatively with parenteral nutrition. Some will require total pancreatectomy. Eradication of the pancreaticojejunostomy and the pancreas does *not* lower operative mortality. In most series, total pancreatectomy operative mortality is still 10 to 15 percent. The operative mortality for a Whipple procedure with an experienced surgeon can be reduced to 5 percent or less (Table I).

Recall Crile's comment that someone who does a Whipple procedure should be able to do so with less than a 10 percent operative mortality. That clearly has been accomplished. Recall, too, Shapiro's comment that a Whipple procedure probably would be better palliation if an operative mortality of under 5 percent could be obtained.

TABLE I. OPERATIVE MORTALITY

REPORT	TOTAL PANCREATX		WHIPPLE	
Brooks 1976	13%	2/16	21%	2/11
Brooks 1982	12%	4/34		
Ihse	17-23%			
Lawrence	16%		15%	
Moossa	9%	4/45	5%	1/19
Longmire	17%		12%	
Lahey	10%			
Mayo 1981	17-15%		21%	0/29
Trede 1985	8%	2/27	1%	1/91
Braasch 1984				0/36
Howard 1968				0/41

Lastly, does total pancreatectomy *improve* survival in pancreatic head carcinoma? The answer is NO. In a review of 898 patients with adenocarcinoma of the pancreas who were treated with a Whipple operation, Jordan[26] showed a 6.5 percent 5-year survival. I think that is a fair figure. The most favorable 5-year survival following a Whipple procedure is up to 25 percent, and many series with 0 percent 5-year survival can be found. I think probably a 6.5 percent 5-year survival in a large series of patients is not unreasonable.

In his book *Surgery of the Pancreas,* Brooks[14] includes a table with an amazing 11 percent 5-year survival following total pancreatectomy for ductal carcinoma of the pancreas (Table II). Looks pretty good, doesn't it? Two series, one by Brooks and one by Moossa, account for nine of the sixteen 5-year survivors of total pancreatectomy.

Brooks' series compares 35 total pancreatectomies with 11 earlier Whipple procedures. By grouping Stage I and Stage II cancers together, he was able to find a significant difference in survival for the two operations. He found no differences for Stage III cancers; i.e., nodal involvement—those whom he, I think, would hope to help with a total pancreatectomy. However, it is unclear if the previous Whipple procedures were all done with curative intent. The only 5-year survivors were Stage I cancers. This suggests, as do other studies such as those by Moossa and Kummerle, a difference in curative potential between Stages I and II. Brooks does not tell us what percent of the two operations falls into each stage in his series.

Moossa and colleagues[10] reported on 51 head of the pancreas carcinomas. Eighteen were treated with a Whipple procedure; 33 with total pancreatectomy. There is no mention of staging. Moossa himself says that comparison of survival data from the two operations probably is not valid. Moossa, elsewhere, has written, "the superiority of total pancreatectomy over the Whipple operation has not been demonstrated significantly in retrospective institutional series."[27]

Now go back and look at Brooks' data claiming an 11 percent 5-year survival. It is an erroneous figure! It is obtained by averaging the percent survivals! It is *not* ob-

TABLE II. SURVIVAL RATE AFTER TOTAL PANCREATECTOMY FOR DUCTAL CARCINOMA*

	NUMBER	MORTALITY (%)	SURVIVAL				
			1 YR (%)	2 YR (%)	3 YR (%)	5 YR (%)	6 YR (%)
Brooks	29	13	44	36	28	16	4
ReMine	51	14	54	29	9	5	—
Ihse	58	17	44	30	30	3	—
Lawrence	15	16	20	7	—	—	—
Moossa	28	7	—	—	35	17	4
Fortner	36	15	47	20	—	—	—
White	14	7	—	—	—	15	7
Longmire	6	17	50	50	—	16	—
Lahey	11	10	—	—	—	0	—
	248	13	43	29	26	11	5

*From Brooks, J.R.: Cancer of the pancreas. In Surgery of the Pancreas. J.R. Brooks (ed.). Philadelphia: W.B. Saunders, 1983, p. 287.

tained by calculating the percentage of *total* survivors versus the *total* number operated on. If that is done, there are actually 16 patients surviving, 212 operated on, for 7.5 percent survival. Brooks also misquotes Ihse as having an 8 percent 5-year survival when he actually had a 3 percent 5-year survival (Table III).[15]

Listen to Longmire, one of the founders of pancreatic surgery. In 1979 he supports total pancreatectomy because of decreased morbidity and better survival in a study of six patients.[28] By 1981 he says, "It is difficult to accept total pancreatectomy as a routine procedure. Total resection diminishes the palliation such operations provide."[29] In his Founder's Lecture in the 1984 American Journal of Surgery, he says, "Our limited results with partial pancreatic excision when the margins of the resection have been found to be free of tumor have been equal to our results with total pancreatectomy. Partial resection has the advantage of being a lower risk procedure and does not produce diabetes."[30] In 1984 he says, "We believe the subtotal pancreatoduodenectomy is the procedure of choice in most cases."[19]

There is one good study that does stage pancreatic head cancer and compares total pancreatectomy with the Whipple procedure.[31] This is the staging: T-1, tumor limited to the pancreas; T-2, tumor extended beyond the pancreas; T-3, tumor invading adjacent organs. Note Table IV showing T-1 and T-2 stages with the Whipple procedure versus total pancreatectomy. Although the numbers are small, total pancreatectomy offers no better and apparently worse survival than a Whipple operation for T-1 and T-2 cancers. With T-3 and N-1 and N-2 cancers, survival rates are similar; although it actually appears by this data that the Whipple procedure is better.

To sum up: *No studies demonstrate a statistically better survival for equal stages of pancreatic cancer using total pancreatectomy.*

The indications for a Whipple operation that are rational and practical are the following:

1. Known periampullary nonpancreatic cancer that is resectable (90 percent of these are resectable);
2. Carcinoma of the head of the pancreas that can be circumscribed by the resection, and
   a. in which frozen section of the margin does not reveal residual and multicentric tumor;
   b. in which the pancreatic duct is of sufficient size and the pancreas of sufficient firmness to permit a pancreaticojejunostomy; and
   c. in the 85 percent of cases in which insulin-dependent diabetes is not pre-existent.

   In the absence of a, b, and c, total pancreatectomy is indicated.
3. A jaundice-producing mass in the head of the pancreas without a tissue diagnosis of cancer. The sensitivity and specificity of various tests have not been discussed. With a small cancer that has a high curability rate—if anything does—obtaining an adequate tissue specimen positive for carcinoma may be extremely difficult. In these cases, if the surgeon is experienced, if the patient is over 50 years of age and not alcoholic, and if an impacted stone, penetrating ulcer, and benign tumor of the duct or ampulla can be ruled out, it is reasonable to proceed with resection.

TABLE III. SURVIVAL RATE AFTER TOTAL PANCREATECTOMY FOR DUCTAL CARCINOMA, WITH NUMBER OF 5-YEAR SURVIVORS*

	NUMBER	MORTALITY (%)	SURVIVAL					
			1 YR (%)	2 YR (%)	3 YR (%)	5 YR (%)	6 YR (%)	5 YR‡ (#)
Brooks	29	13	44	36	28	16	4	5
ReMine	51	14	54	29	9	5	—	2
Ihse	58	17	44	30	30	3 :8	—	2
Lawrence	15	16	20	7	—	—	—	0
Moossa	28	7	—	—	35	17	4	4
Fortner†	~~36~~	15	47	20	—	—	—	—
White	14	7	—	—	—	15	7	2
Longmire	6	17	50	50	—	16	—	1
Lahey	11	10	—	—	—	0	—	0
	212 ~~248~~	13	43	29	26	~~11~~	5	16 = 7.5%

*Modified from Brooks, J.R.: Cancer of the pancreas. In Surgery of the Pancreas. J.R. Brooks (ed.). Philadelphia: W.B. Saunders, 1983.
† Fortner's study does not include 5-year survival data. Thus 36 has been subtracted from the total number of patients.
‡ This column was added by the present author.

TABLE IV.   STAGING OF PANCREATIC HEAD CANCER*

Total Pancreatectomy Versus Whipple Procedure

TNM classifications in 51 patients undergoing partial pancreatico-duodenectomy up until 1977.

	N_0M_0		N_1M_0		N_2M_0	
	No.	%	No.	%	No.	%
T_1	17	33	0		0	
T_2	10	20	6	12	0	
T_3	15	29	2	4	1	2

TNM staging of 62 patients undergoing total pancreaticoduodenectomy.

	N_0M_0		N_1M_0		N_2M_0	
	No.	%	No.	%	No.	%
T_1	6	10	0		0	
T_2	13	21	7	11	0	
T_3	25	40	11	18	0	

Median survival time in 74 patients undergoing a Whipple procedure for pancreatic carcinoma.

TNM STAGING	NO.	MONTHS
$T_1N_0M_0$	13	28
$T_2N_0M_0$	7	16
$T_3N_0M_0$	10	11
$T_{1-3}N_1M_0$	5	12
$T_{1-3}N_{1-2}M_0$	39	14

Median survival time in 92 patients undergoing total pancreatectomy for cancer of the pancreas.

TNM STAGING	NO.	MONTHS
$T_1N_0M_0$	6	8
$T_2N_0M_0$	9	8
$T_3N_0M_0$	15	14
$T_{1-3}N_1M_0$	14	7
$T_{1-3}N_{1-2}M_0$	48	8

*From Kummerle, F. and Ruckert, K.: Surgical treatment of pancreatic cancer. World J. Surg., 8:890–891, 1984.

4. Chronic calcareous pancreatitis with uncontrollable pain. Removing the pancreatic head, uncinate process, and part of the body eradicates the most common site of pancreatitis and of multiple small blocked areas in the ductile system. Frequently, even a 10 to 15 percent pancreatic remnant will stave off diabetes.[14]
5. Pseudocysts of the pancreatic head that cannot otherwise be drained.
6. Severe traumatic disruption of the pancreatic duct and duodenum.

There is no doubt that a Whipple procedure is a procedure of major proportions performed by a surgeon who is not timid upon a cancer that is very aggressive with a very low chance of cure. However, as Lord Smith of Marlow said, no man is an average. I think the best way that one has to approach pancreatic cancer is by way of the French proverb: "Aux grands maux, les grands remedes."

REFERENCES

1. Pasquali, E., Capriolo, F., Pietrarota, P., and Giezia, M.: Operative management of acute pancreatitis. Ital. J. Surg. Sc., 12:285–293, 1982.
2. Crile, G., Jr.: The advantages of bypass operations over radical pancreaticoduodenectomy in the treatment of pancreatic carcinoma. Surg. Gynecol. Obstet., 130:1049–1053, 1970.
3. Gudjonsson, B., Livstone, E.M., and Spiro, H.M.: Cancer of the pancreas: Diagnostic accuracy and survival statistics. Cancer, 42:2494–2506, 1978.
4. Shapiro, T.M.: Adenocarcinoma of the pancreas. A statistical analysis of biliary bypass versus Whipple resection in good risk patients. Ann. Surg., 182:715–721, 1975.
5. Warren, K.W., Choe, D.S., Plaza, J., and Relihan, M.: Results of radical resection for periampullary cancer. Ann. Surg., 181:534–540, 1975.
6. Moossa, A.R. and Levin, B.: The diagnosis of "early" pancreatic cancer: The University of Chicago experience. Cancer, 47:1688–1697, 1981.
7. Tsuchiya, R., Noda, T., Harada, N., et al.: Collective review of small carcinomas of the pancreas. Ann Surg., 203:77–81, 1986.
8. Pollard, H.M., Anderson, W.A.D., Brooks, F.P., et al., Cancer of the Pancreas Task Force: Staging of cancer of the pancreas. Cancer, 47:1631–1637, 1981.
9. Longmire, W.P., Jr., and Shafey, O.A.: Certain factors influencing survival after pancreaticoduodenal resection for carcinoma. Am. J. Surg., 111:8–12, 1966.
10. Moossa, A.R., Lewis, M.H., and Mackie, C.R.: Surgical treatment of pancreatic cancer. Mayo Clin. Proc., 54:468–474, 1979.
11. Feduska, N.J., Dent, T.L., and Lindenauer, S.M.: Results of palliative operations for carcinoma of the pancreas. Arch. Surg., 103:330–334, 1971.
12. Sarr, M.G. and Cameron, J.L.: Surgical palliation of unresectable carcinoma of the pancreas. World J. Surg., 8:906, 1984.
13. Lord Smith of Marlow: Surgery of cancer of the pancreas. In The Exocrine Pancreas. H.T. Harwat and H. Sarles (eds.). Philadelphia: W.B. Saunders, 1979, p. 220.
14. Brooks, J.R.: Cancer of the pancreas. In Surgery of the Pancreas. J.R. Brooks (ed.). Philadelphia: W.B. Saunders, 1983, pp. 263 ff.
15. Ihse, I., Lilja, P., Arnesjo, B., and Bengmark, S.: Total pancreatectomy for cancer: An appraisal of 65 cases. Ann. Surg., 186:675–680, 1977.
16. DelPrato, S., Tiengo, A., Baccaglini, U., et al.: Effect of insulin replacement on intermediary metabolism in diabetes secondary to pancreatectomy. Diabetologia, 25:252–259, 1983.
17. Horie, H., Matsuyama, T., Namba, M., et al.: Responses of catecholamines and other counterregulatory hormones to insulin-induced hypoglycemia in totally pancreatectomized patients. J. Clin. Endocrinol. Metab., 59:1193–1196, 1982.
18. Grant, C.S. and vanHeerden, J.A.: Anastomotic ulceration following subtotal and total pancreatectomy. Ann Surg., 190:1–5, 1979.
19. Longmire, W.P.: Cancer of the pancreas: Palliative operation, Whipple procedure, or total pancreatectomy. World J. Surg., 8:872, 1984.
20. Braasch, J.W., Gongliang, J., and Rossi, R.C.: Pancreaticoduodenectomy with preservation of the pylorus. World J. Surg., 8:900, 1984.
21. Levin, B., ReMine, W.H., Hermann, R.E., et al.: Panel discussion: Cancer of the pancreas. Am. J. Surg., 135:185, 1978.
22. Edis, A.J., Kiernan, P.D., and Taylor, W.F.: Attempted curative resection of ductal carcinoma of the pancreas: Review of Mayo Clinic experience, 1951–1975. Mayo Clin. Proc., 55:531–536, 1980.

23. Tryka, A.F. and Brooks, J.R.: Histopathology in the evaluation of total pancreatectomy for ductal carcinoma. Ann. Surg., 190:373–381, 1979.
24. vanHeerden, J.A., ReMine, W.H., Weiland, L.H., et al.: Total pancreatectomy for ductal adenocarcinoma of the pancreas: Mayo Clinic experience. Am. J. Surg., 142:308–311, 1981.
25. Fortner, J.G.: Surgical principles for pancreatic cancer: Regional, total, and subtotal pancreatectomy. Cancer, 47:1712–1718, 1981.
26. Jordan, G.I.: Surgical management of pancreatic cancer. In Gastrointestinal Cancer. Stroehlein, Ronnsdahl (eds.). New York: Raven Press, 1981.
27. Moossa, A.R., Scott, M.H., and Lavelle-Jones, M.: The place of total and extended total pancreatectomy in pancreatic cancer. World J. Surg., 8:895–899, 1984.
28. Forrest, J.F. and Longmire, W.P.: Carcinoma of the pancreas and periampullary region. Ann. Surg., 189:129–138, 1979.
29. Longmire, W.P. and Traverso, L.W.: The Whipple procedure and other standard operative approaches to pancreatic cancer. Cancer, 47:1706–1711, 1981.
30. Longmire, W.P.: The vicissitudes of pancreatic surgery. Am. J. Surg., 147:17–24, 1984.
31. Kummerle, F. and Ruckert, K.: Surgical treatment of pancreatic cancer. World J. Surg., 8:889–894, 1984.
32. Piorkowski, R.J., Blievernicht, S.W., Lawrence, W., et al.: Pancreatic and periampullary carcinoma: Experience with 200 patients over a 12-year period. Am. J. Surg., 143:189, 1982.
33. Trede, M.: The surgical treatment of pancreatic carcinoma. Surgery, 97:28, 1985.
34. Howard, J.M.: Pancreaticoduodenectomy: Forty-one consecutive Whipple resections without an operative mortality. Ann. Surg., 168:629, 1968.

IX-B: A WHIPPLE OPERATION IS IMPERFECT AND IRRATIONAL

FRANCIS L. SHANNON, M.D.

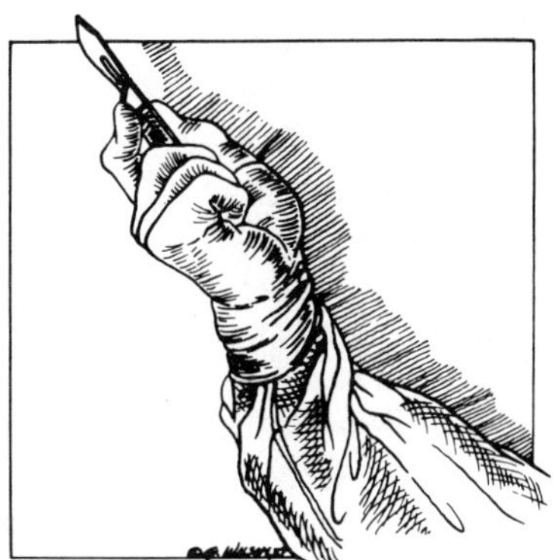

In this era of major surgical accomplishment, the Whipple procedure remains as a stark reminder of our failure to devise safer and more effective treatment for periampullary cancers and other neoplasms of the pancreas. Although recently the operative mortality has become more acceptable, subtotal pancreatectomy is still an ineffective and intrinsically morbid operation. This discussion will demonstrate that the classic Whipple procedure alone is irrational therapy for pancreatic cancer and that it is an intrinsically imperfect operation for other diseases involving the head of the pancreas.

HISTORICAL PERSPECTIVE

Although Allen Oldfather Whipple is credited with defining the essential elements of radical resection of the pancreas and duodenum, Codivilla in Europe was the first surgeon to perform the procedure for periampullary cancer in 1898. Following his lead, Desjardins formulated the anatomical plan of attack on cancers in this region that made resection without excessive blood loss feasible. Halsted and others followed this blueprint but incurred an unacceptable operative mortality of 40 percent in the early 1900s.[1]

Theorizing that jaundice caused systemic complications, Whipple, Parsons, and Mullins[2] in 1935 proposed that a two-stage pancreatic resection might be safe. Thus, the first operation for periampullary obstructive cancers consisted of biliary gastroduodenal decompression with a Roux-en-Y choledochojejunostomy and gastrojejunostomy. When the patient was less jaundiced and better nourished, en bloc subtotal pancreatic and total duodenal resection with simple oversewing of the pancreatic remnant could be done with less operative risk. Through bitter experience, however, it became apparent to Whipple that the consequences of pancreatic fistula were lethal. Furthermore, he eventually found no advantage to performing the operation in two stages.

Thus, in 1942, Whipple[2] advocated a one-stage resection with attachment of the pancreatic remnant to the Roux-en-Y limb. His only subsequent modifications of the procedure involved different routes of establishing gastrointestinal continuity and methods of preventing marginal ulceration. No less than 20 modifications of the classic Whipple procedure have been published over the subsequent 40 years. Despite these changes, one out of every four patients died in the postoperative period. In addition, few patients lived long enough without cancer to suffer the chronic morbidity of the procedure. Much like the Marines after securing a beachhead, pancreatic surgeons were grateful to secure postoperative survival. In retrospect, it has taken 40 years for a small cadre of dedicated surgeons to execute radical resection of the pancreas and duodenum with a tolerable incidence of operative casualties.

TECHNICAL DEFINITION

For the sake of our discussion, I will define the essence of the classic Whipple procedure. The resection involves removal of approximately 45 percent of the head and body of the pancreas, the distal common bile duct, and the pyloroantral region of the stomach. Regional lymph nodes around the head and body of the pancreas are removed en bloc after preresection biopsy of choledochal and celiac nodes. GI continuity is restored by Roux-en-Y jejunal anastomosis to the pancreatic tail, proximal common bile duct, and gastric pouch.

Analysis of this operation as it is used for pancreatic cancer discloses two major problems in terms of its rationale and efficacy.

1. Straddled by the confluence of the superior mesenteric and portal veins, dissection of the neck of the pancreas can incur significant blood loss and compromise the en bloc nature of the resection if tumor extends outside of the pancreatic capsule. In up to 30 percent of pancreatic resections for cancer, the cleavage plane between these vessels and the pancreas is infiltrated with tumor.[3,4]
2. The zone of lymph nodes around the body and tail of the pancreas as well as the nodes at the base of the transverse colon mesentery and in the hilum of the spleen are not removed and may be involved with metastatic disease. Clearly, positive nodes in this region make a patient unresectable for cure according to standard criteria. However, the extended total pancreatectomy results reported by Fortner[5] show that a significant amount of nodal cancer can be left behind by the classic Whipple resection.

Solutions to these anatomic problems require more extensive surgical operations.

Conversely, a total pancreatectomy allows more complete nodal clearance of the region. Regional total pancreatectomy as described by Fortner[5] involves en bloc resection of the portal vein, distal bile duct, and all periaortic and celiac nodes. The relative therapeutic merits of these resectional alternatives in comparison to the classic Whipple operation will be discussed later.

Thus, these anatomic features of the Whipple procedure make it an irrational cancer operation because potential (and frequent) areas of regional spread are left behind.

USES OF THE WHIPPLE PROCEDURE

Over the years, the Whipple resection has been used for nonpancreatic periampullary carcinomas, for chronic pancreatitis confined to the proximal portion of the gland, for severe pancreatic and duodenal trauma, and, unwittingly, for benign causes of obstructive jaundice believed to be due to cancer. I will review briefly the results of the Whipple operation for these diseases.

Periampullary Cancers.   Outnumbered by pancreatic cancers two to one, cancers of the duodenum, ampulla of Vater, and distal common bile duct have been resected successfully but with a rather high operative mortality. Fortunately, the 5-year survival for patients surviving the initial operation exceeds the number of patients succumbing to surgery.[6] However, the prognosis of these cancers is favorable because they usually are present before widespread regional infiltration and metastasis have occurred. Furthermore, these tumors do not tend to involve the entire pancreas. For these reasons, I will concede that a properly performed Whipple procedure is acceptable surgical therapy for nonpancreatic ampullary cancer (Table I).

Chronic Pancreatitis.   The results of the Whipple procedure for chronic pancreatitis constitute a useful assessment of its physiological consequences among patients with moderate to severe disease of the entire pancreas. Collating the results of 11 studies involving 580 patients, I found that at least one-third of the patients did not meet the criteria for resection formulated by Moreaux.[7] Disregarding this point, the overall operative mortality was approximately 8 percent. This risk of death seems rather high for a chronologically young population seeking relief of chronic pain. Furthermore, the absolute utility of preserving a remnant of diseased gland is questionable in view of the 12 percent incidence of *new* malabsorption, 30 percent incidence of *new* diabetes mellitus, and 6 percent incidence of cholangitis (Table II).

TABLE I.   PERIAMPULLARY CANCERS (AMPULLA, DUODENUM, BILE DUCT)

AUTHOR	YEAR	MORTALITY	5-YEAR SURVIVAL
Brooks[13]	1982	18.8%	29.3%
Williams[19]	1979	11.0%	27.0%
Jones[20]	1985	5.0%	24.0%
Tarazi[6]	1986	8.2%	33.0%

TABLE II.   CHRONIC PANCREATITIS*

Overall operative mortality:	7.5%
Long-term morbidity:	
Exocrine insufficiency	12.0%
Diabetes mellitus	30.0%
Marginal ulcer	10.0%
Cholangitis	6.0%

*From Brooks, J.R.: Cancer of the pancreas. Chronic pancreatitis. In Surgery of the Pancreas. J.R. Brooks (ed.). Philadelphia, W.B. Saunders, 1983.

TABLE III. ERAS OF OPERATIVE MORTALITY*

YEARS	N	RESECTABLE	MORTALITY
1950–1970	1056	15%	20%
1971–1978	226	21%	18%
1979–1984	215	19%	4%

*From Brooks, J.R.: Cancer of the pancreas. Chronic pancreatitis. In Surgery of the Pancreas. J.R. Brooks (ed.). Philadelphia, W.B. Saunders, 1983.

The long-term ulcerogenic potential of the Whipple resection is demonstrated by the 10 percent incidence of marginal ulceration. Furthermore, pain has recurred in at least one-third of the survivors; and nearly 40 percent of the patients with benign disease died within five years of operation.[7] The contribution of the operation to their demise cannot be ascertained, but the risk-benefit ratio seems rather narrow.

Benign Disease. The impact of the Whipple operation on patients with benign disease was assessed by Cohen and colleagues[8] in a review of the world literature in 1983. They found that 11 percent of the patients with benign jaundice, but perceived cancers, died as a result of surgery. Another group of patients with chronic pancreatitis had an acceptable 5 percent operative mortality. Among patients with combined pancreatic and duodenal trauma, excluding victims with persistent hemorrhagic shock, a 30 percent hospital mortality rate was observed. This combined study underscores the intrinsically lethal nature of the Whipple procedure.

These retrospective reviews of the consequences of the Whipple procedure among patients with reversible disease emphasize the physiological and technical imperfections. In 1987, it would appear inappropriate to perform an operation with a minimum 5 to 10 percent operative mortality, 12 percent incidence of malabsorption, 30 percent incidence of diabetes, 10 percent incidence of marginal ulceration, and 6 percent incidence of cholangitis. Taken together, a Whipple procedure performed for benign disease has a 60 percent chance of chronic complications.

Pancreatic Ductal Cancer. When used for pancreatic cancer, the Whipple procedure has the same limitations, but, in addition, may be an inadequate cancer operation.

EXCESSIVE OPERATIVE MORTALITY

Cumulative review of operative outcomes in terms of eras of technical advancement shows that improved critical care and anesthetic skills have reduced the operative mortality from 20 to 4 percent (Table III). The cumulative all-time low, however, is skewed by a 1 percent mortality rate emanating from a series of 145 patients reported by Trede[9] in Germany. Excluding this extraordinary series, an average operative mortality of 7 percent is obtained.

Analysis of recent deaths shows that over 40 percent of the mortality is due to either pancreatic leaks or infectious sequelae of doing a big operation in older, debilitated patients (Table IV). In addition, one-half of the deaths from exsanguination were due to free intraperitoneal bleeding from untied vessels and the other half were due to major GI hemorrhages. Thus, 70 percent of the deaths result from techni-

TABLE IV.   WHIPPLE MORTALITY ANALYSIS*

CAUSE OF DEATH	% DEATHS
Hemorrhage	31
Pancreatic Fistula	22
Sepsis	22
Cardiopulmonary	13
Miscellaneous	12

*Data compiled from references 1, 3, 6, 7, 8, 10, 13, 15, 21, and 23

cal and conceptual imperfections of the operation rather than from the patient's disease.

Whipple Complications.   Despite the four-fold reduction in operative mortality, the frequency of technical complications has remained relatively constant. Surprisingly, the incidence of pancreatic fistulae has increased; but the mortality of this complication has declined with the advent of parenteral alimentation. Advances in supportive care, however, have not been sufficient to reduce the mortality of major hemorrhage or intraabdominal sepsis. Clearly, no other cancer operation used in 1987 has a similarly consistent profile of hazard as does the Whipple procedure.

Age-Related Mortality.   A factor contributing to the mortality of the Whipple procedure is the age of the patient (Table V). Patients over 70 years of age have a 2 to 10 times greater risk of dying from surgery than their younger resected counterparts. Furthermore, this increased risk is imposed without providing improved mean survival over a simple palliative bypass. This distressing age-related mortality and life-expectancy would appear to further restrict the utility of the Whipple procedure. In the Mayo Clinic series, at least 25 percent of patients with resectable pancreatic cancer were 70 years or older.[10] Thus, the intrinsic stress of a pancreatic resection is too great for one-fourth of the population who might potentially benefit from curative therapy.

Surgeon-Dependent Mortality.   The learning curve for doing safe pancreatic resections is steep. It has been only within the last 10 years that isolated series have shown that the Whipple procedure can be done with less than 10 percent mortality.[9] A novice pancreatectomist incurs a minimum 20 percent operative mortality.

TABLE V.   AGE-RELATED SURVIVAL

	OPERATIVE MORTALITY		
	YEAR	AGE < 70 Y/O	AGE > 70 Y/O
Andren[21]	1984	24%	58%
Obertop[22]	1982	3%	27%
	MEAN SURVIVAL		
Forrest[3]	1979	16.2 mo.	7.6 mo.

Technical Mortality. Measurable indices of experience that correlate with operative mortality are total operating time and operative blood loss. As Gilsdorf and Spanos[11] noted, long operations have higher mortality rates (Table VI). Furthermore, the systemic and immunologic stress of major operative blood loss influences short-term survival and probably affects long-term freedom from recurrent cancer.

Intrinsic Operative Risks. Best estimates of the current operative risk of a Whipple procedure show that postoperative death is still a significant possibility for the patient with limited pancreatic cancer. Furthermore, the major complications of pancreatic fistula, major GI or intraperitoneal hemorrhage, and sepsis from intraabdominal sources occur in a minimum of 10 percent of patients. This relatively low incidence of postoperative complications is incurred by experienced pancreatic surgeons operating at major centers on carefully selected patients. When compared to the risks of open heart surgery or abdominal aneurysm resection, a Whipple procedure is a very threatening venture. In inexperienced hands, the Whipple procedure is comparable to jumping the Snake River on a motorcycle.

INADEQUATE CANCER OPERATION

Considering the risks involved, one would hope that the operation at least would achieve local control of the cancer. Retrospective assessment following total pancreatectomy shows that pancreatic cancer tends to be a multicentric tumor.[12] These figures do not include studies in which pancreatic ductal hyperplasia was found as well. Thus, regardless of the endocrinological consequences, truly curative surgery for pancreatic cancer demands total pancreatectomy.

The Whipple procedure is inadequate because the major draining lymphatics cannot be excised without a more extensive pancreatic resection. Although occult nodal metastasis has been regarded as a sign of a more biologically aggressive cancer, the minimum objective of complete tumor removal frequently is not accomplished with the Whipple procedure. As Fortner[5] demonstrated by regional total pancreatectomy, microscopic lymph node metastases are found in nearly 90 percent of patients. When compared to series of Whipple resections, almost 50 percent of microscopic disease must be left behind by subtotal pancreatectomy.

TABLE VI. TECHNICAL MORTALITY*

OPERATION DURATION	N	PERCENT OP. MORTALITY
< 8 hours	20	0
8–10 hours	35	17
> 10 hours	26	50
BLOOD LOSS		
< 2500 cc	63	11
≥ 2500 cc	18	52

*Adapted from Table 10: Gilsdorf, R.B. and Spanos, P.: Factors influencing morbidity and mortality in pancreaticoduodenectomy. Ann. Surg., 177:336, 1973.

Finally, the surgeon's assessment of his resection margins misses 20 percent of cancers that have microscopically invaded grossly normal tissue around the head of the pancreas. The areas most subject to such "invisible" spread are the blood vessels adjacent to the neck of the pancreas and the body of the pancreas along which subtotal resection is accomplished.[3]

Thus, the classic Whipple procedure is not sufficiently radical to remove residual cancer in regional lymph nodes, around the tumor mass itself, or multicentric disease in the remainder of the pancreas.

Precarious Pancreatic Anastomosis. The problem of pancreatic leaks following resection has plagued surgeons since such operations were performed. As Whipple noted when he simply oversewed the pancreatic remnant, fistulae develop in 70 percent of patients. When attempting to sew bowel to the cut end of the pancreas, however, a variety of techniques have been devised to reduce the incidence of such leaks.

Review of recent series shows that bowel mucosa to pancreatic duct mucosa approximation is essential to minimize leakage. The utility of stents placed across the pancreaticojejunal anastomosis is difficult to assess. However, anastomotic stenting for six weeks seems prudent when the adequacy of the anastomosis is doubtful.

Regardless of the technique used, however, the pancreatic anastomosis is sufficiently treacherous that I wonder if the benefits of pancreatic tissue preservation justify accepting an obligatory 6 to 10 percent incidence of fistulae with its associated mortality of 20 percent.

Long-Term Exocrine Insufficiency. It has been shown convincingly that 90 percent of patients with pancreatic cancer have secretin- and pancreozymin-stimulated deficiencies in digestive enzyme and bicarbonate secretion. Furthermore, 25 percent have steatorrhea prior to surgery.[13] Among this subset, the role of pancreatic ductal obstruction from cancer cannot be quantified. However, patients with pancreatic cancer have diffuse exocrine dysfunction that precludes significant benefit from saving a pancreatic remnant.

Among the few long-term survivors of the Whipple procedure for pancreatic cancer, Longmire theorized that at least 50 percent had symptoms of exocrine insufficiency due to anastomotic stricture.[14] Among the same group, definite steatorrhea was present in 25 percent; and a 12 percent incidence of steatorrhea was noted among patients having a Whipple resection for chronic pancreatitis.

In terms of endocrine function, 20 percent of patients with pancreatic cancer are diabetic prior to surgery. Furthermore, all patients with pancreatic cancer have abnormal glucose tolerance. Thus, the tendency towards a requirement for exogenous insulin exists. Following total pancreatectomy, several patients have died due to iatrogenic hypoglycemia. However, centers with experience in managing these patients report negligible morbidity and no mortality from glucose control in recent years.[12] Thus, the endocrine benefit of preserving a proportion of islet cells is questionable.

Dismal Long-Term Survival. The 5-year survival for patients who do not succumb to the surgery itself or its attendant physiologic ravages is only 4 percent (Table VII). Furthermore, Grace and colleagues[15] have reported three patients who died of recurrent pancreatic cancer within three to six months of achieving 5-year survivorship.

TABLE VII.　DISMAL LONG-TERM SURVIVAL

			SURVIVAL	
	YEAR	N	5-YEAR	> 5-YEAR
Brooks[13]	1983	1005	4%	—
vanHeerden[10]	1981	141	2%	0
Grace[15]	1986	73	3%	0
Forrest[3]	1979	51	4%	0

In vanHeerden's retrospective review of the Mayo Clinic experience,[10] he found three patients who were alive at five years; but they did not have pancreatic cancer when their original pathology specimens were reviewed. Thus, the Whipple procedure has no impact on survival.

OPTIMISTIC SERIES CRITIQUE

In looking at other studies which extol the "modern" merits of the Whipple procedure, the following study deficiencies are readily apparent:

1. Only the series of Tarazi and colleagues[6] from the Cleveland Clinic re-reviewed the original pathology specimens to confirm the diagnosis among survivors. Thus, the German series showing 14 to 28 percent 5-year survival for pancreatic cancer must be questioned.
2. In the fine print of earlier studies, adjuvant chemotherapy or radiation therapy was given randomly to a selected group of patients undergoing Whipple resection. No effort is made in these papers to acknowledge such therapy as a variable capable of influencing survival.
3. Braasch and associates[16] recently *predicted* that 17 percent of their patients with pancreatic cancer undergoing a pyloric-preserving Whipple would survive five years. In point of fact, only one patient in this series has lived five years; and the remaining four survivors are only *predicted* to survive.
4. Operative deaths are routinely excluded from the calculation of 5-year survival statistics. This was done initially to minimize the impact of 20 percent operative mortality rates on ultimate outcome. However, we must be honest with ourselves and with our patients when we predict the probability of surviving both the operation and the cancer.

PALLIATIVE BYPASS VERSUS WHIPPLE OPERATION

Even proponents of subtotal pancreatectomy will concede that it is not curative but they propose improved palliation (with the "possibility" of cure). With nearly 70 percent of the deaths following operation occurring within two years of surgery, assessment of resection as a more radical form of palliative therapy can be accomplished.

Shapiro,[17] at the University of Chicago, randomized 48 patients who met the criteria for definitive resection to palliative bypass only or Whipple resection. The expected higher operative morbidity and mortality was observed in the Whipple group. However, the quality of palliation was superior in the bypass group. The bypassed patients had a lower reoperation rate and rehospitalization rate than the Whipple group, while both groups enjoyed comparable mean survival.

Critical Survivor Review. Taking Shapiro's study one step further, Gudjonsson and associates[18] reviewed the world's literature to ascertain the characteristics of published survivors. Surprisingly, they found that eight patients survived five years or more after having received only palliative bypass. This fact implies that either a diagnostic error was made or that the biological characteristics of the cancer determine ultimate survival rather than the type of surgery performed.

Overall, however, resection has a mean survival of 14 to 18 months versus four to six months survival for palliative bypass. Buried in this statistic is the fact that patients with more advanced disease typically are relegated to the bypass group.

Total Pancreatectomy. If we persist in performing pancreatic resections for patients deemed to have resectable pancreatic cancer, I suggest that total regional pancreatectomy be done by a dedicated pancreatic surgeon who can offer adjuvant chemoradiation therapy. If I am fortunate enough to have cancer confined to the head of the pancreas or duodenal wall, I should enjoy forty good months of postoperative survival (Table VIII).[12] If I am unfortunate enough to have regional lymph node metastases, I would be better off having a palliative bypass alone.

PHILOSOPHICAL PERSPECTIVE

In conclusion, I want to leave you with Hertzburg's recent comment on the realistic objective of our aggressive surgical therapy: "It is irrational to use a limited operation that has imperfect physiological results for a disease that knows no invasive limits."[10]

TABLE VIII.　TOTAL PANCREATECTOMY*

	COMPARISON WITH WHIPPLE	
	MEAN SURVIVAL	
PROCEDURE	STAGES I and II	STAGE III
Whipple	13 mos.	6 mos.
Bypass	6 mos.	6 mos.
Total	40 mos.	7 mos.

*From Brooks, J.R.: Operative approach to pancreatic cancer. Semin. Oncol., 6:357–367, 1979.

REFERENCES

1. Moossa, A.R., Scott, M.H., and LaVelle-Jones, M.: The place of total and extended total pancreatectomy in pancreatic cancer. World J. Surg., 8:895–899, 1984.
2. Maingot, R.: Pancreatic tumors and periampullary carcinomas. In Abdominal Operations. Norwalk; Appleton-Century-Crofts, 1980, pp. 921–949.
3. Forrest, J.F. and Longmire, W.P.: Carcinoma of the pancreas and periampullary region. Ann. Surg., 189:129–138, 1979.
4. Matsuno, S. and Sato, T.: Surgical treatment for carcinoma of the pancreas. Experience in 272 patients. Am. J. Surg., 152:499–504, 1986.
5. Fortner, J.G.: Regional resection of cancer of the pancreas: A new surgical approach. Surgery, 73:307–313, 1973.
6. Tarazi, R.Y., Hermann, R.E., Vogt, D.P., et al.: Results of surgical treatment of periampullary tumors: A thirty-five year experience. Surgery, 100:716–722, 1986.
7. Moreaux, J.: Long-term follow-up studies of 50 patients with pancreaticoduodenectomy for chronic pancreatitis. World J. Surg., 8:346–353, 1984.
8. Cohen, J.R., Kuchta, N., Geller, H., et al.: Pancreaticoduodenectomy for benign disease. Ann. Surg., 197:68–71, 1983.
9. Trede, M.: The surgical treatment of pancreatic carcinoma. Surgery, 97:28–35, 1985.
10. vanHeerden, J.A.: Pancreatic resection for carcinoma of the pancreas: Whipple vs. total pancreatectomy—an institutional perspective. World J. Surg., 8:880–888, 1984.
11. Gilsdorf, R.B. and Spanos, P.: Factors influencing morbidity and mortality in pancreaticoduodenectomy. Ann. Surg., 177:332–337, 1973.
12. Brooks, J.R.: Operative approach to pancreatic cancer. Semin. Oncol., 6:357–367, 1979.
13. Brooks, J.R.: Cancer of the pancreas. Chronic pancreatitis. In Surgery of the Pancreas. J.R. Brooks (ed.). Philadelphia: W.B. Saunders, 1983.
14. Longmire, W.P. and Traverso, L.W.: The Whipple procedure and other standard operative approaches to pancreatic cancer. Cancer, 47(S):1706–1711, 1981.
15. Grace, P.A., Pitt, H.A., Tompkins, R.K., et al.: Decreased morbidity and mortality after pancreaticoduodenectomy. Am. J. Surg., 151:141–149, 1986.
16. Braasch, J.W., Gongliang, J., and Rossi, R.L.: Pancreaticoduodenectomy with preservation of the pylorus. World J. Surg., 8:900–905, 1984.
17. Shapiro, T.M.: Adenocarcinoma of the pancreas: A statistical analysis of biliary bypass versus Whipple resection in good risk patients. Ann. Surg., 182:715–721, 1975.
18. Gudjonsson, B., Livstone, E.M., and Shapiro, H.M.: Cancer of the pancreas: Diagnostic accuracy and survival statistics. Cancer, 42:2494–2506, 1978.
19. Williams, J.A., Cubilla, A., Maclean, B.J., and Fortner, J.G.: Twenty-two year experience with periampullary carcinoma at Memorial Sloan-Kettering Cancer Center. Am. J. Surg., 138:662–665, 1979.
20. Jones, B.A., Langer, B., Taylor, B.R., and Girotti, M.: Periampullary tumors: Which ones should be resected? Am. J. Surg., 149:46–52, 1985.
21. Andren-Sandberg, A. and Ihse, I.: Factors influencing survival after total pancreatectomy in patients with pancreatic cancer. Ann. Surg., 198:605–610, 1983.
22. Obertop, H., Bruining, H.A., Eeftinck, M., et al.: Operative approach to cancer of the head of the pancreas and the peri-ampullary region. Br. J. Surg., 69:573–576, 1982.
23. Braasch, J.W. and Gray, B.H.: Considerations that lower pancreaticoduodenectomy mortality. Am. J. Surg., 133:480–484, 1977.

DEBATE X

Are Pulmonary Artery Catheters Valuable And Safe?

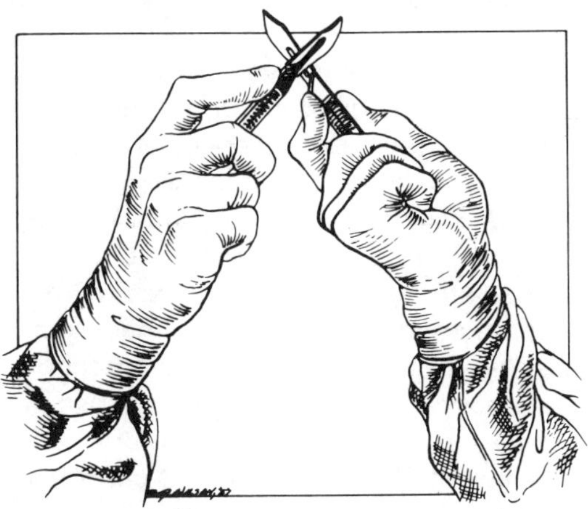

The right and left heart function as two separate organs. Frank and Starling initially described the remarkable capacity of each ventricle to pump independently. Beat to beat, with an increase in venous return, there is an increase in filling pressure resulting in an increased end diastolic volume and ultimately augmented stroke volume. During normal ventilation, right and left ventricular output are not synchronized and vary considerably. The axiom that "the most common cause of right heart failure is left heart failure" is true.

The ventricles can, however, fail independently. Florid pulmonary edema is certainly possible with a normal central venous pressure. Additionally, in the Surgical Intensive Care Unit or operating room, things happen quickly. It is not permissible to wait for rales, infiltrates by x-ray, or right heart failure in order to diagnose left heart decompensation.

Dr. Butler argues that a pulmonary artery catheter provides invaluable hemodynamic data. This data cannot be gathered in any other more responsive or precise fashion. He demonstrates that parameters derived from a pulmonary artery catheter either dictate or change management in up to 50 percent of patients monitored.

Any invasive device must be examined relative to the morbidity of its insertion and use. Dr. Butler reports that surgeons are becoming much more facile with the Swan-Ganz catheter and that the catheter is safe even now.

Dr. Bell disagrees. He points out that it is a long way anatomically and physiologically from the pulmonary capillary wedge position to inferences and approximations concerning left ventricular end diastolic volume, wall stress, and stroke volume. Even in a rigorously controlled physiology laboratory (which a Surgical Intensive Care Unit is not), measurements are dependent on catheter patency, appropriate zeroing/calibration, and ventilatory cycle. Diseases commonly encountered by surgeons, such as COPD, pulmonary embolism, pulmonary artery hypertension, or mechanical ventilation (with PEEP), may dissociate the measured pulmonary artery pressure from left-sided phenomena.

Dr. Bell explains how the pulmonary catheter tip is in continuity with a column of blood leading to the left atrium *only* in West's Zone III lung. When floating a Swan-Ganz catheter in ventilated patients, less than one-third of catheters ultimately will reside in Zone III. Thus, the pulmonary artery wedge pressure may not reflect left ventricular preload.

In addition, a change in preload or left ventricular end diastolic pressure relates directly to end diastolic volume and cardiac output only if ventricular compliance is static. But—compliance is not static. Compliance varies with chronic volume overload, acute volume overload, myocardial ischemia, pericardial effusion, heart rate, positive pressure ventilation, sepsis, trauma, and shock. Thus, even if the measured pulmonary artery wedge pressure did relate to left ventricular preload, this parameter would not characterize stroke volume or indicate cardiac output.

The insertion of a pulmonary artery catheter has been associated with fatal arrhythmias, pulmonary artery peptide, pulmonary infarction, deep venous thrombosis, tricuspid valvular endocarditis, catheter site sepsis, and pulmonary embolism.

Upon reflection, the advent of a catheter that can measure pulmonary artery pressures and flow has been a huge advance to the science of critical care medicine. The opportunities for misapplication, misadventure, and misinterpretation of this invasive devise are equally intimidating.

X-A: SWAN-GANZ CATHETERS ARE VALUABLE AND SAFE

LARRY J. BUTLER, M.D.

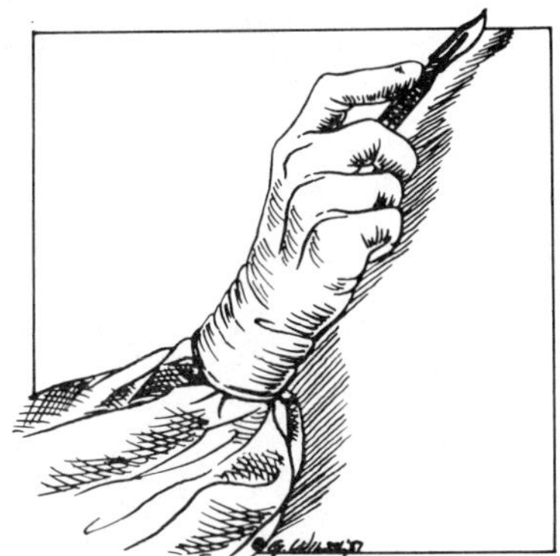

The use of pulmonary artery catheters has become common in surgical intensive care units across the United States. This discussion will focus on the utility and the documented clinical value of this catheter and will reveal the safety of this invasive procedure.

The first central venous catheterization was performed by Verner Forsmann[1] in 1929. Then a 25-year old surgical resident, Forsmann exposed a vein in his own left arm and advanced a urethral catheter into his venous system. The first description of the pulmonary artery wedge pressure was by Dexter[2] who proposed that this pressure reflected the left atrial pressure. Lategola and Rahn[3] first used balloon-directed catheters in dogs in 1955; but it was not until 1970 that Swan, Ganz, and colleagues[4] published the first clinical results of flow-directed pulmonary artery pressure measurements in humans. During the ensuing decade, over two million of these catheters have been placed, and the frequency of their use is increasing.

Very early, it became apparent that there was a difference between central venous pressure and pulmonary artery wedge pressure in critically ill patients. In 1972 Civetta and colleagues[5] published their data on the relationship between central venous pressure and wedge pressure in patients with Swan-Ganz severe multisystem injury, decompensated cirrhosis, and peritonitis. The relationship found in their patients is shown in Figure 1, with the linear relationship representing the normal relationship and the scatter points showing the wide variability of central venous pressure and wedge pressure in this type of surgical patient. Toussaint and colleagues[6] published further data showing the discrepancy between central venous pressure and pulmonary wedge pressure in critical surgical illness.

Figure 2 displays the correlation between central venous pressure and pulmonary wedge pressure in 13 patients with a history of cardiorespiratory disease. This is in clear contrast to the more consistent relationship between central venous pressure and wedge pressure seen in the normal population (Figure 3). There is a clear discrepancy between pulmonary artery wedge pressure and central venous pressure in critically ill patients. This still left the question of the clinical utility of the pulmonary artery cathether and whether having this additional hemodynamic data affected the management of patients.

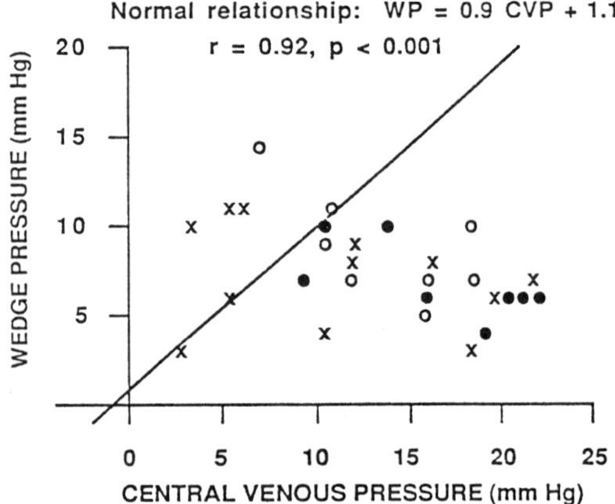

FIGURE 1.   Modified from Civetta, J.M. and Gabel, J.C.: Flow-directed pulmonary artery catherization in surgical patients: Indications and modifications of technique. Ann. Surg., 176:753–756, 1972.

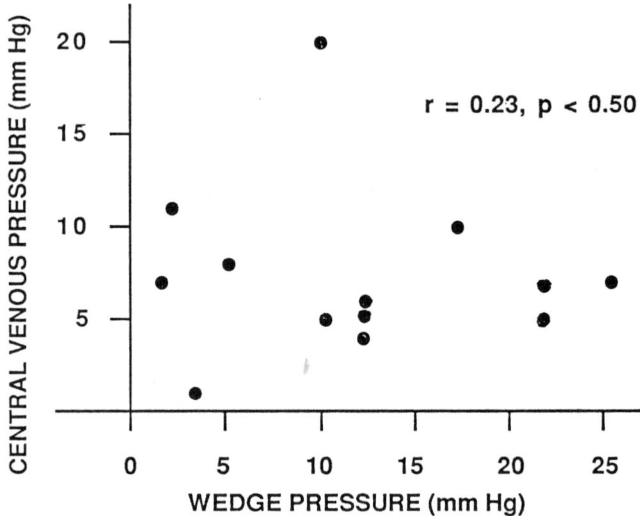

FIGURE 2.   Correlation between CVP and PWP in 13 patients with a history of cardiorespiratory disease. There is a poor correlation between CVP and PWP in this group of patients. Modified from Toussaint, G.P.M., Burgess, J.H., and Hempson, L.G.: Central venous pressure and pulmonary wedge pressure in critical surgical illness: A comparison. Arch. Surg., 109:265–268, 1974.

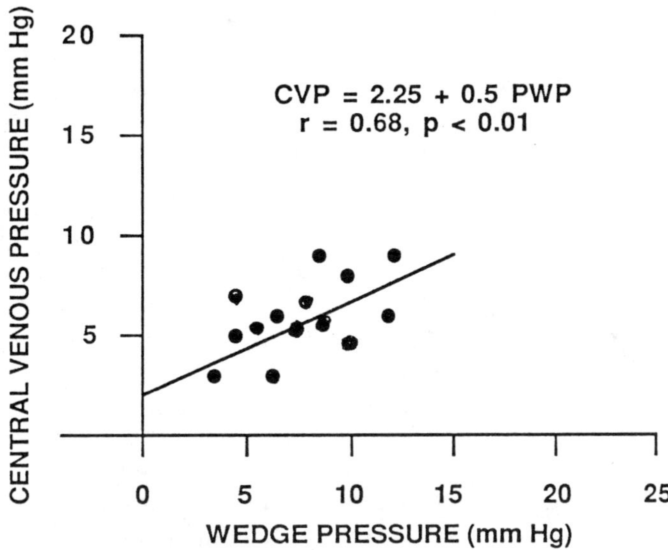

FIGURE 3. Correlation between CVP and PWP in 14 patients with no history of cardiorespiratory disease. There is a significant correlation between CVP and PWP in this group of patients. From Toussaint, G.P.M., Burgess, J.H., and Hempson, L.G.: Central venous pressure and pulmonary wedge pressure in critical surgical illness: A comparison. Arch. Surg., 109:265–268, 1974.

Does pulmonary artery pressure data affect patient management? In 1984 Eisenberg and colleagues[7] prospectively studied 103 pulmonary artery catheterizations and compared the clinical hemodynamic predictions with the actual parameters obtained by the Swan-Ganz catheter. In this study, therapeutic plans were made prior to insertion of the pulmonary artery catheter; and then, compared to the actual therapeutic management, pulmonary pressures were obtained. This study showed that the planned therapy was altered in 58 percent of the 103 patients; and in 30 percent of those 103 patients, some unanticipated therapy was added. The indications for catheterization in these patients are shown in Table I with 57 patients catheterized for interpretation of a pulmonary infiltrate.

In 1983 Conners and colleagues[8] published data comparing the clinical impression with the measured pulmonary artery hemodynamic parameters. This group

TABLE I. INDICATIONS FOR CATHETERIZATION*

CLINICAL PROBLEM	NUMBER OF PATIENTS
Pulmonary infiltrates*	57
Septic shock	18
Cardiogenic shock	16
Hypotension (other)	7
Myocardial infarction	13
Azotemia (intravascular volume status)	11
Other*	14

*Modified from Eisenberg, P.R., Jaffe, A.S., and Schuster, D.P.: Clinical evaluation compared to pulmonary artery catherization in the hemodynamic assessment of critically ill patients. Crit. Care Med., 12:549–553, 1984.

evaluated 62 patients without an acute myocardial infarction who required pulmonary artery catheterization. They compared the clinical evaluation by physical examination to the measured hemodynamic data and found that clinical predictions were accurate in approximately 40 to 50 percent of the cases. An additional surprise was that the clinical predictions of pressure data were no better when generated by attendings and fellows in comparison to the house staff and students.

Again, in this study, therapeutic change was mandated by pulmonary artery catheter data in 48.4 percent of the patients. Complications in this series included a single superior vena cava thrombosis, two hematomas, and one arrhythmia that required treatment. There were no catheter-related deaths.

Fein and colleagues[9] studied 70 ICU patients with pulmonary edema. The patients were judged clinically to have either cardiac (high pressure) or pulmonary (low pressure) edema prior to the insertion of the Swan-Ganz catheter. They found that permeability (low pressure) edema could be predicted clinically 85 precent of the time, but cardiac edema was predicted in only 62 percent of their cases. The significance of this decision is obvious as the treatment for these types of pulmonary edema is different, and the data gathered by the pulmonary artery catheter was critical in determining the correct diagnosis.

Davies and colleagues[10] studied 220 surgical patients. The preinduction pulmonary artery wedge pressure dictated some type of therapeutic action in 41 percent of these patients. The central venous pressure in these patients reflected a change in pulmonary artery pressure in only one-half of the patients, so that there was a documented benefit of pulmonary artery wedge pressure over central venous pressure in 20 percent of patients. This was even more pronounced in patients undergoing cardiopulmonary bypass, in which 62 percent of the patients had a discrepancy in pulmonary artery wedge pressure versus central venous pressure that dictated treatment. This group had reported their morbidity related to pulmonary artery catheterizations (Table II). There was a 3.6 percent incidence of carotid artery puncture with no neurologic sequelae. There was a 25 percent incidence of arrhythmias that required no treatment and a 1.8 percent incidence of sepsis.

Similarly, Babu and colleagues[11] examined 75 elderly patients undergoing peripheral vascular surgery. A pulmonary artery catheter was placed to monitor each patient hemodynamically. Only one-third of these patients had normal left ventricular function. Two-thirds of the patients in this series required some type of therapeutic intervention prior to their operative procedure. Twenty-seven percent required an in-

TABLE II.*

COMPLICATIONS	PATIENTS
A. Of Route of Insertion	
Carotid artery puncture	8 (3.6%)
B. Of Catheterization	
Arrhythmias	56 (25%)
Septicemia	4 (1.8%)
Pulmonary infarct	1 (0.5%)
Balloon rupture	1 (0.5%)

*From Davies, M.J., Cronin, K.D., and Domainque, C.M.: Pulmonary artery catheterization: An asséssment of risks and benefits in 220 surgical patients. Anaesth. Intens. Care, 10:9–14, 1982.

crease in preload by volume administration, 17 percent required inotropic support, and 13 percent required the addition of afterload reduction. In 9 percent of the patients a combination of these therapeutic interventions was used. These investigators found that they could optimize successfully left ventricular function in 96 percent of the patients. Sixteen percent of the patients—roughly one in six—had a modified or lesser surgical procedure as a result of the hemodynamic data. In this series there was one operative death and no catheter-related deaths.

Finally, Quinn and Quebbemann[12] studied 50 general surgical patients and found that the pulmonary artery wedge pressure led to a therapeutic change in 26 percent of this group. They reported no deaths related to pulmonary artery catheterization and again documented the previously noted poor correlation between central venous pressure and pulmonary artery wedge pressure.

The safety of pulmonary artery catheters has been demonstrated repeatedly. Indeed, there are a host of complications that have been described (Table III[13]) and are either insertion related or catheter related. While these complications undeniably occur, their incidence is very low.

In the largest prospective study in the literature, Sise and colleagues[14] studied 320 pulmonary artery catheterizations in 219 patients who were studied for complications. The predominant route of insertion was the subclavian veins, with the internal jugular and femoral approaches being less common. Major complications occurred in 3 percent of the patients, with pneumothorax occurring in 1.8 percent, treatment-requiring arrhythmias occurring in 0.9 percent, and subclavian vein thrombosis occurring in 0.3 percent (a single patient). One patient died, for a catheter-related mortality of 0.3 percent. Minor complications also were noted, including transient arrhythmias, arterial puncture, venous bleed, cellulitis, and catheter-related sepsis.

TABLE III. COMPLICATIONS ASSOCIATED WITH PULMONARY ARTERY CATHETERS*

INSERTION RELATED	CATHETER RELATED
Thoracic:	*Embolic:*
Pneumothorax	Catheter
Hemothorax	Air
Hydrothorax	Blood
Chylothorax	*Septic:*
Traumatic:	Phlebitis
Arterial	Vegetative
Venous	Positive blood culture
Brachial plexus	Positive catheter culture
Measurement related:	*Dysrhythmic:*
Pulmonary infarction	Atrial
Pulmonary arterial rupture	Ventricular
Balloon rupture/	*Perforation:*
fragmentation	Atrial
Air embolism	Ventricular
Bacterial shower	*Miscellaneous:*
	Knotting
	Looping
	Mechanical failure

*From Bodai, B.I. and Holcroft, J.W.: Use of the pulmonary artery catheter in the critically ill patient. Heart and Lung, 11:406–416, 1982.

This study of complications is contrasted with a huge retrospective series of pulmonary artery catheterization complications published by Shah and colleagues.[15] In this series, the internal jugular vein was used for access in 95 percent of the patients. Access complications included carotid artery puncture in 1.9 percent. No patient had neurologic sequelae. The incidence of pneumothorax was 0.5 percent, and transient dysrhythmias were noted in nearly two-thirds of the patients. Persistent PVCs were noted in 3.1 percent of patients. The late complications consisted of four patients with pulmonary artery rupture and minor pulmonary infarcts. There was a single catheter-related mortality in this series, for a catheter-related mortality of 0.016 percent.

A pulmonary artery catheter does add data that cannot be obtained from a central venous line. The catheter does alter the therapeutic plans. Additionally, the Swan-Ganz catheter is, in fact, quite safe. The final and major question to be answered is, "Do we improve survival by the use of this catheter?"

If we simply make minor therapeutic changes related to the data with no impact on survival, then the argument can be made that the catheter is not worth the associated risk and discomfort. Several studies do indicate that the data obtained by the catheter and changes made thereof do influence mortality in our patients.

Rao and associates[16] studied the influence of aggressive hemodynamic monitoring on the mortality in noncardiac surgery patients with a history of myocardial infarction. They found a dramatic reduction in the reinfarction rate associated with the addition of aggressive hemodynamic monitoring. The reinfarction rate dropped from 7.7 percent prior to the use of pulmonary artery pressure monitoring to 1.9 percent.

Moore and associates[17] studied patients with left main coronary artery stenosis and used the hemodynamic data from the pulmonary artery catheter to intervene pharmacologically pre- and perioperatively. The mortality was decreased from 20 percent in this group prior to the use of the catheter to 3 percent in the group who was managed with a pulmonary artery catheter. The perioperative myocardial infarction rate also dropped from 10 percent to 3.6 percent. In this study, the hemodynamic data from the pulmonary artery catheter led to intervention in 57 percent of monitored patients.

Whittemore and associates[18] studied 110 elective and urgent abdominal aortic aneurysm patients and established left ventricular performance curves preoperatively. They then maintained an optimal pulmonary artery wedge pressure in the perioperative period. There was no operative mortality compared to historic controls of 3 to 9 percent. Their perioperative myocardial infarction rate dropped to 3 percent as contrasted to much higher rates in series of similar patients without pulmonary artery catheters.

In a final series, Del Guercio and Cohn[19] prospectively evaluated 148 elderly patients who were cleared for major surgery by standard assessment. These patients all had invasive monitoring, including pulmonary artery and arterial catheters. Their patients were categorized into four stages with Stage 1 patients having normal hemodynamic, respiratory, and oxygen transport. This represented 13.5 percent of their elderly population, however. Stages 2 and 3, which represented the majority (nearly two-thirds) of these patients, had mild (but correctable) aberrations of hemodynamic, respiratory, or oxygen transport. Finally, Stage 4, which represented nearly one-fourth of the patients, had advanced defects that could not be corrected. There were no major complications related to the pulmonary artery catheterizations in this series. There is a clear difference between the mortality of 0 percent in Stage 1 patients and the 100 percent mortality in the Stage 4 patients. For patients in the intermediate stages who could be corrected, there was still an 8.5 percent mortality. In the Stage 4 patients, 8 underwent the planned operation with 100 percent mortality. In 19 patients a nonsurgical therapy was instituted, and in seven patients lesser operations under local anesthesia were performed without mortality. This demonstrates that even in Stage 4 patients the additional data obtained by pulmonary artery catheterization were extremely valuable in determining or limiting the operative procedure in patients who had been cleared for major surgery by routine clinical assessment.

REFERENCES

1. Forsmann, W.: Die sondierung des rechten herzens. Klin. Wschr., 8:2085–2087, 1929.
2. Dexter, L., Haynes, F.W., Burwell, C.S., et al.: Studies of congenital heart disease. J. Clin. Invest., 26:554–560, 1947.
3. Lategola, M. and Rahn, H.: A self-guiding catheter for cardiac and pulmonary catheterization and occlusion. Proc. Soc. Exp. Biol. Med., 84:667–668, 1953.
4. Swan, H.J.C., Ganz, W., Forrester, J., et al.: Catheterization of the heart in man with the use of a flow-directed balloon-tipped catheter. N. Engl. J. Med., 283:447–451, 1970.
5. Civetta, J.M. and Gabel, J.C.: Flow-directed pulmonary artery catheterization in surgical patients: Indications and modifications of technique. Ann. Surg., 176:753–756, 1972.
6. Toussaint, G.P.M., Burgess, J.H., and Hampson, L.G.: Central venous pressure and pulmonary wedge pressure in critical surgical illness: A comparison. Arch. Surg., 109:265–269, 1974.
7. Eisenberg, P.R., Jaffe, A.S., and Schuster, D.P.: Clinical evaluation compared to pulmonary artery catheterization in the hemodynamic assessment of critically ill patients. Crit. Care Med., 12:549–553, 1984.
8. Conners, A.F., McCaffree, D.R., and Gray, B.A.: Evaluation of right-heart catheterization in the critically ill patient without acute myocardial infarction. N. Engl. J. Med., 308:263–267, 1983.
9. Fein, A.M., Goldberg, S.K., Walkenstein, M.D., et al.: Is pulmonary artery catheterization necessary for the diagnosis of pulmonary edema? Am. Rev. Respir. Dis., 129:1506–1509, 1984.
10. Davies, M.J. Cronin, K.D., and Domainque, C.M.: Pulmonary artery catheterization: An assessment of risks and benefits in 220 surgical patients. Anaesth. Intens. Care, 10:9–14, 1982.
11. Babu, S.C., Sharmg, P.U.D., Raciti, A., et al.: Monitor-guided responses: Operability with safety is increased in patients with peripheral vascular surgery. Arch. Surg., 115:1384–1386, 1980.
12. Quinn, K. and Quebbemann, E.J.: Pulmonary artery pressure monitoring in surgical intensive care unit. Arch. Surg., 116:872–876, 1981.
13. Bodai, B.I. and Holcroft, J.W.: Use of the pulmonary artery catheter in the critically ill patient. Heart and Lung, 11:406–416, 1982.

14. Sise, M.J., Hollingsworth, P., Brimm, J.E., et al.: Complications of the flow-directed pulmonary artery catheter: A prospective analysis in 219 patients. Crit. Care Med., 9:315–318, 1981.
15. Shah, K.B., Rao, T.L.K., Laughlin, S., et al.: A review of pulmonary artery catheterization in 6,245 patients. Anesthesiology, 61:221–225, 1984.
16. Rao, T.L.K., Jacobs, K.H., and E.-Etr, A.A.: Reinfarction following anesthesia in patients with myocardial infarction. Anesthesiology, 59:499–505, 1983.
17. Moore, C.H., Lombardo, T.R., Allums, J.A., et al.: Left main coronary artery stenosis: Hemodynamic monitoring to reduce mortality. Ann. Thor. Surg., 26:445–451, 1978.
18. Whittemore, A.D., Clowes, A.W., Hechtman, H.B., et al.: Aortic aneurysm repair: Reduced operative mortality associated with maintenance of optimal cardiac performance. Ann. Surg., 192:414–419, 1980.
19. Del Guercio, L.R.M. and Cohn, J.D.: Monitoring operative risk in the elderly. J.A.M.A., 243:1350–1355, 1980.

X-B: SWAN-GANZ CATHETERS ARE DANGEROUS AND OVER-RATED

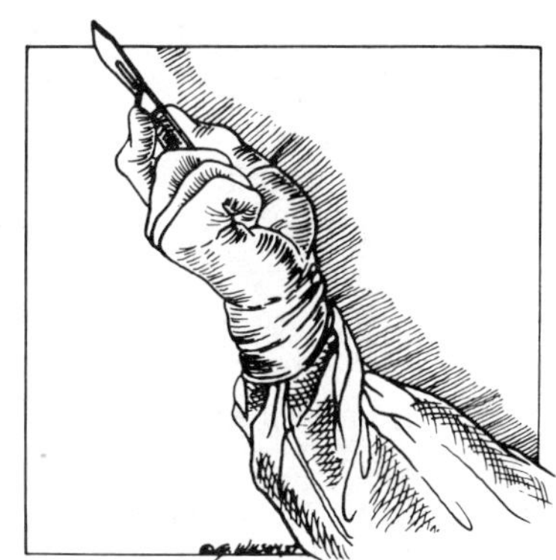

REGINALD C. W. BELL, M.D.

In *The Rape of Lucretia,* William Shakespeare wrote, " . . . and now this pale swan in her watery nest begins the sad dirge of her certain ending." In classical poetic and zoologic tradition, swans were held to be mute until just prior to their death.

Dr. Butler is wrong. Swan-Ganz catheters are dangerous and unreliable. What do pulmonary artery catheters measure? They measure the central venous pressure, pulmonary artery pressures, the pulmonary capillary wedge pressure, and cardiac output. They can be used to obtain mixed venous gases, and they can obtain dysrhythmia data. A plastic catheter with a latex balloon that can be inflated by air is inserted into the central venous system. It is carried by flow out into the right ventricle and out into the pulmonary arterial system. At this point, the balloon should occlude a pulmonary artery leaving a continuous column of blood via the pulmonary capillary system to the pulmonary vein and into the left atrium. If this balloon is completely occlusive so that no pulmonary artery wave form is transmitted and if this tube is completely patent through the capillary system, the venous system, and into the left atrium, then the pressure here will reflect the pressure in the left atrium. This is pulmonary capillary wedge pressure.

Thus, the standard pulmonary artery catheter can measure pulmonary artery wedge pressure, pulmonary artery pressures, and right atrial (central venous) pressure. A temperature probe at the catheter tip will allow an integration of temperature change over time following the injection of cold saline and a calculation of a thermodilution cardiac output. Blood gases drawn from the distal port turn out to be more accurate in obtaining mixed venus oxygen saturation than gases drawn either from the superior or inferior vena cava.[1] Lastly, EKG data can be derived by putting a bipolar electrode on the end of this balloon catheter.

What is the role of the Swan-Ganz catheter in critically ill patients? Most importantly, it is used to help assure adequate tissue oxygen delivery. It also can be used to decrease the risk of pulmonary venous congestion, to diagnose the cause of pulmonary edema, or to protect failing, dying myocardium through interventions that help to decrease wall tension.

What is the diagnostic potential of a pulmonary artery catheter? The primary diagnostic value is in distinguishing cardiogenic from hypovolemic shock. In hypovolemic shock, low filling pressures are associated with a low cardiac output. In cardiogenic shock, the myocardium does not function well in spite of elevated filling pressure.

The catheter can be helpful in diagnosing cardiac tamponade. The hallmark of cardiac tamponade is equalization of diastolic pressures in the right atrium, right ventricle, pulmonary artery, and pulmonary capillary wedge position. The other features of cardiac tamponade, of course, are elevated venous pressures and exaggerated pulsus paradoxus.

The Swan-Ganz catheter also can be useful in diagnosing the etiology of a new systolic murmur. The catheter permits differentiation between a ruptured interventricular septum in which there is a step-up in oxygen saturation across the right ventricle and new mitral regurgitation in which there should be V-waves in the pulmonary artery (PA) wedge tracing. However, new mitral regurgitation can be present without V-waves and may be associated with an apparent oxygen "step-up."[2]

A Swan-Ganz catheter may be helpful in diagnosing pulmonary embolism. The pulmonary artery diastolic pressure is acutely greater than the pulmonary capillary wedge pressure (PCWP). Right ventricular infarction may be diagnosed. In the setting in which right atrial pressures are elevated in relation to the pulmonary artery diastolic pressure, right ventricular infarction should be suspected and an inferior myocardial infarction confirmed by EKG.[3]

Although the Swan-Ganz catheter appears useful at times, it is imprecise and unreliable. It is unreliable because of the series of approximations made equating the pulmonary artery diastolic or wedge pressure to the left ventricular end diastolic volume. We assume that an elevation in the wedge pressure corresponds to an increase in the left ventricular end diastolic volume with consequent increase in stroke volume and resultant increase in cardiac output. These are major assumptions. A long series of approximations is necessary in getting from the pulmonary artery side of the system to the end diastolic volume of the left ventricle.

The pulmonary artery diastolic pressure does not equal the wedge pressure in common clinical situations of pulmonary hypertension, pulmonary embolism, COPD, or mechanical ventilation. The wedge pressure measured at end expiration on a graphic readout often is not equal to the digital readout, especially during mechanical ventilation or during extremes of ventilatory drive. The left ventricular end diastolic pressure may not equal the left atrial pressure, especially in instances of left ventricular dysfunction or during mitral and some aortic valve disease. The left ventricular end diastolic volume may not be proportional to the left ventricular end diastolic pressure during acute hemodynamic alterations. The cardiac output measured by thermodilution probably varies more than 10 percent in most bedside settings. Measured cardiac output also varies with respiration. To be at all valuable, mixed venous gases require correct catheter placement and sample timing.[4]

Pulmonary artery diastolic (PAD) pressure will not reflect the wedge pressure in pulmonary hypertension. Often the PAD is used because the catheter will not wedge or one is hesitant to inflate the balloon due to the risk of pulmonary artery rupture. Normally, in the pulmonary venous system, there is such a low pulmonary vascular resistance that at the end of diastole there is equilibration of pressures between the pulmonary artery diastolic pressure and the left atrial end diastolic pressure. However, with tachycardia or in association with a high cardiac output, equilibration may not be achieved even in the absence of pulmonary hypertension.[5] During those instances, the PAD may be an unreliable reflection of left-sided events. With pulmonary vascular hypertension, elevation in pulmonary vascular resistance and loss of pulmonary capillary reserve causes PAD to overestimate the PCWP.[6-8] The PAD can be very unreliable in a patient who has respiratory insufficiency, who is developing a pneumonia, who has developed ARDS, or who has thrown a pulmonary embolism.[6]

Mammana and colleagues[9] have studied patients after coronary artery bypass surgery. This group found that the PAD, or the pulmonary artery pressure, and pulmonary capillary wedge pressure are significantly dissociated as pulmonary hypertension develops. The pulmonary capillary wedge pressure may not equal the digital readout (Figure 1), especially during mechanical ventilation.

During agitated breathing, the digital readout also may be in error.[10] The true filling pressure of the left ventricle is the intracardiac pressure minus the juxtacardiac (pleural) pressure. To minimize the influence of juxtacardiac pressures, the convention has been to read the pulmonary capillary wedge pressure at end expiration (functional residual capacity) at a time when intrapleural pressures are minimized.[11] However, by definition, PEEP will alter end expiratory pressures and, therefore, LV end diastolic pressure. As a rough approximation, an increase in airway pressure of 10 cm will alter the juxtacardiac pressure by approximately 5 cm. However, this is de-

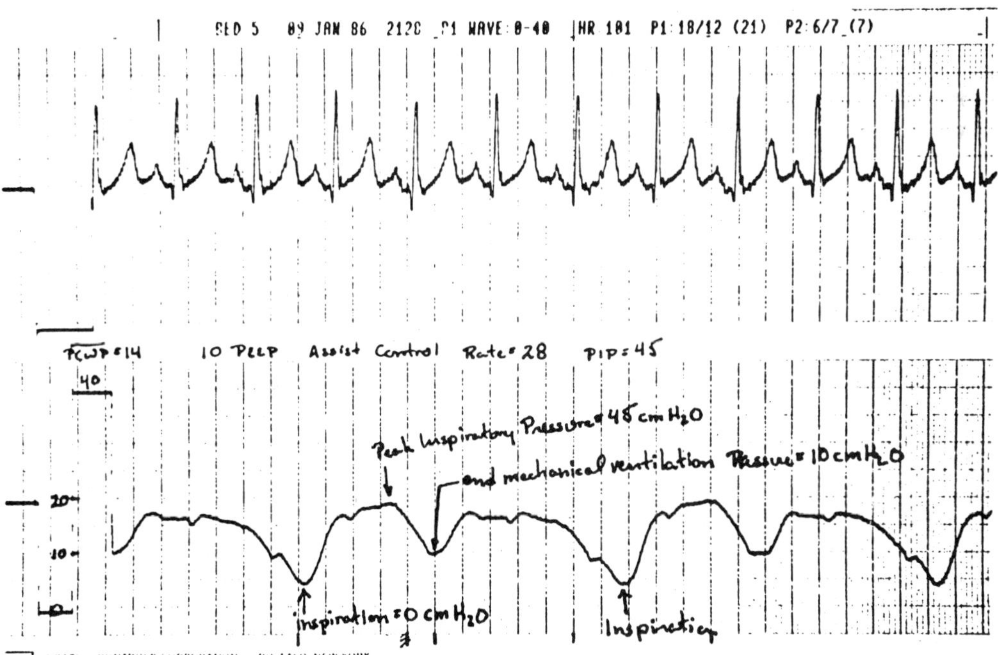

FIGURE 1.

pendent on the compliance (or elasticity) of the lungs and may vary considerably as a patient develops respiratory failure.[10]

It is true also that the pulmonary capillary wedge pressure may not equal the pulmonary venous pressure, especially during PEEP or hypovolemia. How does this happen? A brief review of the functional lung zones as described by West is appropriate.[12] In Zone I, with the patient upright, in the superior lung zones the alveolar pressure is greater than either the pulmonary arterial or venous pressure. By virtue of the hydrostatic gradient from the superior to inferior lung zones, the wedge pressure measurement will reflect the alveolar pressure and neither of the other pressures. In Zone II, the alveolar pressure is indeed greater than the venous pressure but is less than pulmonary arterial pressure. Forward flow is allowed but is rather like a one-way valve. Once forward flow is stopped by the Swan-Ganz balloon, there can be no transmission of pressure backwards from the venous system because the alveolus is occlusive. In neither of these two lung zones will the wedge pressure reflect the pulmonary venous pressure. The circuit is no longer open. The pulmonary artery catheter must be in lung Zone III where the alveolar pressure is less than both arterial and venous pressures to have an open circuit so that the wedge pressure may reflect the pulmonary venous pressure.

When alveolar pressure increases, Zone III moves further inferiorly down the lung. Therefore, PEEP and positive airway pressure will increase Zones I and II and decrease Zone III. With progressive hypovolemia, Zone III also will decrease. How can a good tracing be identified? There are a couple of guidelines. If the catheter tip is in the wrong lung zone—Zone I or II—the traces tend to be relatively free of cardiac pulsation. They exhibit pronounced respiratory variation.[13] The measured pressure may be greater or less than the alveolar pressure (or the airway pressure). Measured pressures are suspect whenever the wedge pressure is greater than the pulmonary artery diastolic pressure.[14] They are also suspect if the change in the wedge pressure is more than one-half the change in PEEP.[15]

Do these problems really occur, especially in a supine patient? In a study done on post-coronary artery bypass patients,[16] the left atrial pressures were measured and compared to wedge pressures (Figure 2). A lateral portable chest x-ray was used to determine how far above or below a left atrial marker the pulmonary artery catheter was placed. Was it in a dependent lung zone, in which case it is most likely in Zone III; or was it in a ventral or anterior lung zone, in which case it very well might be in lung Zone I or II? If the catheter tip is above a left atrial marker or the left atrial pressure is over 7 mm/Hg, as PEEP is induced, the difference between the wedge and the left atrial pressures increases. Even without PEEP, there can be more than a 2 mm/Hg pressure difference. If the catheter tip is within 1 cm of the left atrial marker, then the wedge pressure probably is accurate at zero PEEP. However, by the time 5 cm H_2O PEEP is applied, there will be more than a 6 mm/Hg discrepancy in pressures.

Suppose the catheter tip is within 1 cm of the left atrial marker, but the left atrial pressure is high. Then, what happens if the catheter tip is within or just outside the mediastinum? If it is within the mediastinum, there is an approximate 4 mm/Hg between the wedge and the left atrial pressure. If the catheter tip is beyond the mediastinum, then there may be fairly good correlation between wedge and left atrial pressures even up to 10 cm of water PEEP.

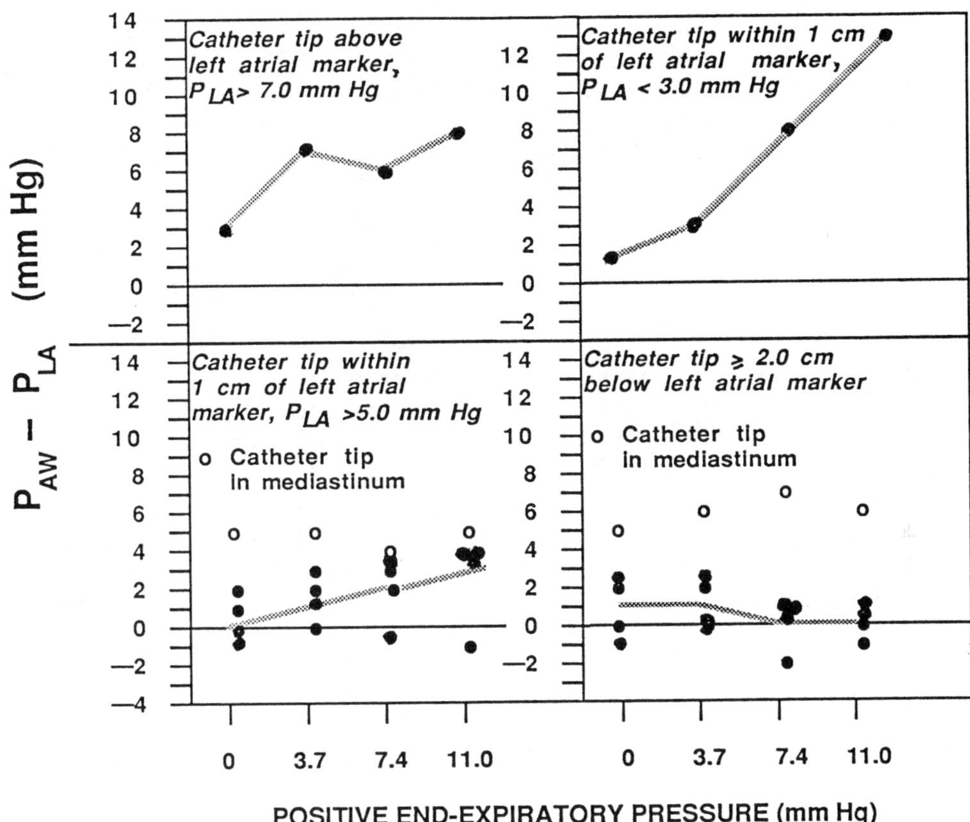

FIGURE 2. Change in difference between left atrial and pulmonary artery wedge pressure at different levels of PEEP and for different catheter locations and left atrial pressures. Redrawn from Shasby, D.M., Dauber, I.M., Pfister, S., et al.: Swan-Ganz catheter location and left atrial pressure determine the accuracy of the wedge pressure when positive end-expiratory pressure is used. Chest, 80(6):668, 1981.

To recapitulate, the pulmonary catheter tip must be more than 2 cm below the left atrial marker to provide an accurate Zone III tracing. But, where do most catheters go? In our own series,[16] of approximately 30 catheters placed, only nine were more than 2 cm below the left atrial marker; and six, almost 20 percent, were *above* the left atrial marker. Thus, when floating a pulmonary artery catheter, there is about a one-third chance of placement in the proper lung zone and about a two-thirds chance of misplacement.

Though rare, large pulmonary venous obstruction can occur. Large pulmonary vein obstruction can result from fixed lesions, such as tumors or mediastinal fibrosis, and perhaps from functional compression of large veins during low flow states with high intrathoracic or pericardial pressures.[12] This is rare. However, it must be kept in mind that a continuous column of blood from the wedged balloon catheter tip to the left atrium is necessary to get a reliable wedge pressure.

It also turns out that the left ventricular end diastolic pressure does not equal the mean left atrial pressure in cases of left ventricular dysfunction or mitral valve disease. Braunwald and Frahm[17] demonstrated that, in cases of left ventricular dysfunction, the atrial kick is crucial to left ventricular filling and that the left ventricular end diastolic pressure is higher than the mean left atrial pressure. A mean difference of approximately 7 mm/Hg between an elevated LV end diastolic pressure and a falsely low left atrial mean pressure was characteristically noted.

In addition, with mitral valvular dysfunction, there may be a failure to equilibrate between the mean left atrial pressure and the left ventricular end diastolic pressure. The mean left atrial pressure will be higher in mitral stenosis.[18] It also will be spuriously elevated in cases of acute mitral regurgitation where the LV systolic pressures are a component of the mean left atrial pressure. Again, V-waves may not be seen during mitral regurgitation.[19] Lastly, in aortic regurgitation, if there is premature closure of the mitral valve and subsequent aortic filling of the ventricle, the left ventricular end diastolic pressure will be higher than the mean left atrial pressure.

Suppose one is able to surmount all these hurdles and can actually get a PAD that fortuitously is fairly close to the left ventricular end diastolic pressure. Now, in acute hemodynamic alterations, the left ventricular end diastolic volume is not proportional to the pressure. Braunwald[20] defines heart failure as an inability of the ventricles to deliver adequate oxygenated blood to the metabolizing tissues either at rest or during normal activity. How is adequate oxygen delivery assessed? The physical examination may be used to examine extremity temperature, mucosal color, and the mental status. We can look at urine output or the products of ischemic metabolism, such as serum lactate, pH, and carbon dioxide.[21] We can measure oxygen consumption or, more simply, the oxygen content of mixed venous blood. As has been stated, the ability to increase cardiac output correlates with increased survival in the critically ill patient.[22]

How can cardiac output be increased? Firstly, the heart rate can be increased. This is an effective technique primarily in the younger patient. The other way to increase cardiac output is to increase stroke volume. This is done by altering preload, contractility, and afterload. Starling's law of the heart defines preload in the following way: "The mechanical energy set free on passage from the resting to the contracted state is a function of the muscle fiber length."[23] Starling's law indicates that stroke volume is related to the end diastolic volume. We often speak of a descending limb of Starling's curve, and we talk as if we want to maximize cardiac output by positioning ventricular filling at the apex of this curve. It turns out that a filling pressure of about 40 mm/Hg or more is necessary to approach the descending limb of Starling's curve in most clinically relevant situations. This rarely occurs.[20]

Secondly, the Starling curve relates stroke volume and end diastolic volume. Compliance is the change in volume relative to a change in pressure and is defined by the slope of the pressure-volume curve. This is a nonlinear curve. Even mild myocardial ischemia results in a stiffer ventricle.[24] Thus, a big change in pressure produces only a small change in volume. The important point is that a change in end diastolic pressure does not necessitate a change in end diastolic volume if the compliance has been altered. Compliance is not static in the critically ill patient.[22]

Decreased left ventricular compliance occurs during chronic volume overload, myocardial ischemia, right ventricular volume overload, pericardial effusion, and increased afterload. It varies with the rate of ventricular filling, PEEP, and hypovolemic shock. Any critically ill patient will exhibit altered left ventricular compliance. Afterload reduction and relief of ischemia will improve LV compliance. Early in the course of chronic volume overload, the ventricle gets flabby but not much bigger. Later the ventricle is bigger, but the muscle may hypertrophy; and the compliance curve stiffens up. Thus, preload cannot be linearly associated with stroke volume and cardiac output.[22,24,25]

Similarly, as a patient becomes progressively tachycardic, the left ventricular pressure volume curve shifts upwards decreasing compliance. Isoproterenol will decrease diastolic filling time while increasing the rate of filling and shift the curve upwards.

Woods and Harken[26] have reported that pulmonary artery temperature varies significantly during the respiratory cycle. Thus, injectate timing may have a substantial influence on calculated thermodilution cardiac output due to normal pulmonary artery temperature changes during respiration.

To summarize, pulmonary artery (Swan-Ganz) catheters are unreliable for the following reasons:

1. The pulmonary artery diastolic pressure may not equal the wedge pressure.
2. The wedge pressure may not equal the observed digital readout.
3. The venous pressure may not equal the wedge pressure during PEEP and hypovolemia in lung Zone I or II.
4. The left atrial pressure may not equal the pulmonary venous pressure if there is venous obstruction.
5. The left ventricular end diastolic pressure may not equal the mean left atrial pressure in association with LV dysfunction or mitral valve disease.
6. The left ventricular end diastolic volume is not proportional to the left ventricular end diastolic pressure in acute hemodynamic alterations.
7. The measured cardiac output probably varies more than 10 percent because it is not typically timed with respiration.

The Swan-Ganz cathether also is dangerous. Insertion may provoke fatal or refractory dysrhythmias, fatal pulmonary artery rupture, serious pulmonary infarction, deep venous thrombosis of the upper extremities, pulmonary embolism, and endocarditis.[27]

The assumption that a pulmonary artery catheter can give data that are reliable and easily interpreted about the efficacy, or possible value, of hemodynamic interventions in the critically ill patient overrates its capabilities. The correlation of mean pulmonary wedge pressure with LV end diastolic pressure is fraught with hazard, especially in the patient with changing pulmonary status. The correct interpretation of pressures and cardiac output when they may not be obtained reliably demands a working knowledge of the effects of altered ventricular compliance on transmural cardiac pressures. The benefits, unreliable and obscure as they are, may not outweigh the risks of this invasive technique.

REFERENCES

1. Horovitz, J.H., Carrico, C.J., and Shires, G.T.: Venous sampling sites for pulmonary shunt determinations in the injured patient. J. Trauma, 11(11):911–914, 1971.
2. Buchbinder, N. and Ganz, W.: Hemodynamic monitoring: Invasive techniques. Anesthesiology, 45:146–155, 1976.
3. Russell, R.O., Jr., and Rackley, C.E.: Hemodynamic Monitoring in a Coronary Intensive Care Unit. New York: Futura Publishing Company, 1981, pp. 226–228.
4. Suter, P.M., Lindauer, J.M., Fairley, H.B., and Schlobohm, R.M.: Errors in data derived from pulmonary artery blood gas values. Crit. Care Med., 3(5):175–181, 1975.
5. Kaltman, A.J., Herbert, W.H., Conroy, R.J., and Kossman, C.E.: The gradient in pressure across the pulmonary vascular bed during diastole. Circulation, 34:377–384, 1966.
6. Zapol, W.M. and Snider, M.T.: Pulmonary hypertension in severe acute respiratory failure. N. Engl. J. Med., 296:476–480, 1977.
7. Fishman, A.P.: Chronic cor pulmonale. Am. Rev. Respir. Dis., 114:775–794, 1976.
8. Rahimtoola, S.H.: Left ventricular end diastolic and filling pressure in assessment of ventricular function. Chest, 63:858–860, 1973.
9. Mammana, R.B., Hiro, St., Levitsky, S., et al.: Inaccuracy of pulmonary capillary wedge pressure when compared to left atrial pressure in the early postsurgical period. J. Thorac. Cardiovasc. Surg., 84:420–425, 1982.
10. Maran, A.G.: Variables in pulmonary capillary wedge pressure: Variation with intrathoracic pressure, graphic and digital recorders. Crit. Care Med., 8:102–105, 1980.
11. Berryhill, R.E., Benumof, J.L., and Rauscher, L.A.: Pulmonary vascular pressure reading at the end of exhalation. Anesthesiology, 49(5):365–368, 1978.
12. West, J.B., Dollery, C.T., and Naimark, A.: Distribution of blood flow in isolated lung; relation to vascular and alveolar pressures. J. Appl. Physiol., 19:713–724, 1964.
13. Tooker, J., Huseby, J., and Butler, J.: The effect of Swan-Ganz catheter height on the wedge pressure-left atrial pressure relationship in edema during positive-pressure ventilation. Am. Rev. Respir. Dis., 117:721–726, 1978.
14. Shin, B., McAslan, T.C., and Ayella, R.J.: Problems with measurement using the Swan-Ganz catheter. Anesthesiology, 43:474–476, 1975.
15. Marini, J.J., O'Quin, R., Culver, B.H., and Butler, J.: Estimation of transmural cardiac pressures during ventilation with PEEP. J. Appl. Physiol., 53:384–391, 1982.
16. Shasby, D.M., Dauber, I.M., Pfister, S., et al.: Swan-Ganz catheter location and left atrial pressure determine the accuracy of the wedge pressure when positive end-expiratory pressure is used. Chest, 80(6):666–670, 1981.
17. Braunwald, E. and Frahm, C.J.: Studies on Starling's law of the heart. IV. Observations on hemodynamic functions of the left atrium in man. Circulation, 44:633–642, 1961.
18. Hugenholtz, P.G., Ryan, T.J., Stein, S.W., and Abelman, W.H.: The spectrum of pure mitral stenosis. Hemodynamic studies in relation to clinical disability. Am. J. Cardiol., 10:773–784, 1962.
19. Roberts, W.C., Braunwald, E., and Morrow, A.G.: Acute severe mitral regurgitation secondary to ruptured chordae tendineae: Clinical, hemodynamic, and pathologic considerations. Circulation, 33:58–70, 1966.
20. Braunwald, E. (ed.): Heart Disease: A Textbook of Cardiovascular Medicine, 2d ed. Philadelphia: W.B. Saunders, 1984, p. 447, 433–434.
21. Shah, D.M., Browner, B.D., Dutton, R.E., et al.: Cardiac output and pulmonary wedge pressure. Arch. Surg., 112:1161–1164, 1977.

22. Sibbald, W.J.: Myocardial function in the critically ill: Factors influencing left and right ventricular performance in patients with sepsis and trauma. Surg. Clin. North Amer., 65(4):867–893, 1985.
23. Starling, E.H.: The Linacre lecture on the law of the heart. London: Longmans, Green and Company, Ltd., 1918.
24. Gaasch, W.H., Levine, H.J., Quinones, M.A., and Alexander, J.K.: Left ventricular compliance: Mechanisms and clinical implications. Am. J. Cardiol., 38:645–653, 1976.
25. Glantz, S.A. and Parmley, W.W.: Factors which affect the diastolic pressure-volume curve. Circ. Res., 42(2):171–180, 1978.
26. Woods, M., Scott, R.N., and Harken, A.H.: Practical considerations for the use of a pulmonary artery thermistor catheter. Surgery, 79:469–475, 1976.
27. Pace, N.L.: A critique of flow-directed pulmonary arterial catheterization. Anesthesiology, 47(5):455–465, 1977.

DEBATE XI

Radical Versus Local Surgical Therapy
For Breast Cancer

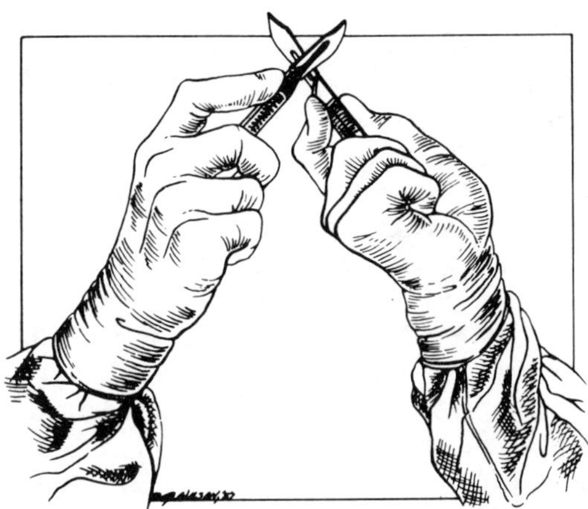

"I panicked. Night was the worst time for me. I was alone with my thoughts. All I knew was that I had cancer and four or five lymph nodes were involved, which meant that the cancer had traveled to a certain extent. I was going to have to go through chemotherapy."[1]

Breast cancer is perhaps the penultimate surgical disease. Almost all surgical controversies can be incorporated into the total therapy of cancer of the breast. Breast cancer is very common. Surgical therapy is effective. The natural history is well-defined. But, the philosophic basis upon which a surgical procedure is selected remains emotional rather than scientific.

Radical surgery derives from the Halstedian view that all cancer begins with a single cell and that the neoplastic cell then divides and grows. Initial spread occurs in an orderly and predictable fashion to local and then regional nodes. The lymph node filters become loaded with malignant cells. When the nodal barriers are overwhelmed, tumor cells escape and spread systemically. If, at any stage of progression, the surgical extirpation is sufficiently radical to encompass *all* malignant disease, then the surgery will be curative.

Conversely, the alternative view of cancer has been championed by Fisher. Here the premise is that cancer initially is a systemic disease characterized by immunoincompetence. We all "catch" cancer several times each day. Every time an ugly cell degenerates in a malignant fashion, however, our competent immune system recognizes the foreign cell and kills the offender. Therefore, in order for a malignant cell to gain a foothold, the patient's immune system must be dysfunctional. This view dictates that radical surgery consequently is misdirected, disfiguring, and silly. There is no way to excise a systemic problem. The primary tumor alone should be removed and regional nodes sampled to determine the necessity of systemic anticancer therapy—systemic therapy for systemic disease.

Dr. Gutman evaluates modified radical mastectomy relative to long-term survival, incidence of local-regional failure, adequacy of staging, morbidity, mortality, cosmesis, and cost. He concludes that a modified radical mastectomy remains the procedure of choice for patients with Stages I and II carcinoma of the breast.

Dr. Gutman points to many long-term studies that chronicle the success of radical surgery. Thirty years following radical mastectomy, many patients remain free of disease. Therefore, breast cancer never was systemic. Similarly, if cancer initially is systemic, then prognosis should not relate to initial tumor size—but it does. Dr. Gutman critiques the available comparative studies and concludes that we are endangering the lives of American women by our current fettish for breast conservation.

Conversely, Dr. Haug challenges the Halsted paradigm. He refers to early work by Fisher demonstrating that radiolabeled tumor cells seem to pass freely through regional lymph nodes. He cites many standard variations in local-regional therapy that do not ultimately influence survival. Whether the primary has been controlled by lumpectomy or the most aggressive of procedures, the prognosis depends not on surgical technique but on the more global host-tumor relationship.

To date, more than 10,000 women have been included in studies of breast cancer therapy. Almost 3,500 have participated in randomized, controlled trials. Dr. Haug restricts his discussion to the most rigorous of prospective, randomized series. The World Health Organization trial conducted between 1972 and 1980 revealed no survival advantage for mastectomy over lumpectomy—acknowledging superior cosmetic results with the latter. The NIH trial (1979–1984) identified no difference between modified mastectomy and lumpectomy with axillary sampling plus radiotherapy. Between 1976 and 1984, Fisher coordinated a national collaborative trial that suggested a survival *advantage* for conservative therapy over mastectomy. Similarly, 12-year follow-up of the Veronesi trial in Milan indicated "conclusively" that total ablative breast procedures are *"not* justified."

Conservative physicians and surgeons historically have been suspicious of and refractory to change. We have focused on a myriad of technical modifications of the mastectomy procedure itself. Substantive advances in this very common disease will result only from a better understanding of host-tumor immunobiology.

REFERENCE

1. Hill, A.F., Hamilton, P.K., and Ringer, L.: I'm a Patient, Too. In CanSurmount. New York: Nick Lyons Books, 1986, p. 60.

XI-A: BREAST CANCER—THE NEED FOR RADICAL SURGERY

JEFFREY J. GUTMAN, M.D.

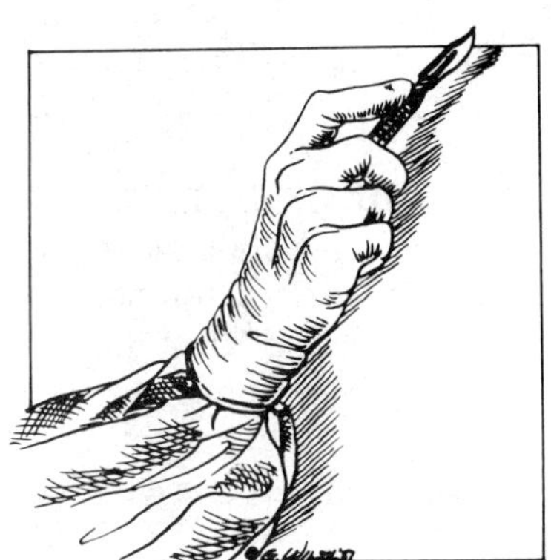

Breast cancer is now the second leading cause of cancer death in women in the United States. It will affect one out of nine women—120,000 new cases will be diagnosed this year.[1] The current controversy concerning the approach to the treatment of breast cancer is whether breast-sparing procedures are as good as or better than radical surgery. It can be shown today that, if one considers the long-term survival, incidence of local-regional failure, adequacy of staging, morbidity, mortality, cosmesis, and cost efficiency, radical surgery clearly is the optimal operation for patients with Stages I and II carcinoma of the breast.

The controversies involving radical versus conservative treatment of breast cancer stem from two divergent views on the natural course of breast cancer.[2] The radical view is that of Halsted.[3] He believed that breast cancer begins with a single cell and that it grows to a critical mass, at which time it metastasizes in an orderly and predictable route to the axillary lymph nodes. Surgery that encompasses all tumor and metastasis should be curative. At one point, Halsted even suggested doing a total hip disarticulation and shoulder disarticulation en bloc to cure metastases that were found in bone.

The conservative, or alternative, view is that which has been championed by Bernard Fisher.[2] He believes that breast cancer is a systemic disease at its inception and that local surgery has a limited effect on outcome. There are multiple problems with this alternative theory of Fisher. It ignores the diverse nature of breast cancer.[4] It is not one disease. An inflammatory cancer is a fatal disease with early dissemination. Any local treatment will have little influence on survival. A cystosarcoma phylloides is a locally invasive carcinoma with no spread to the axilla and very late hematogenous spread. Local therapy is curative.

Of the adenocarcinomas, there is also a spectrum from the aggressive scirrhous carcinoma to the indolent colloids, tubular, and medullary carcinomas. Patient's age and hormone status play a role in determining final outcome. To state that breast cancer is a systemic disease at inception is a grave error as it is not a single disease. The Fisher hypothesis also ignores the fact that there are numerous large studies with long-term follow-up—to as much as 30 years—which document that breast cancer is a curable disease by local radical surgery and that these patients go on to survive and match the survival of women without breast cancer (Table I).

The studies of Adair and colleagues,[5] Brinkley and Haybittle,[6] Duncan and Kerr,[7] and Haagensen and Bodian[8] chronicle more than 4,000 patients with follow-up of 20 to 47 years. These investigations have documented that breast cancer is, in fact, a curable disease with radical surgery. The alternative view also rejects the fact that prognosis declines as a cancer grows. A tumor found at less than 1 cm has a far better prognosis than one greater than 3 cm.

Duncan and Kerr[7] and Takuma and colleagues[9] classified tumor survival versus size. With each 1 cm increase in tumor size, long-term survival decreased significantly (Table II). If one believes the alternative view that breast cancer is a systemic disease at its inception, then one would expect to see no change in survival based on the primary

TABLE I

	PATIENTS	YEARS FOLLOW-UP
Adair[5]	1,458	30.6
Brinkley[6]	704	25.0
Duncan[7]	988	20.0
Haagensen[8]	1,036	47.0

TABLE II. FIVE-YEAR CURE RATES BY SIZE OF TUMOR AND STATUS OF AXILLARY NODES*

	AXILLARY NODES NEGATIVE			AXILLARY NODES POSITIVE		
	TOTAL	% CURED	% CURE	TOTAL	% CURED	% CURE
0.1–0.5 cm	107	88	82.2	42 (28%)**	22	52.4
0.6–1.0 cm	744	533	71.6	241 (24%)	131	54.3
1.1–2.0 cm	2742	1877	68.4	1416 (34%)	644	39.1
2.1–3.0 cm	2107	1330	63.1	1561 (43%)	611	39.1
3.1–4.0 cm	987	603	61.1	983 (50%)	321	32.6
4.1–5.0 cm	506	299	59.1	663 (57%)	172	25.9
5.1 + cm	456	259	56.8	829 (65%)	177	21.3
Unknown	1257	812	64.6	2097 (63%)	706	33.7
Total	8906	5801	65.1	7832	2784	35.5

Exclusions as in Table 6 of source.
*From Nemoto, T., Vana, J., Bedwani, R.N., et al.: Management and survival of female breast cancer: Results of a national survey by the American College of Surgeons. Cancer, 45: 2922, 1980.
**Frequency of axillary node positive patients.

size. The alternative view also ignores the fact that survival decreases as the number of involved lymph nodes increases. Numerous investigations have documented that survival is related directly to the number of lymph nodes involved. The SEER data from the American College of Surgeons, which derived from more than 20,000 cases of breast cancer, documented the improved survival in patients with less than four nodes involved compared to the poor prognosis of patients with greater than four nodes involved.[10]

I believe that the above long-term studies with large numbers of patients document that, when breast cancer begins as a local disease, its outcome is determined by the size of the primary lesion and the extent of local disease and survival can be affected by local therapy. Which is superior—radical surgery, breast sparing alone, or breast sparing in conjunction with radiation therapy? This is a difficult controversy to interpret. There are multiple long-term studies with 20 to 40 years follow-up documenting the efficacy of radical surgery. However, these studies are all retrospective, selective, and non-randomized without controls. In fact, they are case histories with one author and one surgeon. What these studies do is to document the remarkable efficacy of radical surgery.

Table III shows the American College of Surgeons' data on 1,147 cases of breast cancer followed for 10 years and gives the 10-year survival with no evidence of disease following radical surgery for Stages 0, I, and II disease.[10] Stage 0 disease can expect a 96 percent, no-evidence-of-disease 10-year survival; Stage I, 73 percent no-evidence-of-disease 10-year survival; Stage II, 43.1 percent no-evidence-of disease 10-year survival. This averages to 64.8 percent 10-year survival with no evidence of disease. These values should be taken as the historical controls for the efficacy of radical surgery.

Table IV compares different approaches to tumor stage and survival. Crile has been an advocate of minimal surgery followed by radiation therapy.[11] He reported a 10-year survival of 45 percent with a recurrence rate of 7 percent. Conversely, Urban[12] from Sloan-Kettering has been an advocate of extended radical surgery with the excision of the internal mammary nodes. He reported a 10-year survival of 61 percent and a local recurrence rate of 7.7 percent. Leis[13-15] is an advocate of selective surgery or modified radical mastectomy. He reports a 10-year survival of 62.1 per-

TABLE III. TEN-YEAR ABSOLUTE NED SURVIVAL RATES (1147 MASTECTOMIES)*

Stage 0		
Noninvasive	84/85	98.8%
Invasive	67/72	93.1%
Total	151/157	96.2%
Stage I	403/552	73.0%
Stage II	189/438	43.1%
Total	743/1147	64.8%
% Invasive	1062/1147	92.6%
Invasive survival	659/1062	62.1%

*From Leis, H.P.: Update in primary potentially curable breast cancer treatment. Cont. Surg., 26:21, 1985.

TABLE IV.   POTENTIALLY CURABLE INVASIVE BREAST CANCERS (COMPARATIVE RESULTS)†

	NUMBER PATIENTS	TEN-YEAR SURVIVAL	LOCAL RECURRENCE
Conservative selective surgery (Crile—Cleveland Ohio)	453	45.0% (revised to)	7.0%* 12.0%
Radical selective surgery (Urban—Memorial Sloan-Kettering)	564	61.0%	7.7%
Moderate selective surgery (Leis—New York Medical College)	1062	62.1%	7.9%**
Primary radiotherapy (Calle—Foundation Curie)	514	51.0% S_1 S_2	12.0%*** 55.0%
NSABP—National Cancer Institute (Predominantly radicals) (Limited adjuvant chemotherapy)	826	46.0%	

*Axillary recurrences not included
**N.E.D.—Skin grafts 2.1%
***33% Secondary mastectomies
†From Leis, H.P.: Update in primary potentially curable breast cancer treatment. Cont. Surg., 26:22, 1985.

cent and local recurrence of 7.9 percent. Radiation therapy alone, championed by Calle,[16] produces a 51 percent survival at ten years with a 12 percent recurrence of the initial tumor in Stage I disease; whereas radiation therapy of Stage II disease is associated with a 55 percent rate of recurrence.

Fisher[17] coordinated the National Surgical Adjuvant Breast Project and reported a 10-year survival of 46 percent. This study began in 1971 and involved 34 centers throughout the United States and Canada. It compared radical mastectomy to complete axillary dissection to simple mastectomy without axillary dissection. Patients who subsequently were found to have positive nodes were randomized to axillary dissection versus radiation therapy. At the end of ten years, no significant difference in the 10-year survival in any of the forms of therapy was appreciated.

This study should be looked at cautiously. To begin with, the 10-year survival following radical surgery is significantly less than that reported by the standard historical controls (Table 1). For instance, there is a minimum of 10 to 15 percent worse survival than reported by Haagensen and Bodian,[8] Donegan,[18] and Urban,[12] whose 10-year survivals were all greater than 60 percent. It makes one wonder whether this study[17] suffers from a Type I error; namely, that there is a flaw in its basic design. There was no standardization of what was to be considered a modified radical mastectomy. If ten surgeons were to perform a "modified radical mastectomy," they might carry out ten different operations. Such operations could range from Urban's radical procedure in which the internal nodes are taken to a simple mastectomy with axillary sampling alone. Yet, they all may be classified as the same operation.

One must also wonder about the small numbers of procedures being performed at some of the centers. This study involved 34 centers, and there were more than 100 surgeons involved. Of the 1,660 patients randomized in this study, only one-third—approximately 550—received a modified radical mastectomy. With 100 surgeons in this study, that calculates to only five procedures each.

This study also suffers from a Type II error in which the numbers were inadequate to find a significance at the 95 percent confidence level. For a disease that must be followed for a minimum of ten years, it is estimated that a minimum of 2,000 patients would be required to identify a 10 percent difference in therapy. This study involved only 1,660 patients. If this study is, in fact, in error, if the trend in the United States has shifted to conserving breasts, and if in the long-term results there is a 10 to 15 percent penalty or loss of life by switching to the more conservative therapies, then thousands of women could lose their lives. In a 10-year period of time, estimating only a 10 percent devaluation in surgical therapy, 120,000 women will lose their lives needlessly.

Another issue concerning conservative therapy is whether a tumorectomy or quadrantectomy is adequate surgery. Can the breast be left in place? The answer is clearly no. To begin with, local procedures ignore the multicentric origin of breast cancer. In up to 50 percent of patients, breast cancer has been documented as multifocal.[19,20]

Sir Headley Adkins and colleagues[21] published a study in 1972 comparing wide excision to radical surgery for Stage I disease. Following tumorectomy, only randomized patients were taken immediately to the operating room and underwent radical surgery. They compared the survival with Stage I disease and found that the survival was 10 to 15 percent better for radical surgery. With Stage II disease, survival following radical surgery was greater than 60 percent at 10 years compared to less than 20 percent for lumpectomy. Clearly, local surgery alone is inadequate.

Hayward[22] published a study in 1981 that compared radical mastectomy to wide excision looking at local recurrence rates, distant disease, and survival at 8 years. Again, the survival rate for local surgery was significantly worse than that for radical surgery.

Rosen and colleagues[23] had independent surgeons perform what the surgeons considered to be an adequate tylectomy procedure. These patients then were taken immediately to the operating room for a completion radical mastectomy. Pathological studies then were performed on the breast tissue to determine the efficacy of local excision. For tumors less than 2 cm in size, 26 percent of specimens had positive margins; for tumors greater than 2 cm in size, 38 percent had residual tumor. Rosen and associates also compared quadrantectomy to radical surgery. With central lesions in which quadrantectomy was performed, 80 percent of the specimens had persistent tumor. When all other quadrants were combined, 25 to 35 percent of patients had positive margins. This study demonstrates that neither tylectomy nor quadrantectomy can be relied upon to remove all local disease.

The second question that must be answered is, "How much axillary dissection is necessary?" To begin with, physical examination is totally inadequate for staging.[10,18,23] There is a false-positive to false-negative rate of 30 to 40 percent based on physical examination alone. This was shown by the SEER data of Smart and colleagues[10] (Table V). These studies documented that fingers could not be trusted to determine the extent of disease in the axilla.

Is axillary sampling enough? The answer again is clearly no. Ten percent of patients will have skip metastases in which the Level 1 nodes will be negative but the Level 2 or 3 will be positive.[24,25] Axillary sampling will result in a false-negative rate of 10 to 15 percent. Complete axillary dissection should be performed to provide accurate staging.

The next question is whether local surgery can be combined with radiation therapy to equal or improve the results of modified radical mastectomy. The answer is clearly no. It is recognized that radiation therapy will delay the occurrence of local-regional recurrences but will not prevent them. Radiation will have no documentable benefits on survival. Problems also exist with radiation therapy. To begin with, it is not a benign procedure[26] (Table VI). It can lead to significant early and late morbidity in 10 to 20 percent of patients. This is a complication rate that is actually greater than that of the currently performed modified radical mastectomy.

Radiation therapy must be preceded by a complete axillary node dissection.[24-28] Complete dissection is necessary for adequate staging. Radiation therapy must be preceded by some type of local tumor therapy.[16,29] One-third of breast cancers are totally radioresistant. Radiation therapy to tumors greater than 3 cm in size also provides poor cosmetic results due to the fibrosis and scarring of the breast tissue, and the benefit of a breast-sparing procedure is lost.[30-32] Radiation therapy is also carcinogenic.[33,34]

Radiation therapy decreases the immune competency of the host and the patient's tolerance to chemotherapy. Fisher believes that the axillary lymph nodes should be left in place to maintain immune competence. However, if the axilla is radiated, one loses that benefit as these nodes are no longer functional. Radiation therapy requires a specialty center. It is time-consuming. It requires daily therapy five days a week for a minimum of five weeks and booster doses to large local tumors for additional weeks. This is fine if one lives close to a big city in which a radiation center is located, but it is obviously impractical for patients from rural areas. The modified radical mastectomy obviates the need for radiation therapy, and patients go home within one week of surgery with only routine follow-up.

Radiation therapy is expensive. At the University of Colorado Health Sciences Center in 1987, radiation therapy averages $1 per rad. A minimum of 5,000 rads are required, and frequently a booster dose of 2,000 rads to the primary site is required. This is an additional cost of almost $7,000, which far exceeds the cost of a modified radical mastectomy alone. One must also include the cost for the initial procedure—a lumpectomy-quadrantectomy with axillary dissection. When cost alone is figured, a modifed radical mastectomy clearly is a cost-efficient therapy.

Since there are clearly no advantages to radiation therapy, what are the advantages of modified radical mastectomy? The advantages are:

1. It has the lowest rate of axillary and local recurrences.
2. It treats the multicentric origin of the disease.
3. It allows for adequate staging.
4. It is proven effective in long-term studies.
5. It has low morbidity and mortality.
6. It is cost efficient.

TABLE V. SEER BREAST CANCER DATA 1975.*
PHYSICAL VS. PATHOLOGIC EXAMINATION OF AXILLARY LYMPH NODES

CLINICAL ASSESSMENT	NO. CASES	PERCENT	PATHOLOGY REPORT ON AXILLARY LYMPH NODES		
			POSITIVE	NEGATIVE	NO INFORMATION
No palpable nodes	3645	(55.0%)	1259 (34.5%)	2335 (64.1%)	51 (1.4%)
Palpable but *not* involved	105	(1.5%)	33 (31.4%)	72 (68.6%)	0
Palpable and involved	414	(6.2%)	358 (86.5%)	51 (12.3%)	5 (1.2%)
Palpable and not stated	681	(10.3%)	434 (63.7%)	242 (35.5%)	5 (0.7%)
Palpable and fixed	30	(0.5%)	28 (93.3%)	2(6.6%)	0
No information	1753	(26.4%)	623 (35.5%)	1091 (62.2%)	39 (2.2%)
TOTAL	6628	(100%)	2735 (41.3%)	3793 (57.2%)	100 (1.5%)

*From Smart, C.R., Myers, M.H., and Gloeckler, L.A.: Implications from SEER data on breast cancer management. Cancer, 41:789, 1978.

TABLE VI. RADIATION COMPLICATIONS*

EARLY
Atrophy and shrinking
Fibrotic bands and thickening
Pneumonitis
Supraclavicular thickening
Telangiectasis and pigment changes
Dermatitis and ulcers
Edema of the arm and breast
Chest wall and arm pain
Bone and joint damage (rib fractures)

SUBTLE DELAYED
Nerve damage (brachial plexus)
Large blood vessel damage
Myocardial damage
Spray radiation to opposite breast
Other radiation induced cancers

*From Leis, H.P.: Update in primary potentially curable breast cancer treatment. Cont. Surg., 26:19, 1985.

7. It avoids the cost and inconvenience of radiation therapy.
8. It allows for good cosmetic results.

The morbidity and mortality of modified radical mastectomy are far less than that of the classic Halsted radical mastectomy. In *Cancer Principles and Practice of Oncology*, Harris and Fisher state that "infrequent incidence of surgical complications as accompanied the abandonment of the Halsted radical mastectomy eliminates that consideration as a factor in deciding upon the operation to use."[4] The mortality rate of the modified radical mastectomy is less than 1 percent. Wound complications, such as flap necrosis, infection, and edema, are less than 5 percent. Arm edema, when accompanied by radiation therapy, is less than 5 percent. The complication rate of the modified radical mastectomy is no greater than that of the quadrantectomy and axillary sampling with radiation therapy.

The currently performed modified radical mastectomy preserves the musculature and shape of the chest wall. It uses thicker skin flaps and allows immediate reconstructive surgery to be performed at the initial operation.[35-40] This can be performed as simply as placing an implant below the pectoralis major. Of the less than 10 percent of women who undergo this procedure, 95 percent are satisfied with the results.[41,42] They feel that they have a good reconstruction and look good in revealing clothing, such as evening wear, swim wear, and active wear. If one looks at those with breast-sparing operations combined with radiation therapy for Stage I disease, only 72 to 90 percent are satisfied with the results. With Stage II, 51 to 65 percent are satisfied.[30] Radiation therapy also gives very poor cosmetic results when the initial tumor is greater than 3 cm in size and is left in place. This requires an increased dose of radiation therapy, which results in increasing fibrosis and deformities of the breast. Also, women with very large or very small breasts have poor cosmetic results with quadrantectomy. This also creates a breast that is more difficult to reconstruct than that following a modified radical mastectomy. There also are many women who are not candidates for radiation therapy, such as women with large or small breasts or centrally or medially located lesions.

In conclusion, the modified radical mastectomy provides the best long-term survival. It has the lowest incidence of local-regional recurrences. It allows the best staging and indications for adjuvant chemotherapy. It is not carcinogenic. It is cost effective and convenient to the patient. It is time-saving. It has low morbidity and mortality. It allows good reconstructive procedures that can be performed at the initial surgery. In short, it is the operation of yesterday, the operation of today, and will continue to be the procedure of choice in the future.

REFERENCES

1. American Cancer Society. Cancer Facts and Figures, 1986. New York: American Cancer Society, 1986.
2. Fisher, B.: A commentary on the role of the surgeon in primary breast cancer. Breast Cancer Res. and Treat., 1:17–26, 1987.
3. Halsted, W.S.: The results of radical surgery for cure of cancer of the breast performed at the Johns Hopkins Hospital. Ann. Surg., 20:497, 1894.
4. Harris, J.R., Helman, S., Camillio, G., and Fisher, B.: Cancer of the breast. In Cancer Principles and Practices of Oncology. V.T. Devita, S. Helman, and S.A. Rosenberg, (eds.). Philadelphia: J.B. Lippincott Company, 1985, 1119–1179.
5. Adair, F., Berg, J., Joubert, L., and Robbins, G.F.: Long-term follow-up of breast cancer patients: The 30-year report. Cancer, 33:1145–1150, 1974.
6. Brinkley, D. and Haybittle, J.L.: The curability of breast cancer. Lancet, 2:95–97, 1975.
7. Duncan, W. and Kerr, G.R.: The curability of breast cancer. Br. Med. J., 2:781–783, 1976.
8. Haagensen, C.D. and Bodian, C.: A personal experience with Halsted's radical mastectomy. Ann. Surg., 199:143–150, 1984.
9. Nemoto, T., Vana, J., Bedwani, R.N., et al.: Management and survival of female breast cancer: Results of a national survey by the American College of Surgeons. Cancer, 45:2917–2924, 1980.
10. Smart, C.R., Myers, M.H., and Gloeckler, L.A.: Implications from SEER data on breast cancer management. Cancer, 41:787–789, 1978.
11. Crile, G., Jr.: Results of conservative treatment of breast cancer at 10 and 15 years. Ann. Surg., 181:26–30, 1975.
12. Urban, J.A.: Surgical management of palpable breast cancer. Cancer, 46:983–987, 1980.
13. Leis, P.: Modified radical mastectomy. In Moderate Selective Surgical Approach in Breast Cancer. Current Diagnosis and Treatment. S.A. Feig, and R. McLelland, (eds.). New York: Masson Publishing Co., 1983, 445–461.
14. Leis, H.P., Jr.: Selective moderate surgical approach for potentially curable breast cancer. In The Breast. H.S. Gallager, H.P. Leis, Jr., R.K. Snyderman, and J.A. Urban, (eds.). St. Louis: C.V. Mosby Co., 1978, 232–247.
15. Leis, H.P., Jr.: Selective and reconstructive surgical procedures for carcinoma of the breast. Surg. Gynecol. Obstet., 148:27–32, 1979.
16. Calle, R., Pilleron, J.P., Schlienger, P., and Vilcoq, J.R.: Conservative management of operable breast cancer: Ten years experience at the Foundation Curie. Cancer, 42:2045–2053, 1978.
17. Fisher, B.: Ten-year results of a randomized clinical trial comparing radical mastectomy and total mastectomy with or without radiation. N. Engl. J. Med., 312:674–681, 1985.
18. Donegan, W.L.: Surgical clinical trials. Cancer, 53:691–699, 1984.

19. Schwartz, G.F., Patchesfsky, A.S., Feig, S.A., et al.: Multicentricity of non-palpable breast cancer. Cancer, 45:2913–2916, 1980.
20. Rosen, P.P., Braun, D.W., Jr., and Kinne, D.E.: The clinical significance of preinvasive breast carcinoma. Cancer, 46:919–925, 1980.
21. Atkins, Sir Hedley, Hayward, J.L., Klugman, D.J., and Wayte, A.B.: Treatment of early breast cancer. A report after 10 years of a clinical trial. Br. Med. J., 2:423–429, 1972.
22. Hayward, J.: The surgeon's role in primary breast cancer. Breast Can. Res. Treat., 1:27–32, 1981.
23. Rosen, P.P., Fracchia, A.A., Urban, J.A., et al.: Residual mammary carcinoma following simulated partial mastectomy. Cancer, 35:739–747, 1975.
24. Stenkvist, B., Bengtsson, E., Dahlquist, B., et al.: Predicting patient cancer recurrence. Cancer, 50:2884–2893, 1982.
25. Pigott, J., Nichols, R., Maddox, W.A. and Balch, C.M.: Metastases to the upper levels of the axillary nodes in carcinoma of the breast and its implications for nodal sampling procedures. Surg. Gynecol. Obstet., 158:255–259, 1984.
26. Fisher, B.: A commentary on the role of the surgeon in primary patient care. Breast Can. Res. Treat., 1:17–26, 1981.
27. Leis, H.P.: Update in primary potentially curable breast cancer treatment. Cont. Surg., 26:13–43, 1985.
28. Lichter, A.S.: Current status of primary breast cancer treatment with local excision plus radiation. Curr. Concepts Oncol., 5:17, 1983.
29. Veronesi, U., Saccozzi, R., DelVecchio, M., et al.: Comparing radical mastectomy with quadrantectomy, axillary dissection, and radiotherapy in patients with small cancers of the breast. New Engl. J. Med., 305:6–11, 1981.
30. Harris, J.R., Beadle, G.F., and Hellman, S.: Clinical studies on the use of radiation therapy as primary treatment of early breast cancer. Cancer, 53:705–711, 1984.
31. Bataini, J.P., Picco, C., Martin, M., and Calle, R.: Relationship between time-dose and local control of operable breast cancer treated by tumorectomy and radiotherapy or by radiotherapy alone. Cancer, 42:2059–2065, 1978.
32. Stehlin, J.S., Evans, R.A., Gutierrez, A.E., et al.: Treatment of carcinoma of the breast. Surg. Gynecol. Obstet., 149:911–922, 1979.
33. Tokunaga, M., Norman, J.E., Asano, M., et al.: Malignant breast tumors among atomic bomb survivors, Hiroshima and Nagasaki, 1950–1974. J. Nat. Canc. Inst., 62:1347–1359, 1979.
34. Kim, J.H., Chu, F.C., Woodard, H.Q., et al.: Radiation-induced soft-tissue and bone sarcoma. Radiology, 129:501–508, 1978.
35. Baral, E.: Breast cancer following irradiation of the breast. Cancer, 40:2905–2910, 1972.
36. Dean, C., Chetty, U., and Forrest, A.P.M.: Effects of immediate breast reconstruction on psychosocial morbidity after mastectomy. Lancet, 1(8322): 459–462, 1983.
37. Dinner, M.I. and Dowden, R.V.: Breast reconstruction: State of the art. Cancer, 53:809–814, 1984.
38. Frazier, T.G. and Noone, R.B.: Immediate reconstruction in the treatment of primary carcinoma of the breast. Surg. Gynecol. Obstet., 157:413–414, 1983.
39. Georgiade, G.S.: Immediate reconstruction of the breast following modified radical mastectomy for carcinoma of the breast. Clin. Plast. Surg., 2:383–388, 1984.
40. Georgiade, G., Georgiade, N., McCarty, K.S., Jr., and Seigler, H.F.: Rationale for immediate reconstruction of the breast following modified radical mastectomy. Ann. Plast. Surg., 8:20–28, 1982.
41. Goldberg, P., Stolzman, M., and Goldberg, H.M.: Psychological considerations in breast reconstruction. Ann. Plast. Surg., 13:38–43, 1984.
42. Noone, R.B., Frazier, T.G., Hayward, C.Z., and Skiles, M.S.: Patient acceptance of immediate reconstruction following mastectomy. Plast. Reconstr. Surg., 69(4):632–640, 1982.

XI-B: BREAST CANCER—LUMPECTOMY IS ONLY RATIONAL THERAPY

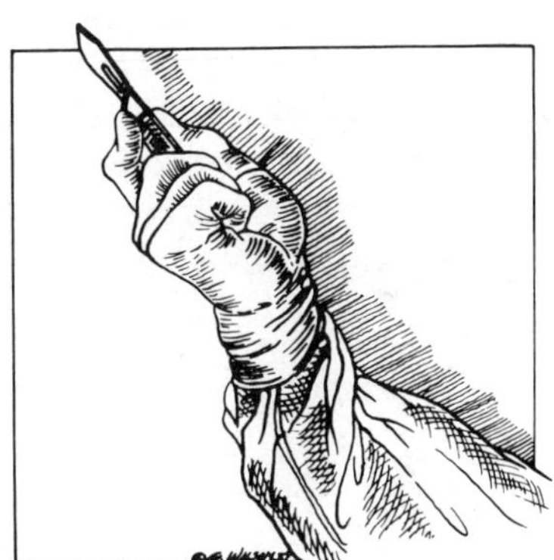

CRAIG E. HAUG, M.D.

Perhaps a more straightforward title for this debate would be "Breast Preservation versus Breast Amputation." Ancient surgeons studied and treated breast cancer. As such a highly visible, surgically accessible, and long-studied disease, one would think that by now the treatment of breast cancer would be the least controversial of all cancers. One would be wrong.

Almost a century ago, Halsted formulated the principles of cancer treatment recognized as Halstedian. In the case of breast cancer, those principles had their expression in the icon of breast cancer surgery—the radical mastectomy. Breast cancer was perceived to be a local disease, surgically "curable" until that unknown moment when distant metastases occurred. No matter how small the tumor, the entire breast and a section of chest were summarily removed.

It may be surprising to realize that the first challenges to the radical mastectomy came about not because of skepticism with the Halsted paradigm but because of doubts on the part of true believers as to the ability of the radical mastectomy to fulfill all its tenets faithfully. Since even radical mastectomy left lymph nodes behind, groups began to flirt with various methods that might embody Halsted's principles even more vigorously, such as radical radical mastectomy and lesser operations combined with radiotherapy.

While trying to buttress the Halsted paradigm, these benevolent revolts actually paved the way for lumpectomy. They showed that:

1. Survival was unrelated to the radicality of operation.
2. A certain percentage of very early breast cancers seemed to slip by the outflanking maneuver of radical surgery.
3. Patients indeed could survive for many years free of disease following mere local excision and radiotherapy.
4. Local recurrence after lumpectomy did not have the same poor prognosis as did local recurrence following mastectomy.
5. Seventy to 80 percent of conservatively treated patients had good-to-excellent cosmetic results.

The full importance of this last point concerning cosmesis goes beyond psychological health, however. Although conservative surgery has not been designed primarily to improve the cure rate over mastectomy, by providing greater incentive to women for self-screening and early reporting, the conservative approach may lead indirectly to improved prognosis because the patient then more likely can choose a procedure to spare her breast. So, given the findings of these early trials, the stage was set for a parting of the ways with Halsted.

TUMOR BIOLOGY

The prospective clinical data support lumpectomy. Before reviewing these data, a brief discussion of why lumpectomy should be effective in terms of tumor biology seems appropriate.

Is breast cancer a local or a systemic disease? If it is local as Halsted thought, then the radical operation, which attempts to outflank the tumor, makes sense. If it is systemic, no radical operation can be radical enough.

According to Halsted, there is an orderly pattern of tumor cell dissemination based on mechanical considerations. This is first by direct extension to regional lymph nodes and only then to distant sites, thus supporting en bloc dissection; i.e., radical mastectomy. In this scenario, the positive node is not only an indicator of tumor spread but also an instigator of more disseminated disease.

The tenets of the alternative hypothesis are diametrically opposed to Halsted's hypothesis. Laboratory work in the 1950s and 1960s, mostly by Fisher,[1] indicated that there was no orderly pattern of tumor cell dissemination. It was found that labeled tumor cells could embolize right through regional lymph nodes and flip back and forth between blood and lymphatics, challenging the philosophy of en bloc dissection. These experiments supported the idea of breast cancer as a systemic rather than local-regional disease—probably from inception.

While Halsted thought a tumor was autonomous of its host, others found evidence that a complex host-tumor relationship affects every facet of the disease and is exemplified by the regional lymph node. The positive lymph node is an indicator of a host-tumor relationship that *permits* development of metastases rather than being the inciter of distant disease.

Fisher[1] also reported that in experimental animals tumor growth will occur at a remote site of tissue injury. Thus, there must be a constantly circulating pool of dormant tumor cells that can latch onto and thrive in the proper remote environment. This experiment elegantly demonstrated both the systemic nature of breast cancer and the host-tumor relationship.

If breast cancer is systemic from the outset, the obvious implication is that variations in local-regional therapy are unlikely to affect survival substantially. The reason for this is not difficult to understand. Once the primary lesion has been controlled, whether by local excision, radiotherapy, or the most radical surgery that surgeons can devise, the patient's fate depends on how long the system has been showered with tumor and the particular host-tumor relationship.

In 1971, Fisher[1] initiated a major prospective, randomized study comparing radical mastectomy versus total mastectomy with and without radiotherapy. In the radical mastectomy group, 40 percent of patients with clinically negative axillary nodes (in other words, Stage I patients) were, in fact, histologically positive. The significance of this is that, since patients were randomized, 40 percent of the clinically negative node patients in both other groups should have had subclinical axillary tumor as well. In the case of those patients receiving only total mastectomy without radiotherapy, these nodes remain both unremoved (no axillary dissection) *and* untreated (no radio-therapy). According to Halsted, leaving these nodes to fester should have done two things:

1. All of these patients eventually should develop clinically positive nodes, and
2. Their fate should be darker.

Neither of these predictions came true. Only about 15 percent, not 40 percent, developed clinically positive nodes; and, after delayed axillary dissection, their risk of distant recurrence and survival after ten years was the same as the other two groups. Deferral of axillary node resection did not jeopardize survival, again supporting the concept that nodal metastases are more an indicator than instigator of generalized disease.

The biological principles embodied in the alternative hypothesis set the stage for the next step, breast-conserving operations.

DEFINITION OF TERMS[2]

Which patients are eligible for breast conservation? Firstly, they should have Stage I or II disease. Stage I patients possess a tumor ≤2cm without clinically evident axillary nodes. Stage II patients can have a tumor up to 5 cm with palpable but non-fixed axillary nodes. This represents more than 80 percent of patients presenting with breast cancer in the United States. Secondly, the woman should care about cosmesis and breast preservation—no problem with this. Ultimately, the prime criterion for patient selection is simply the feasibility of resection of the primary tumor without major cosmetic deformity. This includes those patients with unifocal disease, those patients with tumor not directly under the nipple, and those patients with moderate-sized breasts.

Over the years there have been so many different kinds of extirpative mastec-tomies developed that the nomenclature has become confusing. There is, however, one unifying principle that is not confusing—breast amputation.

Essentially there are only three types of partial mastectomies:

1. Local excision involves simple excision of tumor without regard to micro-scopic margins.
2. Wide excision is the technique most commonly used and encompasses 1 to 2 cm of adjacent breast tissue. This technique is designed to provide clear mi-croscopic margins.
3. Quadrantectomy is the technique used in Veronesi's[3] Milan trial, which removes the involved quadrant of breast.

LUMPECTOMY TECHNIQUE[4]

Radical mastectomy removes not only tumor but also a large section of surrounding muscle. Modified radical mastectomy takes a smaller section of chest. Wide local excision, or lumpectomy, is an excisional biopsy that removes tumor along with a small coating of breast tissue. The end result of lumpectomy is that the patient retains a relatively normal appearing figure after removal of a 3 cm tumor and axillary dissection. Of course, the smaller the tumor, the better the cosmetic result can be. With mastectomy, on the other hand, no matter how tiny the tumor, the end result is always the same.

Certainly breast reconstruction can improve cosmetic results in some. However, if mastectomy is not any better than lumpectomy in treating breast cancer, then a disfiguring mastectomy should not be done, and the results of postmastectomy breast reconstruction becomes a nonissue. For the best cosmetic results, a curvilinear incision right over the tumor along with a separate incision for the axillary dissection generally is recommended rather than radial incisions or a combined breast/axillary incision.

RADIOTHERAPY[4]

Surgery and radiotherapy are complementary in that local tumor control can be achieved by radical surgery alone, radical radiotherapy alone, or by a combination of a moderate amount of both. From a purely cosmetic and functional standpoint, most would agree that a moderate amount of surgery (for removal of gross disease only) coordinated with a moderate amount of radiotherapy (for eradication of local occult disease) is optimal, providing 80 to 95 percent good-to-excellent cosmetic results and a less than 1 percent incidence of significant complications. The point of contention is whether moderation provides optimal survival as well.

PROSPECTIVE STUDIES

Since Halsted, over 10,000 patients have been included in studies focusing on the treatment of primary breast cancer without mastectomy.[5] The controlled randomized trials include almost 3,500 patients. Several controlled trials were aborted because of difficulties in patient recruitment. It is one thing to have a woman agree to a mastectomy after her doctor stresses vehemently that mastectomy is the best treatment. It is another matter to have her agree after her doctor tells her he does not know which therapy is best and asks if she would mind if he flipped a coin.

The retrospective data show survival rates for conservatively treated patients as similar to those of patients treated with variations of the radical mastectomy, even to 30 years. Cosmetic results were judged good to excellent by 81 to 85 percent of patients. The following discussion will consider only the prospective, randomized trials. The prospective, randomized trial has supplanted retrospective, matched, controlled studies, historical controls, and institutional reviews of clincial experience as the most valid means of accumulating data.

The Guy's[6] study was the first prospective trial and, as such, perhaps not surprisingly, the most flawed. Trial I began in 1961 and was terminated for Stage II patients in 1971 when it appeared that conservative treatment in these patients significantly decreased survival. Trial II was a continuation of Trial I minus Stage II patients. Oddly, when Stage I patients were restudied in Trial II, their survival also was decreased, conflicting with Trial I results.

Unfortunately, this study was not only marred by these internal inconsistencies, but also there were other problems. Patients received inadequate radiotherapy (remember this was 1961), no axillary dissection, and no routine policy of operative salvage in cases in which there was local or regional recurrence. At the very least, these results must be viewed as suspect. In fact, to my knowledge, the Guy's trial final report was never published in a journal but rather was published in a general book on breast cancer. Interestingly, the author of that book omits mention of the Guy's trial altogether in a 1986 review article.[7]

The World Health Organization[8] conducted a study between 1972 and 1980 comparing modified radical mastectomy versus tumorectomy combined with axillary dissection and breast irradiation (and boost) in 179 patients with Stages I and II disease (< 2 cm) with a mean follow-up of 4.5 years. The report showed that there was no significant difference in either overall survival (95 percent for lumpectomy versus 91 percent for mastectomy) or relapse-free survival (85 percent for lumpectomy versus 74 percent for mastectomy). There was not a significant difference in either local or distant recurrence, but both trends favored the conservative group. The cosmetic result of conservative treatment was good to excellent in 92 percent of cases.

The NIH prospective study[9] was conducted between 1979 and 1984. It focused on modified mastectomy versus lumpectomy with axillary dissection and breast radiotherapy (and boost) for 124 Stages I and II patients. It found "overall recurrences and patterns of recurrence to be no different in the two groups."

Now we come to the big guns: Fisher's NSABP trial and Veronesi's Milan trial. In 1976, Fisher[10] proceeded to the next test of his alternative hypothesis—a randomized trial comparing total mastectomy versus segmental mastectomy with or without radiotherapy. By 1984, 1,843 patients with Stage I and Stage II disease less than 4 cm had been randomized. All patients underwent axillary dissection, and patients with positive nodes received adjuvant chemotherapy.

Patients treated with segmental mastectomy and radiotherapy had a 5-year disease-free survival that was significantly higher ($p = 0.04$) than that for total mastectomy patients, equal distant disease-free survival, and improved overall survival (that approached significance; $p = 0.07$).

Even segmental mastectomy without radiotherapy provided a disease-free survival and distant disease-free survival no different from total mastectomy, with an advantage that again approached significance ($p = 0.06$) in overall survival. This study actually achieved significance only when patients with negative nodes were included.

Think about this. Conservative therapy did not just sort of hang in there with mastectomy—it was significantly better. Soon it may not only be justified to do a lumpectomy for early breast cancer, but also it may be counterproductive not to do so. Opponents argue that we must wait for the ten-year results. Yes, the ten-year results might be different. In addition to the already significant differences in favor of conservative treatment, by five years *all* the trends might become significant as well.

Comparing just the two lumpectomy groups shows that radiotherapy significantly decreased the incidence of local recurrent disease in the operated breast. Ninety-two percent of patients treated with radiotherapy remained free of breast tumor at five years as compared to 72 percent of those receiving no radiotherapy ($p < 0.001$). Among patients with positive nodes, 98 percent of those treated with radiotherapy and 64 percent of those receiving no radiotherapy remained tumor free ($p < 0.001$).

Fisher states: "We *conclude* that segmental mastectomy, followed by breast irradiation in all patients and adjuvant chemotherapy in women with positive nodes, *is* appropriate therapy for Stage I and II breast tumors $\leqslant 4$ cm provided that margins of resected specimens are free of tumor."[10] Notice that he does not say "maybe we conclude," "looks like it could be," or "as of five years." He believes these results are conclusive for reasons which will be discussed now.

In fact, he has already moved on to such other issues as: can positive margins or tumor recurrence be treated with re-lumpectomy rather than mastectomy? And, which subgroups of patients can forego radiotherapy? Remember, although some 25 percent of patients experience recurrence within five years if radiotherapy is omitted, it is equally true that almost 75 percent of patients do not. Is it possible to identify these patients perhaps by biological, hormonal, or pathological criteria and select patients suitable for local excision only without radiotherapy?

From 1973 to 1980 Veronesi[3] randomized 701 patients with Stage I breast cancer to either Halsted radical mastectomy or to QUART treatment (quadrantectomy, axillary dissection, and radiotherapy). Although not as bold as the Fisher trial, this trial does have longer-term follow-up. However, die-hard mastectomists will be disappointed to know that an analysis for the 12-year experience merely confirms the five-year results. The actuarial disease-free 10-year survival and overall survival rates between the two treatment groups are practically superimposable.

When stratified according to axillary involvement, in patients with positive nodes, QUART treatment was significantly superior in terms of relapse-free survival ($p = 0.03$) and near significance in overall survival ($p = 0.08$).

Veronesi states, "It is reasonable to consider the results as *conclusive*. Total ablative operations are *not* justified."[3]

Of course, there are always going to be those physicians and surgeons who are suspicious of or resistant to change. The primary issue, it seems to me, centers around the question of follow-up time. Opponents cannot argue with the results as they stand now, so they argue over follow-up. It is true that breast cancer can recur any time from 10, 20, 30 or more years after initial therapy, but how long should we wait? 30 years? Not likely. So, where do we draw the line?

1. The switch from radical mastectomy to modified radical mastectomy was made long before 10-year prospective data were available. If five-year data were good enough then, why are they not now? Why suddenly this self-righteous commitment to 10-year follow-up?

2. The Veronesi results are almost ten years out and merely confirm the five-year results.
3. Differences in recurrence rates are expected before differences in survival. Since 95 percent of recurrences occur by four years and since there are no differences in recurrence rates after five years in either the Milan or NSABP trials, no difference in survival is anticipated with further follow-up.
4. There are not even any trends in favor of mastectomy to suggest that with time a significant advantage will emerge. In fact, all trends favor lumpectomy.

RECAPITULATION

1. Both laboratory and clinical data indicate that even early breast cancer is a systemic disease. The many implications of this concept reject the need for mastectomy, which was based on Halsted's anatomic/mechanistic theory of tumor metastasis. There is no operation radical enough to outflank a systemic disease. If micrometastases already exist at the time of treatment and preordain the outcome, at least let us achieve local control with the best cosmetic, functional, and psychological results.
2. Theory aside, from a purely practical viewpoint, the prospective clinical trial data argue very strongly that breast conservation and modern radiotherapy work. Results in terms of local/regional control and survival are at least comparable and in some cases superior to those of mastectomy.
3. Now that we can legitimately *minimize* disfigurement in the treatment of breast cancer, the next step is to *maximize* survival with the development of therapy based on biologic considerations rather than empiricism. Advances in breast cancer therapy are, short of luck, likely to result only from a better understanding of both human and cancer immunobiology.

REFERENCES

1. Fisher, B.: The revolution in breast cancer surgery: Science or anecdotalism? World J. Surg., 9:655–666, 1985.
2. Harris, J.R., Hellman, S., and Kinne, D.W.: Limited surgery and radiotherapy for early breast cancer. N. Engl. J. Med., 313:1365–1368, 1985.
3. Veronesi, U., Banfi, A., DelVecchio, M., et al.: Comparison of Halsted mastectomy with quadrantectomy, axillary dissection, and radiotherapy in early breast cancer: Long-term results. Eur. J. Cancer Clin. Oncol., 22:1085–1089, 1986.
4. Fisher, B., Wolmark, N., Fisher, E.R., and Deutsch, M.: Lumpectomy and axillary dissection for breast cancer: Surgical, pathological, and radiation considerations. World J. Surg., 9:692–698, 1985.
5. Danoff, B.F., Haller, D.G., Glick, J.H., and Goodman, R.L.: Conservative surgery and irradiation in the treatment of early breast cancer. Ann. Intern. Med., 102:634-642, 1985.
6. Hayward, J.L.: The Guy's Hospital trial on breast conservation. In Conservative Management of Breast Cancer. J.R. Harris, S. Hellman, and W. Silen (eds.). Philadelphia: J.P. Lippincott, 1983, pp. 77–90.
7. Harris, J.R.: Management of localized breast cancer. Hosp. Pract., 21:61–72, 1986.

8. Sarrazin, D., Monique, L., Rouesse, J., et al.: Conservative treatment versus mastectomy in breast cancer tumors with macroscopic diameter of 20 millimeters or less. Cancer, 53:1209-1213, 1984.

9. Lichter, A.S., Danforth, D., Lippman, M., et al.: A randomized trial comparing mastectomy versus excisional biopsy plus radiation in the treatment of Stage I and II breast cancer. Int. J. Rad. Oncol. Biol. Phys., 10(suppl. 2):105-106, 1984.

10. Fisher, B., Bauer, M., Margolese, R., et al.: Five-year results of a randomized clinical trial comparing total mastectomy and segmental mastectomy with or without radiation in the treatment of breast cancer. N. Engl. J. Med., 312:665-673, 1985.

DEBATE XII

Ischemic Limb: Primary Amputation
or Distal Bypass?

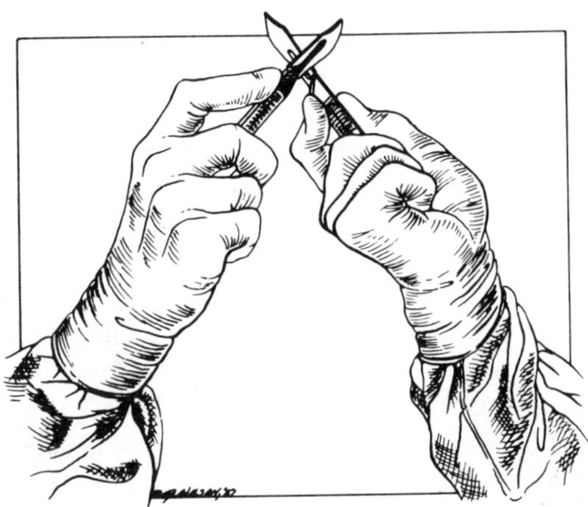

Vascular reconstructive surgery is more sophisticated, surgeons are more proficient, rehabilitative capabilites have developed, and patient expectations have skyrocketed. Amputation, however, is one of the very earliest (and most effective) of surgical procedures. When an appendage is no longer functional, indeed, when an extremity becomes a liability by virtue of pain or sepsis, amputation is a logical and decisive solution. Morbidity and mortality are maximal in the vascular surgical population due to the documented association of peripheral atherosclerosis with cardiopulmonary disease. The rehabilitative rewards of intervention in this elderly and immobile group can be subtle and fleeting. Indeed, on reviewing an arteriogram with no discernible dye below the trifurcation, a vascular surgeon must remember that "It is tough to get blood out of [or into] a stone."

Dr. Brown argues that psychological hang-ups concerning body integrity are functionally counterproductive. As surgeons, our mission is to restore our patient's mobility with biped gait. We can accomplish this more expeditiously following amputation. Time is at a premium. Five years following distal arterial reconstruction, only one-third of patients have a useful extremity and only one-half of them are alive!

Conversely, if we proceed safely and expeditiously with an amputation, the patient will benefit from early ambulation with a prosthesis.

Dr. Brown presents several series in which 90 percent of patients following a below-knee amputation are walking with a prosthesis at five years. Similarly, when these fragile patients are monitored meticulously and managed in an intensive care unit, the operative mortality for above- and below-knee amputations can be as low as 3 percent and 1 percent respectively.

Dr. Haug disagrees. He will describe the recent revolution in vascular surgery permitting infrapopliteal bypass grafting with spectacular results relative to graft patency, limb salvage, rehabilitation, and survival. He will refer to a series of octogenarians undergoing distal bypass procedures with an operative mortality of only

6 percent—equivalent to cumulative series of all age patients undergoing amputation. Indeed, a recent composite analysis of 11 series involving 965 amputations revealed a primary healing rate of 74.9 percent, late healing rate of 82 percent, mortality rate of 6.7 percent, and a rehabilitation rate of only 63.8 percent. Amputation remains a physically and psychologically harrowing procedure.

Dr. Haug also argues that even temporary distal bypass graft patency may permit healing of foot injury/infection with attendant limb salvage, even when the graft ultimately closes.

Even the most broadminded of patients must acknowledge the mutilating nature of an amputation. For many patients, an amputation is both a physically and a psychologically crippling event. Many amputees experience stump pain, and one-third are forced to retire from work.

In reading the surgical literature, one must be specially sensitive to the phenomenon of "denominator shift." Many of the people at Disneyworld are kids with full heads of hair. Only 1 percent of the *people* at Disneyworld—but 50 percent of the *grandfathers*—are as bald as a cue ball. Similarly, the phenomenon of "temporal shift" makes historic comparisons risky. Both prosthesis engineering and vascular surgery are evolving with lightning speed. To compare the computerized fuel injection system of a 1988 Volkswagen to the spark plugs of a 1970 Rolls Royce clearly is unfair. No prospective, randomized studies comparing distal arterial bypass to amputation ever have been, or are likely to be, done. Therefore, in reading the subsequent discussion—or the rest of the surgical literature—watch out!

XII-A: ISCHEMIC LIMB: PRIMARY AMPUTATION

JAMES M. BROWN, M.D.

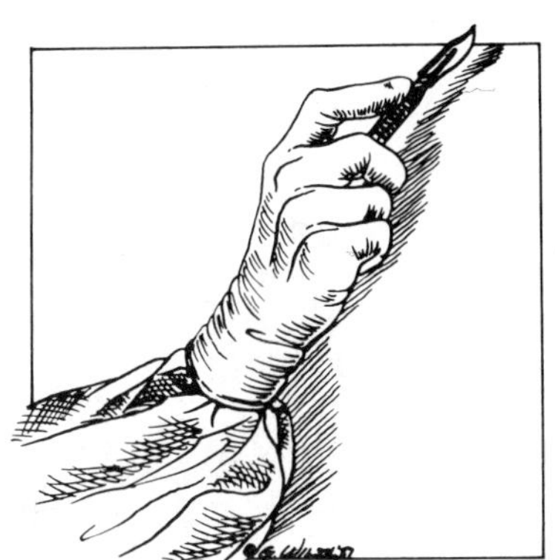

This essay will demonstrate that amputation is a successful surgical procedure with reasonable, attainable results associated with low morbidity and low mortality. Present-day rehabilitation promptly provides the patient with a usable prosthesis permitting bipedal gait. Down time, which is so dangerous in the geriatric patient, is negligible. Conversely, arterial reconstruction with distal bypass is a poor palliative procedure inflicted on a high-risk, poor-prognosis patient. Admittedly, the technical proficiency of present-day vascular surgeons is awesome. Cartier quality, however, requires both Cartier workmanship and Cartier raw materials. Even Willie Shoemaker cannot win the Kentucky Derby atop Old Paint.

Figure 1 is from a paper by Szilagyi and colleagues.[1] Femoropopliteal saphenous vein graft patency is presented with up to 15 years follow-up. This study includes patients presenting with claudication, gangrene, ischemic changes, ischemic ulcerations, or rest pain. At five years, only 50 percent of grafts are patent. In addition, up to one-half of these patients will not be alive at five years. Szilagy took into account not only patients with threatened limbs but also the less ominous group of claudicators. If we examine only patients with threatened limbs, then these data on patency and survival rates are even worse.

Functional palliation is the goal of therapy in the patient with a threatened distal limb. Palliation is "the chance of survival with a functioning limb at a given time after surgery."[2] That means that our surgical goals are to preserve bipedal gait and to give our patient a functional (albeit prosthetic) limb. I will show that this can be done most safely and expeditiously with amputation.

O'Donnell and colleagues[3] studied 79 femoropopliteal and femorotibial bypasses done for limb salvage. They report a 48 percent 5-year patency and only 47 percent 5-year survival. One-half of the patients had patent grafts at five years. One-half of the patients were alive at five years. As defined by Martin,[2] the rate of palliation at four years was 37 percent. One-third of the patients whom they set out to treat four years earlier had a functional extremity at four years. That is not very good. The one-year palliation rate was only 59 percent. The patients in this study were operated on for threatened limb, rest pain, ulceration, or gangrene.

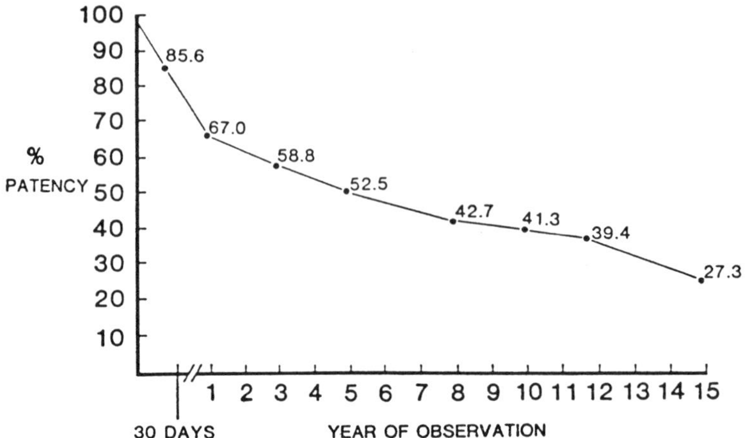

FIGURE 1. Femoropopliteal saphenous vein graft patency. From Szilagy, D.E., Hageman, J.H., Smith, R.F., et al.: Autogenous vein grafting in femoropopliteal atherosclerosis: The limits of its effectiveness. Surg., 86:841, 1979.

Stoney[4] reviewed femorotibial grafts from a conglomeration of studies by Ramsburgh and colleagues,[5] Reichle and Tyson,[6] Morton and associates,[7] and Martin and Foster.[2] The operative mortality for femorotibial grafts was 4 to 6 percent. There was an immediate graft failure rate of 20 to 35 percent. There was a late (greater than one month postoperative) graft failure rate of 30 to 50 percent. Interestingly, the amputation rate in spite of an open graft was 7 to 10 percent. The effective palliation at two years was only 50 percent.

Similarly, in a series by Stoney and colleagues[8] of 80 patients following femoropopliteal bypass grafting, 26 percent of these patients, operated on for leg salvage, were alive with a functioning limb at one year—that is poor, poor palliation.

Ramsburgh and colleagues[5] studied 148 patients following femoropopliteal bypass grafting. The two-year patency rate was 50 percent. Seventy grafts failed. Of these 70 failed grafts, 36 patients required amputation. Not only did they report poor graft patency, but also a failed graft increased the patient's risk of amputation. This series included claudicators. One-fourth of the patients presented for surgery with symptoms of claudication alone.

Reichle and Tyson[6] reviewed 364 patients following femoropopliteal and femorotibial bypass grafting for gangrene, rest pain, claudication, and ulceration. They report a 50 percent 5-year graft patency and a 32 percent salvage failure. One-half of their grafts were not patent at five years, and one-third of the patients operated on for limb salvage required amputation.

DeWeese and Rob[9] reported their experience with lower extremity revascularization. The overall 5-year survival was 24 percent. The operative mortality was greater than 70 percent if the patient was more than 70 years old or had atherosclerotic heart disease or diabetes. If the patient presented with claudication, the 5-year mortality rate was 26 percent. If the patient had rest pain, the 5-year mortality rate was 42 percent! The limb and, indeed, patient, survival following distal arterial reconstructive procedures are horrible.

Now, let me show you that amputation is a successful, low morbidity, low mortality operation in 1987. The goals for amputation are to:

1. remove gangrenous tissue,
2. relieve pain,
3. obtain primary healing, and
4. rehabilitate to ambulation.

Let's look at a study by Roon and colleagues[10] who studied 113 below-knee amputations. This group used xenon blood flow to determine level of amputation. There was a zero percent operative mortality with 91 percent of the patients rehabilitated at five years. Nine out of 10 patients were walking on a prosthetic limb at five years.

Some other values for rehabilitation are shown in Figure 2.[10] In addition, Stoney[4] reports 80 percent of patients are rehabilitated, and Couch and colleagues[11] report 90 percent of patients are walking with a prosthesis. Roon and colleagues[10] indicate that 91 percent of patients following a below-knee amputation are using a prosthesis at five years.

Unlike the protracted vascular reconstructive procedures, an amputation may be performed safely. Bunt and colleagues[12] have reported 253 major amputations, of which 113 were below the knee with an operative mortality of 0.9 percent and 140 were above the knee with an operative mortality of 2.8 percent. These vascular surgeons conscientiously monitored systemic and pulmonary artery pressure. They aggressively used diuresis, nitroglycerin, and dopamine. They packed the amputated extremity in dry ice, and all patients were managed in an intensive care unit following

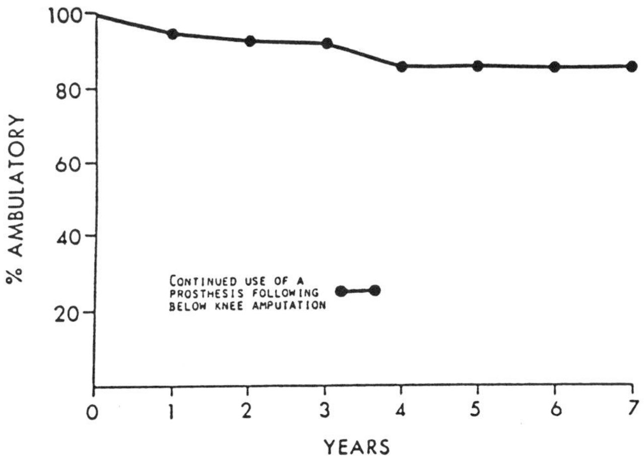

FIGURE 2. Values for rehabilitation. From Roon, A.J., Moore, W.S., and Goldstone, J.: Below-knee amputation: A modern approach. Am. J. Surg., 134:156, 1977.

surgery. Their concern paid off. Amputation, in 1988, does not have the same high operative mortality with which it was associated in the past.

Finally, Kazmers and colleagues[13] prospectively compared 45 matched patients with similar popliteal artery pressures who underwent either below-knee amputation or distal arterial reconstruction. They found that the risk of having an above-knee amputation was substantially greater in the arterial bypass group.

In conclusion, we have seen that distal arterial bypass surgery has a significant operative morbidity/mortality and that the 5-year patient survival and graft patency are poor. On the other hand, amputation carries a gratifying 5-year palliation and rehabilitation rate. In 1988, let's stop deluding ourselves with vascular surgical histrionics. Our patients deserve an expeditious procedure (amputation) that will get them back on their feet (albeit prosthetic) as safely and quickly as possible.

REFERENCES

1. Szilagyi, D.E., Hageman, J.H., Smith, R.F., et al.: Autogenous vein grafting in femoropopliteal atherosclerosis: The limits of its effectiveness. Surgery, 86:836–851, 1979.
2. Martin, C.E. and Foster, J.H.: Factual palliation with femoropopliteal bypass for salvage. J. Surg. Res., 18:215–220, 1975.
3. O'Donnell, J.A., Brener, B.J., Brief, D.K., Alpert, J., and Parsonnet, V.: Realistic expectation for patients having lower extremity bypass surgery for limb salvage. Arch. Surg., 112:1356–1363, 1977.
4. Stoney, R.J.: Ultimate salvage for the patient with limb-threatening ischemia. Am. J. Surg., 136:228–232, 1978.
5. Ramsburgh, S.R., Lindenauer, S.M., Weber, T.R., et al.: Femoropopliteal bypass for limb salvage. Surgery, 81:453–458, 1977.
6. Reichle, F. and Tyson, R.R.: Comparison of long-term results of 364 femoropopliteal or femorotibial bypasses for revascularization of severely ischemic lower extremities. Ann. Surg., 182:449–455, 1975.
7. Morton, D.L., Ehrenfeld, W.K., and Wylie, E.J.: Significance of outflow obstruction after femoro-popliteal endarterectomy. Arch. Surg., 94:592–599, 1967.
8. Stoney, R.J., James, D.R., and Wylie, E.J.: Surgery for femoropopliteal atherosclerosis: A reappraisal. Arch. Surg., 103:548–553, 1971.
9. DeWeese, J.A. and Rob, C.G.: Autogenous venous bypass grafts five years later. Ann. Surg., 174:346–356, 1971.
10. Roon, A.J., Moore, W.S., and Goldstone, J.: Below-knee amputation: A modern approach. Am. J. Surg., 134:153–158, 1977.
11. Couch, N.P., David, J.K., Tilney, N.L., et al.: Natural history of the leg amputee. Am. J. Surg., 133:469–473, 1977.
12. Bunt, T.J., Manship, L.L., Bynoe, R.P., and Haynes, J.L.: Lower extremity amputation for peripheral vascular disease: A low-risk operation. Am. Surgeon, 50:581–584, 1984.
13. Kazmers, M., Satiani, B., Evans, W.E., et al.: Amputation level following unsuccessful distal limb salvage operations. Surgery, 87:683–687, 1980.

XII-B: ISCHEMIC LIMB: DISTAL BYPASS

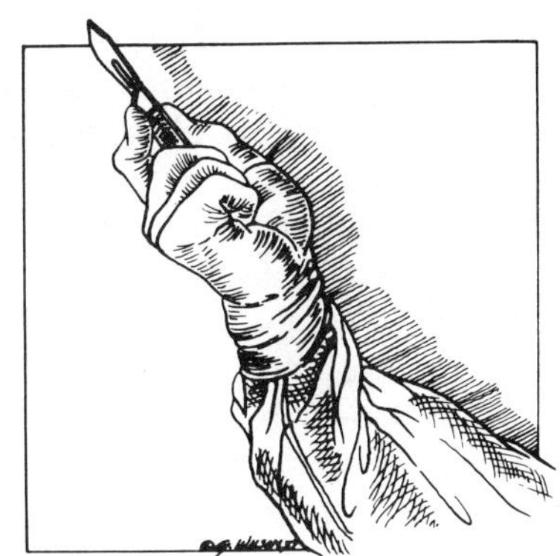

CRAIG E. HAUG, M.D.

Is it better to try to save an ischemic limb threatened by severe atherosclerosis or just to amputate immediately? The catch here is that the limbs to be saved require distal bypass; that is, bypass to the vessels distal to the popliteal. Such an operation is often thought to be fraught with dangers for generally very old and systemically atherosclerosed patients. The mean age of patients undergoing distal bypass is over 70; some are in their 80s and 90s, and more than 60 percent have diabetes.

Hand wringers sometimes advise amputation in these patients, arguing that they are too old or too sick or present too many technical difficulties to undergo distal bypass surgery. They believe it is better to cut the patient's losses short, so to speak. In fact, mortality figures for amputation are consistently much higher than those for bypass. What's more, even if patients survive the operation, the result of amputation even at the below-knee level in this elderly infirm group is often permanent inability to walk with a prosthesis because of poor vision, generalized weakness, or other atherosclerotic problems. Older patients often see amputation as a final disabling event that prevents mobility, self-care, and enjoyment of life. Conversely, almost without exception, age and medical status should not be considered reasons to withhold arterial reconstruction.

In the words of President Reagan, "Don't cut and run." Being fairly old himself, I suppose he figured he had an interest in this subject.

Assessing the risk/benefit ratio of distal arterial bypass versus primary amputation in part depends on one's philosophy and perspective on subjective factors such as quality of life and the ability to live and function independently. However, certain objective parameters are relevant. Probably the two most important for revascularization are graft patency and limb salvage rates. The concept of limb salvage has evolved to include patients whose extremities have been saved even if the graft ultimately occludes. Other issues include whether the level of amputation is endangered by a failed bypass, the advanced age of this patient pool, operative mortality, and cost. Ultimately, what percent of patients achieve bipedal gait with or without a prosthesis following vascular reconstruction or amputation?

I will demonstrate to all but my opponent's satisfaction that vascular bypass is superior to primary amputation in each and every respect. I want to warn, however, that absolute answers are not possible, since there are no prospective, randomized trials that compare the results of distal bypass to primary amputation. Patients would never accept such an experiment. Just imagine saying to a patient, "Well, Mr. Jones, funny thing is we're not really sure which would be better for you—trying to save your leg or simply cutting if off right now. Oh, hey, I tell you what—let's flip a coin."

Distal bypass, also called small vessel or infrapopliteal bypass, is a vascular reconstructive bypass from somewhere on the femoral artery proximally to the arteries beyond the popliteal distally.

The popliteal bifurcates into the anterior and posterior tibial arteries. The perineal artery is the largest branch of the posterior tibial. The anterior tibial artery runs down to the foot where it becomes dorsalis pedis. Even the dorsalis pedis can receive a bypass graft effectively.

Distal bypass is performed when standard femoropopliteal bypass is warranted but not feasible, such as in patients with an extensively diseased popliteal artery or in patients with primarily distal disease. Just as in femoropopliteal patients, femorodistal bypass should be performed only for limb salvage, not claudication; that is, it should be performed only in those patients with severe ischemic rest pain, progressive ischemic ulceration, or impending or frank gangrene. It is in this group that the threat of limb loss is greatest.

Only about 5 to 10 percent of patients should be denied an attempt at revascularization based on this small list of contraindications which includes:

- severe organic mental syndrome (inability to ambulate)
- life-threatening infection
- gangrene and infection proximal to bounds of traditional transmetatarsal amputation

Important principles of treatment include:

1. adequate preoperative or intraoperative arteriography
2. initial correction of the most proximal significant stenosis or occluded segment
3. the use of autogenous vein grafts in preference to prosthetic grafts
4. use of the most distal in-flow site when there is no proximal disease or occlusion
5. completion arteriography (to detect technical surprises)
6. antiplatelet therapy
7. minor amputations or debridements to the foot of devitalized and septic tissue as needed
8. aggressive reoperation if the primary procedure fails early or even late if the limb is still dependent on the graft.

Results of distal arterial bypass procedures are reported in terms of patency and limb salvage, which usually runs 10 to 20 percent higher than patency. The concept of limb salvage has evolved to include patients whose extremities have been saved even if the graft ultimately occludes. In a sense, limb salvage is the most important element because it is the ultimate definable parameter. This concept includes those patients with a functional bypass as well as those whose graft lasts just long enough to get the leg out of trouble. This can happen because the need for revascularization is often precipitated by tissue necrosis secondary to minor trauma, infection, or liquefaction of corns and calluses. Healing of these lesions can be strikingly prompt after bypass and does not necessarily recur after bypass closure. In addition, during the interval natural collaterals have developed.

As shown in Table I, recent studies of distal vascular bypass procedures using primarily reverse saphenous vein have found initial patency rates ranging from 79 to 90 percent, 2-year patency rates between 51 and 92 percent, and 5-year patency rates between 37 and 62 percent. One-year limb salvage rates range from 54 to 89 percent, and 5-year limb salvage rates range between 47 and 75 percent.

Operative mortality figures range from 0 percent to a high of 2.9 percent. Because of patients' advanced age and the systemic nature of atherosclerosis, this figure is surprisingly low and is probably due to the fact that major body compartments are not breached. Failed bypass also does not seem to alter the mortality of subsequent amputation.

Given the discouraging rate of eventual ambulation in the geriatric amputee and the limited life expectancy of these patients, even the worst results with distal vascular bypass represent excellent palliation. The trend is clear. Results have improved significantly over the last eight years.

Table II shows that results with the *in situ* bypass technique generally have been even better than with a reversed vein conduit. In 1981, Buchbinder and colleagues[1] performed a randomized study comparing *in situ* and reverse saphenous vein bypass. At one year the patency rate of 93 percent after *in situ* versus 63 percent after reverse saphenous vein bypass was statistically significant, necessitating termination of the study. Subsequent intermediate term results are equally good with patency rates up to 96 percent at two years for *in situ* grafts.

Interestingly, results by Taylor and colleagues[2] using reverse saphenous vein bypass were just as good. This group reported a 92 percent 3-year primary patency and an 89 percent 2-year limb salvage rate. Figure 1 depicts cumulative patency results for all reverse saphenous vein grafts compared to each site of distal anas-

TABLE I.   REVERSE SAPHENOUS VEIN BYPASS RESULTS

	NO.	PATENCY (%)			LIMB SALVAGE (%)		
		30-DAY	2-YR	5-YR	1-YR	2-YR	5-YR
Maini (1978)[13]	44	79	55	55	—	—	73
Szilagyi (1979)[14]	133	82	51	37	—	—	—
Reichle (1979)[15]	164	—	—	—	54	—	47
Perdue (1980)[16]	40	90	53	49	82	72	67
Veith (1981)[17]	204	77	—	47	—	—	51
Auer (1983)[18]	148	—	—	62	—	—	75
Veith (1986)[19]	106	—	60	—	80	75	—
Cantelmo (1986)[3]	30	—	79	—	89	—	—
Taylor (1986)[2]	76	—	92	—	—	89	—
Buchbinder (1986)*[4]	14	—	92	—	—	—	—

*Popliteal-foot bypass

TABLE II. *IN SITU* VEIN BYPASS RESULTS

		PATENCY (%)			LIMB SALVAGE (%)		
	NO.	30-DAY	2-YR	5-YR	30-DAY	3-YR	5-YR
Buchbinder (1981)[1]	47	—	93*	—	—	—	—
Leather (1984)[20]	245	94	79	62	—	—	—
Levine (1985)[21]	55	96	72	—	—	—	—
Bush (1985)[22]	50	88	94	70**	—	—	—
Buchbinder (1986)[23]	60	93#	91	—	85#	—	—
Buchbinder (1986)[4##]	23		96	—	—	—	—

*1-year patency results
**4-year patency results
 #90-day patency results
##Fem-foot bypass

tomoses and includes popliteal as well as infrapopliteal sites. Results of distal bypass are excellent and even as good as those of above-knee femoropopliteal bypass.

This group claims that the apparent superiority of *in situ* grafts over the last several years is a misperception caused by the use of historical controls. Figure 2 compares the Oregon group's present series to their previous results before 1980.[2] Improved patency can be accounted for almost entirely by a marked decrease in early graft failure. After one month, the slope of the curves are very similar.

These vascular surgical investigators present a strong case that the improvement in patency with *in situ* compared to reverse saphenous vein grafts represents recent

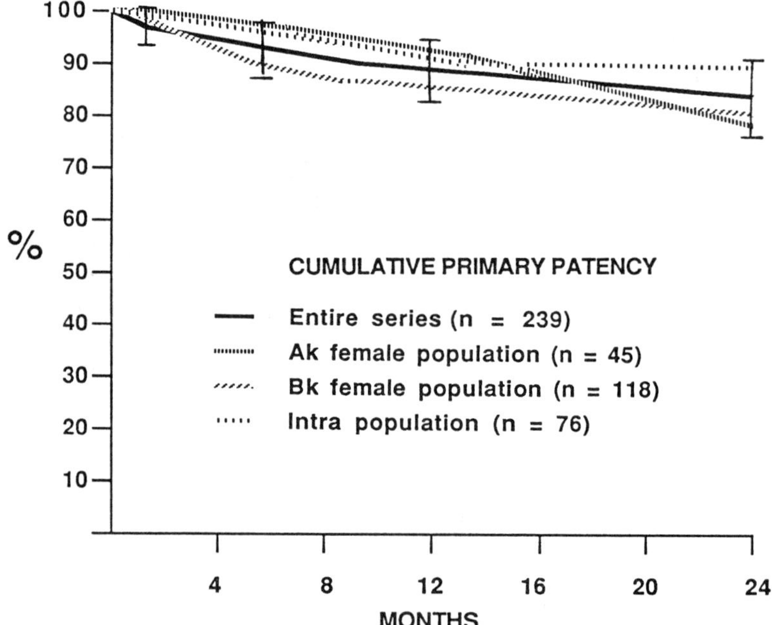

FIGURE 1. OHSU Vascular Service reverse vein grafts. From Taylor, L.M., Phinney, E.S., and Porter, J.M.: Present status of reversed vein bypass for revascularization. J. Vasc. Surg., 3:290, 1986.

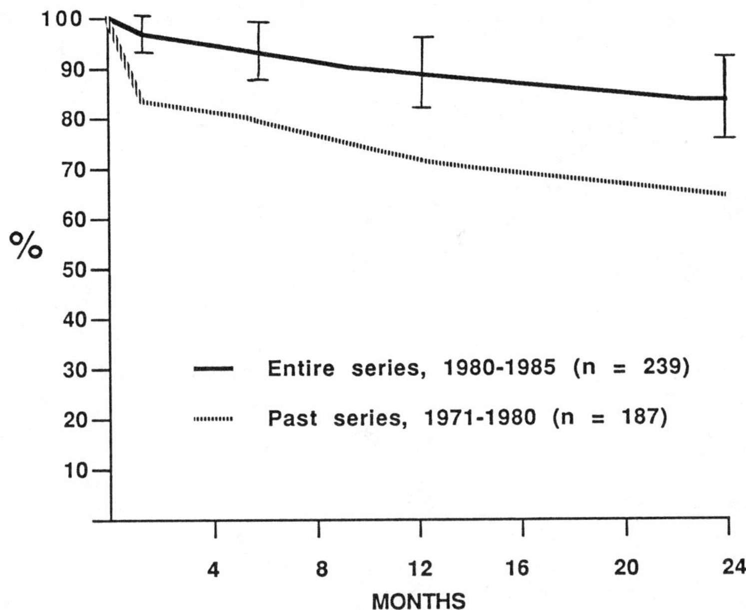

FIGURE 2.   OHSU Vascular Service reverse vein grafts. Patency of present series compared with previous series of similar operations. From Taylor, L.M., Phinney, E.S., and
Porter, J.M.: Present status of reversed vein bypass for revascularization. J. Vasc. Surg.,
3:292, 1986.

general improvements in operative technique and antiplatelet therapy rather than
long-term intrinsic superiority of the *in situ* graft itself. One of these recent improvements in technique involves the use of a more distal graft origin. Using the superficial femoral or popliteal artery rather than the common femoral artery, Cantelmo
and colleagues[3] found an 89 percent and 82 percent limb salvage rate at one and
three years, respectively. They concluded that "Results of distal vein graft reconstruction originating from the superficial femoral or popliteal artery in our patients are
comparable with those of any other group of patients with occlusive disease."

Buchbinder and colleagues,[4] primarily *in situ* vein advocates, found that, by moving the proximal anastomoses distally from the femoral artery to the popliteal, 2-year
patency rates with reverse saphenous veins increased from 42 percent to 92 percent,
comparable to the 96 percent rate using *in situ* vein grafts. They concluded that
"Femoral-foot bypass with *in situ* vein and popliteal-foot bypass with reversed vein
have appreciably increased vein utilization, graft patency, and limb salvage."

Veith and colleagues[5] take this a step further, performing tibiotibial or distal-
distal reverse saphenous vein grafts in patients who did not have longer segments of
usable vein and who faced imminent amputation without reconstruction. Eleven of
14 patients (79 percent) had a patent bypass and functional limb six to 50 months
after operation. Their conclusion was that "These newer short vein bypasses appear
to represent an advance in arterial surgery to affect limb salvage."

As we can begin to see, the work being done in the 1980s is not looking at just
distal bypass anymore, it is looking at extremely distal bypass. Satisfied that distal
bypass can be done with good results, investigators now are pushing out the frontiers,

asking how distal, how old, how far gone can these patients be—and still get good results.

In 1985, Dalsing and colleagues[6] studied patients with established gangrene of the toes or forefoot, eschewing patients with merely rest pain and ischemic ulceration. Limb salvage was 70 percent, 60 percent, and 28 percent at one, three, and five years, respectively, with an operative mortality of 1.7 percent. Conclusion: "The high limb salvage rate, low mortality rate, and low rate of above-knee amputation in the present study appear to warrant attempted limb salvage."

Scher and colleagues[7] studied patients over 80 years old, the oldest being 99 years old, and found vein bypass patency rates of 58 percent at one year and 44 percent at two years. The operative mortality of 6 percent is no higher than the average mortality of all patients undergoing primary amputation. Conclusion: "These data support an aggressive approach to arterial reconstruction in elderly patients and indicate that advanced age alone should not be considered a contraindication to attempts at limb salvage."

Another important issue in this controversy relates to the ability to obtain final amputation healing at the below-knee level in those patients in whom limb salvage has failed. The value of preservation of the knee joint in the ultimate rehabilitation of the amputee is recognized universally.

Raviola and colleagues[8] retrospectively studied patients who underwent distal bypass. A preoperatively predicted amputation level, either below or above knee, was assigned to each patient based on various preoperative clinical criteria. Of those 32 patients predicted to require a below-knee amputation, 18.7 percent received a below-knee amputation after failed bypass, and 21.9 percent required an above-knee amputation instead. Clearly, these patients did not benefit from bypass. On the other hand, almost 60 percent of patients who would have been subjected to a below-knee amputation were able to keep their legs. Of those nine patients who were predicted to require an above-knee amputation, one-third ended up with one after failed bypass. Again, this group did not benefit by bypass. On the other hand, one-third had their amputation lowered to below knee, and one-third escaped major amputation altogether. They concluded that " . . . it appears that the benefits of limb salvage or lowered amputation level greatly outweighed the few cases in which the amputation level was raised."

It is important to point out that by saying 21.9 percent of patients who got an above-knee amputation instead of below-knee amputation were not helped by bypass is not the same as saying that they were hurt by bypass. About 20 percent of primary below-knee amputations eventually are converted to an above-knee amputation as well.

This leads to a related point. Beware if my opponent parades out data comparing the high percentage of above-knee amputations among the subset of failed bypass patients to the 20 percent of above-knee amputations among all patients undergoing primary below-knee amputation—implying that failed bypass raises the amputation level. For example, instead of a 21.9 percent above-knee amputation rate among all patients at risk, he might quote the much higher rate of 54 percent among failed bypass patients. A 54 percent above-knee amputation rate after failed bypass is greater than a 20 percent above-knee amputation rate after primary below-knee amputation. Therefore, failed bypass jeopardizes chances of healing a below-knee amputation, right?

Wrong!

It sounds plausible, but the methodology is unsound. It is not valid to have all patients at risk as the denominator in the primary amputation group and just a small, select subset of patients, those who failed bypass, as the denominator in the other group. The denominator, in both cases, should be *all* patients with a threatened limb who are predicted to be capable of healing a below-knee amputation.

AMPUTATIONS

As late as the 1960s, reported mortality for primary amputation for ischemia ranged as high as 20 to 40 percent. Even today, it is not hard to find amputation mortality figures over 10 percent. A composite analysis of 11 more recent amputation series involving 965 amputations shows a primary healing rate of 74.9 percent, an eventual healing rate of 82 percent, a mortality rate of 6.7 percent, and a rehabilitation rate of *only* 63.8 percent (Table III).[9]

No matter what kind of treatment (bypass or amputation) we offer our patients, our goal must be to provide the patient with the ability to work, so as to postpone chronic illness, maintain vigor, and slow social and psychological involution. A study by Little and colleagues[10] emphasized that these goals often are not achieved. About one-third of the patients were forced to retire from active work by the amputation, about three-fourths reported a serious decline in social activities, only about one-half were really independent with their prosthesis in the long term, one-fourth reported severe and intractable pain related to the amputation stumps, and only about one-fourth felt that the amputation definitely was beneficial. The authors comment that "It cannot be emphasized too firmly that anyone who seeks to carry out a mutilating procedure must explain the matter to the patient with sympathy and honesty and that the disadvantages must not be completely suppressed."

Even under optimal conditions, it is difficult for a patient to accept amputation psychologically if he knows that there is *any* potential for limb salvage. Older patients often see amputation as a final disabling event that prevents mobility, self-care, and the enjoyment of life.

Let's look at cost. If patients are lumped together, both failures and successes, and if all rehabilitation costs are included, the average distal bypass costs about the same as or maybe less than the average amputation. In 1986, Mackey and colleagues[11] showed that the mean total cost during a several year follow-up period was comparable between bypass and amputation—about $40,000. Gupta and colleagues[12] found the mean total cost of small vessel bypass to be about $27,000, including all physician, hospital, reoperation, and rehabilitation costs. The mean total cost of below-knee amputation and in-hospital rehabilitation was also about $27,000. However, when the out-of-hospital care costs of the 26 percent of patients who failed rehabilitation were included, the final cost of amputation was substantively more. They concluded: "Our overall data demonstrate that, although limb salvage pro-

TABLE III. BELOW-KNEE AMPUTATION: CONVENTIONAL TECHNIQUES*

REFERENCE	NUMBER OF AMPUTATIONS	PRIMARY HEALING (%)	EVENTUAL HEALING (%)	MORTALITY RATE (%)	REHABILITATION WITH PROSTHESIS (%)	AVERAGE TIME OPERATION TO REHABILITATION (DAYS)
Warren & Kihn	121	48.8	66.9	4.1	69.4	180–270
Chilvers et al.	53	50.0	67.9	7.5	60.4	—
Robinson	47	77.0	—	17.0	83.0	—
Bradham & Smoak	84	85.7	88.0	—	—**	—
Block & Whitehouse	43	88.0	95.0	0.0†	53.5	120–180
Cranley et al.	101	76.0	86.0	7.0	73.3	—
Lim et al.	55	53.0	83.0	16.0	51.0	70
Leker & Jacobs	69	77.0	85.0	8.7	52.2	201
Wray et al.	174	92.0	—	3.5	70.0	49–77
Nagrendran et al.	174	80.5	91.4	—	—	—
Berardi & Keonin	44	—	61.4	4.5	29.5	111
Averaged Totals	965	74.9	82.0	6.7	63.8	133

*From Malone, J.M., Moore, W.S., Goldstone, J., and Malone, S.J.: Therapeutic and economic impact of a modern amputation program. Ann. Surg., 189:801, 1979.

**Authors commented that very few patients attained ambulation; however, no numbers were given.

†Two patients died before discharge, and were not included as postoperative deaths.

cedures are expensive, they can achieve a high degree of functional limb salvage. Primary BKA may be equally expensive and less satisfactory."

RECAPITULATION

While quality of life cannot be measured, we can take it as axiomatic that most if not all patients would prefer to keep their leg. Let's face it, for one's social life and self-image, a real leg is always better than a fake leg.

Aggressive attempts at limb salvage can achieve graft patency in the majority of patients for several years—at least 50 percent and up to 80 to 90 percent in recent series—provided meticulous technical standards are observed. In fact, latest intermediate-term results of distal bypass are equal to those of femoropopliteal bypass. Functional limb salvage rates clearly are superior to the 63 percent rehabilitation rate in the composite amputation series cited and even compare favorably with the 80 plus percent rehabilitation rate in the very best amputation centers. This is remarkable when you think about it. Distal bypass is no longer a last-ditch, what-have-we-got-to-lose procedure. It has attained parity with amputation in terms of achieving ultimate bipedal gait with a single major operation.

The big difference, of course, is that while both patients have achieved bipedal gait only one is *actually a biped*. This becomes especially important in the 33 percent of patients in whom the opposite leg becomes threatened because of the symmetry of the disease process. If this happens, the patient with the prosthesis must consider bypass next time because the chance of his walking with bilateral prosthesis is slim at best. In other words, along with everything else, primary amputation unnecessarily burns bridges.

As to the issue of amputation level, while attempts at revascularization may raise amputation level in a minority of patients, and I emphasize *may*, there is no "maybe" to the fact that the majority of patients go on to have two legs until they die, whereas they would have had only one without revascularization.

The issue of patient durability is a nonissue. Due to improvements in the treatment of coronary artery disease, longevity has improved significantly in these patients. Fifty to 80 percent of these patients live longer than five years. They still deserve the best we have to offer.

The operative mortality of distal arterial reconstructive procedures is about one-half that of amputation. But, I do not want to make too much of this since randomization is not feasible.

The average costs of the two treatments are about equal—so far. The greater the success rate with bypass, the more the average cost will come down. Already, a single successful bypass costs less than a single successful amputation with rehabilitation.

In conclusion, the high limb salvage rate, low mortality rate, and low rate of above-knee amputations not only encourage limb salvage attempts but also mandate them. Indeed, this is an archaic debate. Amputation should be provided as primary therapy in only about 10 percent of patients. The real issue, instead of focusing on *whether* to bypass, is *how best* to bypass.

REFERENCES

1. Buchbinder, D., Singh, J.K., Karmody, A.M., et al.: Comparison of patency rate and structural change to *in situ* and reversed vein arterial bypass. J. Surg. Res., 30:213–218, 1981.
2. Taylor, L.M., Phinney, E.S., and Porter, J.M.: Present status of reversed vein bypass for revascularization. J. Vasc. Surg., 3:288–297, 1986.
3. Cantelmo, N.L., Snow, J.R., Menzoian, J.O., and Loberfo, F.W.: Successful vein bypass in patients with an ischemic limb and a palpable popliteal pulse. Arch. Surg., 121:217–220, 1986.
4. Buchbinder, D., Pasch, A.R., Rollins, D.L., et al.: Results of arterial reconstruction of the foot. Arch. Surg., 121:673–677, 1986.
5. Veith, F.J., Ascer, E., Gupta, S.K., et al.: Tibiotibial vein bypass grafts: A new operation for limb salvage. J. Vasc. Surg., 2:552–557, 1985.
6. Dalsing, M.C., White, J.V., Yao, J.S.T., et al.: Infrapopliteal bypass for established gangrene of the forefoot or toes. J. Vasc. Surg., 2:669–677, 1985.
7. Scher, L.A., Veith, F.J., Verta, M.J., et al.: Limb salvage in octogenarians and nonagenarians. Surgery, 99:160–165, 1986.
8. Raviola, C.A., Nichter, L., Baxter, J.D., et al.: Femoropopliteal tibial bypass: What price failure? Am. J. Surg., 144:115–123, 1982.
9. Malone, J.M., Moore, W.S., Goldstone, J., and Malone, S.J.: Therapeutic and economic impact of a modern amputation program. Ann. Surg., 189:798–802, 1979.
10. Little, J.M., Petritsi-Jones, D., and Kerr, C.: Vascular amputees: A study of disappointment. Lancet, 1:793–795, 1974.
11. Mackey, W.C., McCullough, J.L., Conlon, T.P., et al.: The costs of surgery for limb-threatening ischemia. Surgery, 99:26–35, 1986.
12. Gupta, S.K., Veith, F.J., Samson, R.H., et al.: Cost analysis of operation for infrainguinal arteriosclerosis. Circulation, 66(suppl. 2):9, 1982.
13. Maini, B.S. and Mannick, J.A.: Effect of arterial reconstruction on limb salvage: A ten-year appraisal. Arch. Surg., 113:1297–1304, 1978.
14. Szilagy, D.E., Hageman, J.H., Smith, R.F., et al.: Autogenous saphenous vein grafting in femoropopliteal atherosclerosis: The limits of its effectiveness. Surgery, 86:836–851, 1979.
15. Reichle, F.A., Rankin, K.P., Tyson, R.R., et al.: Long-term results of 474 arterior reconstruction for severely ischemic limbs: A 14-year follow-up. Surgery, 85:93–99, 1979.
16. Perdue, G.D., Smith, R.B., Veazey, C.R., and Ansley, J.D.: Revascularization for severe limb ischemia. Arch. Surg., 115:168–171, 1980.
17. Veith, F.J., Gupta, S.K., Samson, R.H., et al.: Progress in limb salvage by reconstructive arterial surgery combined with new or improved adjunctive procedures. Ann. Surg., 194:386–401, 1981.
18. Auer, A.I., Hurley, J.J., Binnington, H.B., et al.: Distal tibial vein grafts for limb salvage. Arch. Surg., 118:597–602, 1983.
19. Veith, F.J., Gupta, S.K., Ascer, E., et al.: Six-year prospective multicenter randomized comparison of autologous saphenous vein and expanded polytetra fluoroethylene grafts in infrainguinal arterial reconstructions. J. Vasc. Surg., 3:104–114, 1986.
20. Leather, R.P., Shah, D.M., Corson, J.D., and Karmody, A.M.: Instrumental evolution of the valve incision method of *in situ* saphenous vein bypass. J. Vasc. Surg., 1:113–123, 1984.
21. Levine, A.W., Banoyk, D.F., Bonier, P.H., and Towne, J.B.: Lessons learned in adopting the *in situ* saphenous vein bypass. J. Vasc. Surg., 2:145–153, 1985.
22. Bush, H.L., Nabseth, D.C., Curl, G.R., et al.: *In situ* saphenous vein bypass grafts for limb salvage. A current fad or a viable alternative to reversed vein bypass grafts? Am. J. Surg., 149:477–480, 1985.
23. Buchbinder, D., Rollins, D.L., Verta, M.J., et al.: Early experience with *in situ* saphenous vein bypass for distal arterial reconstruction. Surgery, 99:350–356, 1986.

DEBATE XIII

Surgery For Claudication

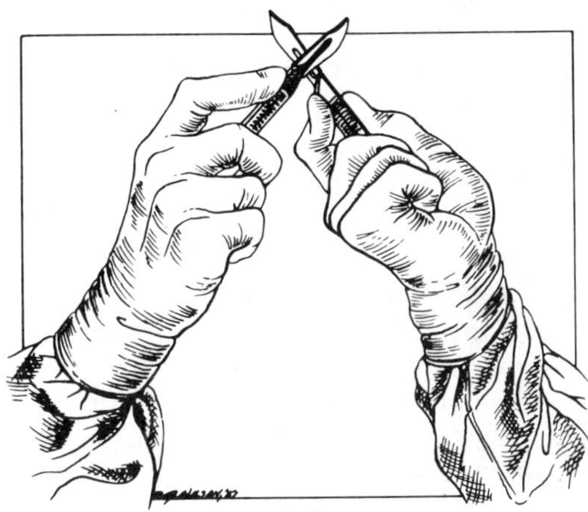

Claudication is a symptom of peripheral vascular atherosclerosis. Symptoms are subjective. As clinicians, we are all familiar with the frighteningly stoic laborer from Maine or Wyoming. Conversely, we all recognize the wimpy malpractice lawyer who requires morphine for a haircut. The purpose of the following discussion is to examine whether a patient who complains of limiting claudication (but no limb threat) should be offered a potentially risky revascularization procedure.

Dr. Piotrowski believes that a sensitive vascular surgeon should offer to rehabilitate any patient with limiting claudication. He supports this premise by exploring the natural history of peripheral vascular disease. In 1987, a patient presenting with claudication has only a 5 percent risk of amputation at five years. That sounds low; but, over and over again in this series of debates we learn that statistics should never be accepted at face value. Dr. Piotrowski points out that claudication is just a manifestation of systemic atherosclerosis. Patients with claudication have a 5- and 10-year mortality of 30 percent and 50 percent, respectively. Thus, the patients with the most aggressive disease do not face amputation—they die! By culling this group out of the numerator, the amputation rate looks spuriously good.

Dr. Piotrowski refers to a large series of nondiabetic claudicators who underwent surgical revascularization. The operative mortality was 0.9 percent. The 5-year patency was 74 percent. The amputation rate was only 0.8 percent in another series of aortoiliac bypass procedures for claudication, and graft patency was 95 percent at five years with no amputations! Overall, the operative mortality of femoropopliteal bypass surgery for claudication is a low 0.4 percent. Even better, the operation works. Seventy percent of patients will have pain-free extremities at five years. The risk of amputation does not increase following surgery. Revascularization can be performed with acceptable morbidity, mortality, and graft patency to achieve excellent palliation of claudication in those patients who request surgery. Humane vascular surgeons should offer a surgical alternative to the disabled patient with claudication.

On the other hand, Dr. Chambers argues that a small group of inappropriately aggressive vascular surgeons is escalating this issue completely out of proportion. In men less than 50 years of age, the prevalence of peripheral vascular disease is only 1 to 1.5 percent. By the age of 60 years, this figure has increased only to 4 to 6 percent. These low figures are even lower for women, whose incidence of claudication seems to lag at least a decade behind men. Additionally, Dr. Chambers presents a compilation of studies indicating that only 25 percent of patients who present with intermittent claudication will experience a progression of symptoms during the rest of their lives! This deterioration in symptoms will occur during the 12 months following initial presentation in only 10 percent of patients. Thus, the issue is small; and surgeons should never rush to confront this overrated nonproblem. When jousting with windmills, forebearance is advisable.

In recommending any surgical procedure, the surgeon weighs the risk of disease against the risk of surgical intervention. There is a consensus within the vascular literature that an operative candidate is less than 65 years old and has only proximal vascular disease. He does not smoke and has no evidence of coronary or cerebrovascular disease or diabetes. Dr. Chambers argues that this patient does not exist; or, if he does exist, he does not have vascular disease either.

Must vascular surgeons, therefore, abandon their patients with claudication? Dr. Chambers eloquently relates the impact of a smoking cessation program on death, amputation, claudication in the opposite limb, myocardial infarction, cerebrovascular accident, and surgery for limb salvage as well as the claudication itself.

Indeed, if O.J. Simpson injures his popliteal artery while leaping over a suitcase in the airport and subsequently develops claudication, he should be offered vascular reconstructive surgery. Other good-risk candidates simply do not exist.

XIII-A: CLAUDICATION REQUIRES SURGICAL INTERVENTION

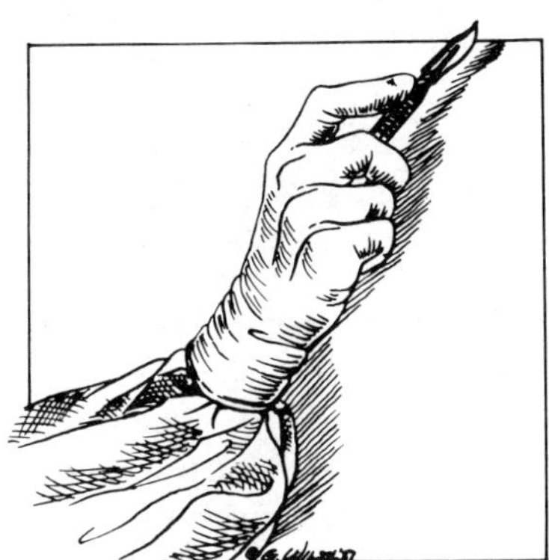

JOSEPH J. PIOTROWSKI, M.D.

As is true of most things in surgery, it is very difficult to defend operating on a patient with minimal symptoms who does not request an operation. However, when a patient does request surgery for a disabling condition such as claudication which he feels is limiting his life style, one must examine the morbidity, mortality, and results of that surgery.

After examining the natural history of lower extremity claudication, alternatives to surgery, and the morbidity and mortality for both aortoiliac and femoropopliteal bypass surgery, it will become apparent that a surgical alternative should be offered patients with claudication.

Claudication is a symptom, not a disease. Atherosclerosis is the disease process. We are not discussing an operation that is going to change the overall prognosis of atherosclerosis. We are considering a procedure that is designed to relieve a symptom. The question is: Can this be done with acceptable morbidity and mortality?

Claudication comes from the Latin word *claudicatio,* which means limping or lameness. An excellent recent review of the natural history of peripheral vascular disease[1] reveals that approximately 75 percent of claudicators will either stabilize or improve over time. Approximately 25 percent will deteriorate, and 21 percent will require surgery for limb salvage. The amputation rate varies, depending on the series quoted. Prior to the era of surgical revascularization procedures, the amputation rate in claudicators was approximately 4 to 12 percent. With the more recent series in which patients developing critical ischemia are revascularized, there currently is a 5 percent amputation rate over five years.

Intuitively, this rate appears low. Due to concomitant coronary artery disease, the apparently low amputation rate is a statistical trick. When a person has peripheral claudication, his 5-year mortality is 30 percent; 10-year mortality is 50 percent; and 15-year mortality is 70 percent! This is increased in diabetics and those who have more extensive distal disease. These patients do not exhibit lower extremity difficulties because their coronary mortality is so high. Thus, the reported amputation rate is spuriously low because patients with lethal cardiovascular disease do not survive to get into the numerator.

What alternatives to surgery exist for patients with disabling claudication? Percutaneous transluminal angioplasty has a complication rate of approximately 4 to 22 percent and requires an operation anyway in over 5 percent of the attempted cases.[2] The technical failure rate is approximately 15 percent. In these cases the catheter or guide wire could not pass the obstruction.

In a "successful" angioplasty, failure to improve the ankle-brachial index occurs in about 25 percent of cases. There is a bias in all these studies. Case selection is such that approximately 10 to 56 percent of patients admitted for some sort of vascular procedure are diverted to percutaneous transluminal angioplasty. When angioplasty is not possible (the vascular "dregs"), patients are offered a surgical procedure.

The length of the stenosis or occlusion is related strongly to angioplasty outcome.[3] When the lesion is less than 3 cm in length, the 5-year patency was 77 percent for occlusive disease and 89 percent with stenotic disease. With lesions greater than 3 cm in length, however, the 5-year patency is 26 percent and 54 percent, respectively. Percutaneous transluminal angioplasty clearly is more useful in short, nonocclusive lesions.

The level of the stenosis or occlusion also determines outcome following angioplasty. At the iliac level, there is an approximate 4 percent technical failure rate, a 74 percent 5-year patency, and a 58 percent 7-year patency. At the femoropopliteal level, there is a 17 percent technical failure rate and only a 63 percent 9-month patency and 23 percent 5-year patency. In fact, in a review article by Rutherford and Kumpe, they indicated that: "Arterial reconstruction is applied to that distinct majority of cases with diffuse, extensive, or multiple occlusive lesions."[2]

What about drug therapy? Pentoxifylline, naftidrofuryl, cinnarizine, flunarizine, buflomedil, cyclandelate, and ketanserin have all been used to improve walking distance in patients with claudication. All have shown an 80 to 100 percent increase in walking distance.

Porter and Barr[4] reported on 26 patients treated with pentoxifylline (Trental). This is a small number of patients. However, the absolute claudication distance increased from 92 meters to 156 meters. These patients are severely limited by their claudication; and even with the increase in walking distance, these patients remain disabled.

What about exercise therapy? Ekroff and colleagues[5] reported 148 patients who were exercised three times a week by a physical therapist for 30 minutes per session. Approximately 13 percent of these patients could not complete the study, and 9 percent subsequently went to surgery after the study was completed. In other words, 22 percent failed or regressed with this treatment. After removing the patients who will make the statistics look bad, the average increase in walking distance was from 300 meters to 700 meters.

Wilson and colleagues[6] reported 53 patients who went through a modified walking program. Approximately 74 percent of them completed the program, and 31 percent stopped smoking. At five years, 45 percent were stable, 25 percent were worse, 19 percent were worse and required surgery, 9 percent died, and 2 percent required an amputation. This is an interesting study in that it related walking program success to the initial ankle-brachial index. When patients had an ankle-brachial index of .6 or above, most of them benefitted from the walking program. Approximately one-half of the patients with an ankle-brachial index of .4 to .6 improved. Patients with an ankle-brachial index less than .4 did not improve; in fact, most of these patients progressed in their disease.

What about the results of surgical revascularization for claudication? Generally, these data are divided into two different areas: the aortoiliac and femoropopliteal groups. Watt and colleagues[7] reported 277 patients who underwent aortobifemoral bypass for claudication. None of these patients was diabetic, and the average age was 51 years. Their operative mortality was 6 percent early in the series, but this improved to 0.9 percent in the last half of the series. The immediate patency was 99 percent, and the 5-year patency was 74 percent. Their amputation rate was 0.8 percent.

Hill and colleagues[8] reported 56 patients who had aortoiliac bypass operations for claudication. This is an interesting study since the relief of claudication was correlated with the patency of the superficial femoral artery (SFA) prior to the aortoiliac bypass procedure. When there was either an open or occluded SFA, the patency rates were similar—approximately 90 percent for both. In other words, the profunda femoris artery allows the graft to remain open. However, when the superficial femoral was open, there was relief of claudication in 86 percent of patients, which was nearly as good as the patency rate. When the superficial femoral was occluded, the relief of claudication by aortobifemoral bypass alone was only 26 percent. Therefore, calf claudication will not be relieved by an aortoiliac bypass procedure alone in the presence of peripheral disease.

Sonnenfeld[9] reported 71 patients who had aortoiliac bypass for claudication. The operative mortality was 3 percent. Mortality at one year was 6 percent and at five years was 15 percent. There was a 9 percent morbidity related primarily to wound complications. Their immediate patency rate was 100 percent, 98 percent at one year, and 95 percent at five years. There were no amputations in this group. Aortoiliac bypass is an effective procedure with good long-term patency. However, this procedure does have associated morbidity and mortality that may not be acceptable in a patient with only claudication.

What about the femoropopliteal data? As shown in Table I, from a series of studies, operative mortality approximates 0.4 percent. Their 5-year mortality was 22 percent, and 10-year mortality was 54 percent, which is the same as the natural history of the disease. As expected, this is not a life-saving procedure. However, it is a low-mortality procedure and does not increase the overall mortality of the patient as the years go by.

What about the effectiveness of femoral popliteal bypass? Table II reveals that immediate patency rates in patients bypassed for claudication are excellent—95 percent. Five-year patency is about 72 percent; 10-year patency is 50 percent. You can tell your patient that, after bypass, there is a 70 percent chance that his limb will be pain free at five years.

What about amputation rate? Does this procedure for claudication increase the risk of amputation? As shown in Table III, the amputation rate over five years averages 2 percent. The natural history of claudication reveals a 5-year amputation rate of 5 percent. It is clear that there is not an increased incidence of amputation in patients who undergo revascularization for claudication. Therefore, surgery does not increase morbidity; but it does relieve symptoms.

TABLE I.   FEMOROPOPLITEAL BYPASS WITH REVERSED SAPHENOUS VEIN

| | | MORTALITY (%) | | |
AUTHOR	PATIENTS	OPERATIVE	5-YEAR	10-YEAR
Darling, 1972[17]	196	0.5	—	—
Cutler, 1976[16]	183	0	18	—
DeWeese, 1977[15]	103	0	20	48
Barker, 1978[14]	85	0	26	—
Szilagyi, 1979[13]	153	0	44	—
Mannick, 1980[12]	43	0	4	—
King, 1980[11]	160	2.5	20	—
Sladen, 1985[10]	100	0	21	61
Total/Averages	1,023	0.4	22	54

TABLE II.   FEMOROPOPLITEAL BYPASS PATENCY

CLAUDICATION DATA IN REVERSED SAPHENOUS FEMORAL POPLITEAL BYPASS

| | | PATENCY (%) | | |
AUTHOR	PATIENTS	IMMEDIATE	5-YEAR	10-YEAR
Darling, 1972[17]	196	97	74	—
Cutler, 1976[16]	183	100	82	—
DeWeese, 1977[15]	103	—	74	45
Barker, 1978[14]	85	—	70	—
Mannick, 1980[12]	43	98	88	—
King, 1980[11]	160	97	67	—
Sladen, 1985[10]	100	86	68	54
Total/Averages	870	95	72	50

TABLE III.   AMPUTATION RATE AFTER FEMORAL POPLITEAL BYPASS FOR CLAUDICATION

AUTHOR	PATIENTS	AMPUTATION 5 YEARS (%)
Darling, 1972[17]	196	0
Cutler, 1976[16]	183	4.0
DeWeese, 1977[15]	103	0
Barker, 1978[14]	85	3.0
Szilagyi, 1979[13]	153	0
Mannick, 1980[12]	43	2.0
King, 1980[11]	160	2.0
Sladen, 1985[10]	100	5.0
Total/Average	1,023	2.0

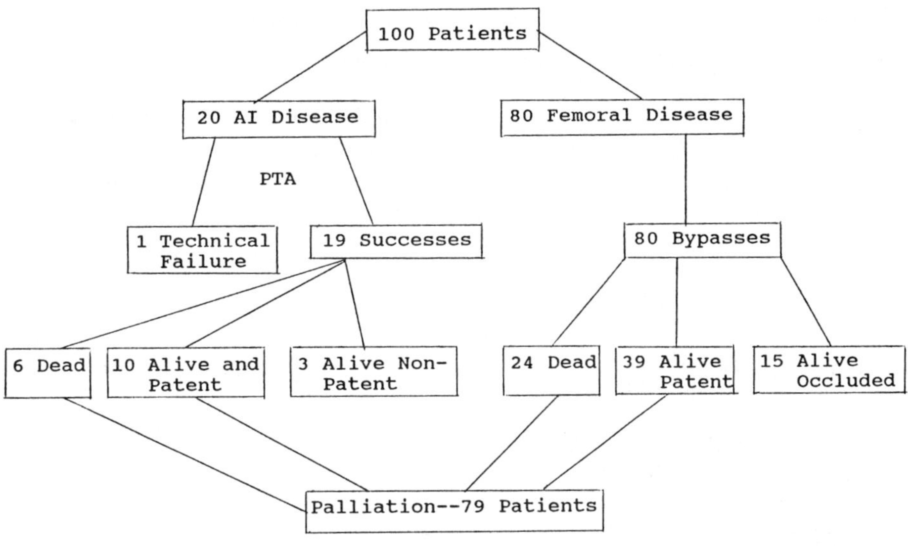

FIGURE 1.

Sladen and Gilmour[10] followed 100 patients after femoral popliteal bypass for ten years with 100 percent follow-up. Mortality was 0 percent operatively, 21 percent at five years, and 61 percent at ten years. Primary patency was 86 percent at 30 days, 68 percent at five years, and 54 percent at ten years. The associated secondary patency was 95 percent, 86 percent, and 78 percent, respectively. Amputation rate was 5 percent over ten years and 2.5 percent at five years. This is the same as the natural history of the disease.

In general, of 100 patients who present with disabling claudication (Figure 1), approximately 20 will have aortoiliac disease and 80 will have strictly femoral disease. With favorable lesions, the aortoiliac lesions deserve a trial of percutaneous transluminal angioplasty. There is a high success rate with this lesion. At five years, six of these patients will be dead, ten will have patent arteries and be symptom free, and three will have nonpatent vessels. Femoropopliteal disease will be present in 80 patients, all of whom should undergo femoropopliteal bypass surgery. At five years, 24 of these patients will be dead, 39 will have patent grafts, 15 will have occluded grafts, and 2 will have required amputation.

Evidently, if a patient is dead at five years, he has not been palliated. However, if his graft remained open until he died, the patient will have been palliated successfully for that period of time. Therefore, 79 of 100 patients will be palliated using this algorithm (Figure 1).

In conclusion:

1. From the natural history of the disease, we know that 25 percent of claudicators will deteriorate and that with surgical salvage the amputation rate is 5 percent.
2. The mortality of patients presenting with claudication at 5, 10, and 15 years is 30, 50, and 70 percent, respectively.

3. Percutaneous transluminal angioplasty is good for stenotic isolated lesions of proximal vessels and should be the procedure of choice only in these cases.
4. Drug therapy and exercise either mildly increase walking distance in those severely impaired or help those who would not ordinarily request surgery.
5. Surgery can be performed with acceptable morbidity, mortality, and graft patency to achieve excellent palliation of symptoms in those patients who request it.

REFERENCES

1. Dormandy, J.A. and Mahir, M.S.: The natural history of peripheral atheromatous disease of legs. In Vascular Surgery: Issues in Current Practice. R.M. Greenhalgh, C.W. Jamieson, and A.N. Nicolaides, (eds.). New York: Grune & Stratton, 1986, pp. 3–17.
2. Rutherford, R.B., Patt, A., and Kumpe, D.A.: The current role of percutaneous transluminal angioplasty. In Vascular Surgery: Issues in Current Practice. R.M. Greenhalgh, C.W. Jamieson, and A.N. Nicolaides, (eds.). New York: Grune & Stratton, 1986, pp. 229–244.
3. Krepel, V.M., vanAndel, G.J., vanErp, W.F.M., and Breslau, P.J.: Percutaneous transluminal angioplasty of the femoropopliteal artery: Initial and long-term results. Radiology, 156:325–328, 1985.
4. Porter, J.M. and Baur, G.M.: Pharmacologic treatment of intermittent claudication. Surgery, 92:966–971, 1982.
5. Ekroth, R., Dahllof, A-G, Gundevall, B., Holm, J., and Schersten, T.: Physical training of patients with intermittent claudication: Indications, methods, and results. Surgery, 84:640–643, 1978.
6. Wilson, S.E., Schwartz, I., Williams, R.A., and Owens, M.L.: Occlusion of the superficial femoral artery: What happens without operation? Am. J. Surg., 140:112–118, 1980.
7. Watt, J.K., Gillespie, G., Pollock, J.G., and Reid, W.: Arterial surgery in intermittent claudication. Br. Med. J., 1:23–26, 1974.
8. Hill, D.A., McGrath, M.A., Lord, R.S.A., and Tracy, G.D.: The effect of superficial femoral artery occlusion on the outcome of aortofemoral bypass for intermittent claudication. Surgery, 87:133–136, 1980.
9. Sonnenfeld, T.: Reconstructive vascular surgery for intermittent claudication. Acta Med. Scand., 212:145–149, 1982.
10. Sladen, J.G. and Gilmour, J.L.: Fate of claudication after femoropopliteal vein bypass: Prospective long-term follow-up of 100 patients. Can. J. Surg., 28:401–404, 1985.
11. King, R.B., Myers, K.A., Scott, D.F., Devine, T.J., Johnson, N., and Morris, P.J.: Femoropopliteal vein grafts for intermittent claudication. Br. J. Surg., 67:489–492, 1980.
12. Donaldson, M.C. and Mannick, J.A.: Femoropopliteal bypass grafting for intermittent claudication: Is pessimism warranted? Arch. Surg., 115:724–727, 1980.
13. Szilagyi, D.E., Hageman, J.H., Smith, R.F., et al.: Autogenous vein grafting in femoropopliteal atherosclerosis: The limits of its effectiveness. Surgery, 86:836–851, 1979.
14. Alinaji, Barker, C.F., Berkowitz, H.D., Chu, J., and Roberts, B.: Femoropopliteal vein grafts for claudication: Analysis of 100 consecutive cases. Ann. Surg., 188:79–82, 1978.
15. DeWeese, J.A. and Rob, C.G.: Autogenous venous graft ten years later. Surgery, 82:775–784, 1977.
16. Cutler, B.S., Thompson, J.E., Kleinsasser, L.J., and Hempel, G.K.: Autologous saphenous vein femoropopliteal bypass: Analysis of 298 cases. Surgery, 79:325–331, 1976.
17. Darling, R.C. and Linton, R.R.: Durability of femoropopliteal reconstruction. Am. J. Surg., 123:472–479, 1972.

XIII-B: SURGERY IS *NOT* NECESSARY FOR CLAUDICATION

JODI A. CHAMBERS, M.D.

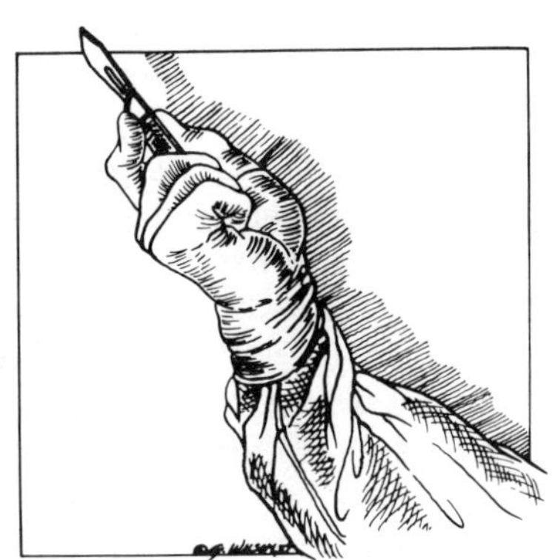

Claudication is a pain in the leg. The topic of claudication concerns the symptom complex of lower extremity pain and fatigue secondary to ischemia. The pain characteristically is experienced at a predictable level of exertion and relieved with rest. The debate centers arount treatment.

Should all patients with claudication undergo revascularization surgery? For those of you who have any doubt as to the answer, let me put your minds at ease early: the answer is no. A small percentage of patients does exist who should be offered the option of arterial reconstruction. As usual, the problem is not black and white and needs to be individualized. Proponents of surgery consider claudication an operative indication when it "impairs occupational performance or the desired lifestyle of an otherwise good-risk patient—providing a favorable anatomic situation for reconstruction exists."[1]

I propose to demonstrate that the majority of patients never need surgery; and, furthermore, few patients meet the above restrictive conditions.

The logical place to begin is with the natural history of the disease. As stated by Boyd, "The critical evaluation of any type of treatment of a disease should be made against the background of the natural course of the disease, particularly in a generalized progressive disease like arteriosclerosis."[2]

For starters, how big is the problem? In their review, Dormandy and Mahir[3] summarized 11 studies dealing with the prevalence of peripheral vascular disease and the incidence of intermittent claudication. These studies varied from a simple questionnaire format to in-depth interview, physical examination, and noninvasive vascular laboratory studies. When the questionnaires were followed-up with in-depth examination, these investigators found an approximate 30 percent false-positive rate of apparent peripheral vascular disease alone. These false positives represent people with arthritis, sciatica, and spinal osteoarthritis rather than claudication from atherosclerosis.

In a population of men less than 50 years old, the prevalence of lower extremity vascular disease is 1 to 1.5 percent. This figure increases with age, such that by the age of 60 the prevalence is 4 to 6 percent. The same is true for incidence of claudication—in men less than 60 years old the figure is 0.5 percent per year; over the age of 60 it increases to 4 percent per year. Although less data are available for women, it would appear that the prevalence of vascular disease is about equal to men and that incidence of claudication appears to lag behind men by approximately ten years.

Is everyone in the population equally at risk or are there certain high-risk subgroups? A number of studies[1,4-6] have shown that there are high-risk subgroups. Patients with coronary artery disease and diabetes mellitus and cigarette smokers are likely to have associated peripheral vascular disease. Controversy still exists regarding the role of hypertension, hypercholesterolemia, and elevated triglycerides. These high-risk factors not only manifest claudication with increased frequency, but also they probably affect the progression and outcome. The cumulative effect of these risk factors also is more than additive. For instance, Hughson and colleagues[4] have reported that in a patient with coronary artery disease, diabetes, and smoking, the 5-year incidence of claudication increased from 2 percent to 11.4 percent per year. They also broke these data down into prevalence-related risk factors. One factor increased the prevalence threefold. All three factors together resulted in a 22-fold increase.

Coronary artery disease in and of itself is associated with a four- to sevenfold increase in the associated likelihood of peripheral vascular disease; diabetes mellitus a three- to sixfold increase; and smoking greater than 15 cigarettes per day had a ninefold increased association. Smoking, the one factor that we would appear to have much control over, is also the factor with the highest associated risk. Now that we have some idea of how many and who are at risk, what happens once they have developed symptoms of claudication?

The eight studies summarized in Table I deal with progression of disease following presentation with claudication to a physician. This progression table shows that overall there is good agreement that approximately 25 percent of patients with intermittent claudication will experience any progression of symptoms in their whole lifetime. Thus, 75 percent stabilize or improve, eliminating three-fourths of the patients from any consideration of operative intervention simply by virtue of our understanding and knowledge of the natural history of the disease.

Of note, in the study by Boyd[2] in which 1,440 patients were followed, only 10 percent of the patients progressed within the first 12 months. This is significant because we, therefore, have the luxury of time for observation and clinical reassessment when confronted with a patient with claudication. Even of those who deteriorate symptomatically, ultimately only 3 to 5 percent will undergo amputation. This is with *or without* surgery.

What about amputation? If one considers all claudicators, the overall amputation rate probably is less than 2 percent. Studies are available to indicate that the combined amputation rate is 2 to 5 percent in patients followed by physicians.[3] As usual, one must be very careful in reading and interpreting data from the surgical literature. For instance, the study by Szilaygi[3] is not representative in that 75 percent of his patients had rest pain and were not true claudicators alone.

Is there any way to predict which patients are at higher risk for limb loss? There definitely are prognosticators of gloom:

TABLE I. INTERMITTENT CLAUDICATION: CLINICAL PROGRESS FROM PRESENTATION TO A DOCTOR*

FIRST AUTHOR (YEAR OF PUBLICATION)	NUMBER OF PATIENTS	FOLLOW-UP (YEARS)	STABLE OR IMPROVED	WORSE
LeFevre (1959)	185	5	74.6	25.4
Bloor (1961)	1476	4-10	71	29
Schadt (1961)	362	9	93.3**	6.7**
Begg (1962)	198	5-13	68.8	31.2
Taylor (1962)	412	3-12	82.7	17.3
Ulrich (1973)	304	0.6-6.4	75	25
Imparto (1975)	104	0.5-8	79	21
Kallero (1981)	193	8.5-11.5	78.8	21.1

*From Dormandy, J.A. and Mahir, M.S.: The natural history of peripheral atheromatous disease of the legs. In Vascular Surgery: Issues in Current Practice. R.M. Greenhalgh, C.W. Jamieson, and A.N. Nicolaides (eds.). New York: Grune & Stratton, 1986, p. 7.
**Survivors only.

1. Age greater than 65 years is associated with an increased amputation rate.
2. Those patients with distal vascular disease have an amputation rate of 7 percent versus 2 percent for patients without distal disease.
3. In a study by Juergens and associates[7] with 5-year follow-up, in those patients who continued to smoke there was 11.4 percent amputation rate versus 0 percent for patients who stopped smoking.
4. Diabetes increases the risk of amputation fivefold.
5. Finally, symptom severity is an apparent prognostic factor. Those patients who have worse claudication tend to have an increased amputation rate. Indeed, the 2 to 3 percent amputation rate in claudicators jumps to 9 percent in those patients with rest pain.

Unfortunately, the patients most at risk for amputation are also those patients considered to be the poorest operative candidates. Unfortunately for the claudicator, the status of his lower extremity is not his only or most major problem.

Malone and associates[1] noted that the life expectancy of patients with symptoms of aortoiliac disease was ten years less than their age-matched controls. The normal 50-year-old male has an 87 percent 5-year expected survival and a 73 percent 10-year survival. If he has cerebral vascular disease, his life expectancy drops to 77 percent and 36 percent at five and 10 years, respectively. If he has claudication, his expectancy is 87 percent and 40 percent. With coronary artery disease, he can expect a 72 percent and 25 percent survival at five and ten years. With diabetes mellitus, he has an 83 percent and 0 percent chance of living five and ten years. The basis for this would not appear to be the claudication but the vascular disease in vital anatomic areas. Coronary artery disease and cerebral vascular disease with claudication have an increased mortality, whereas claudication alone is not significantly more ominous than the control population.

Diabetes mellitus is a bad prognosticator, not only for limb survival but also for total body survival. The poor prognosis of patients with intermittent claudication and diabetes mellitus is well recognized. There was a 100 percent mortality within eight years for diabetic patients undergoing arterial reconstruction for intermittent claudication.[1] Unfortunately, diabetics are not the only subgroup with a decreased life expectancy. Overall, after five, ten, and 15 years of follow-up for patients with claudication, the mean mortality rate is 30, 50, and 70 percent, respectively.

This overall dismal picture must play a critical role in assessing the indications for surgery in patients who present with claudication. Should patients with poor long-term survival, specifically those patients with diabetes mellitus and significant coronary artery disease, risk reconstructive vascular surgery for symptomatic intermittent claudication or should they be reassured that their disease will stabilize? The responsible vascular surgeon should not risk life with surgery unless his patient's limb is at risk from disease.

Malone and associates[1] and Darling[8] have stated that "reconstructive procedures should be in good-risk patients with favorable anatomy." Do candidates who fulfill these criteria exist? As you can see, most of the vascular surgical investigators would prefer that the patient be less than 65 years old, have proximal disease only, be a non-smoker, have no evidence of coronary artery disease, and not have diabetes mellitus. Do any such candidates exist?

What percent of patients with claudication have ominous associated disease? Using history and EKG as screening methods, up to 58 percent of patients with intermittent claudication also have coronary artery disease (Table II).

Although historically 40 to 60 percent of patients with claudication would appear to have coronary artery disease,[9] it may prove to be much higher than this when more invasive methods of delineating coronary anatomy and disease are utilized. It would appear that a minimum of two-thirds of claudicators have objective evidence of coronary artery disease. Disease increases with age. Many of the surgical series[2-4] indicate that only 25 to 30 percent of patients have proximal vascular disease only.

As you can see, the optimal candidates are few in number. As patients get older, the odds get worse.

Figure 1 is perioperative mortality analysis by age for claudicators undergoing reconstructive surgery. In patients over the age of 80 years, the mortality rate is as

TABLE II.   PREVALENCE OF CORONARY ARTERY DISEASE AT PRESENTATION TO A DOCTOR (SELECTED STUDIES)*

FIRST AUTHOR (YEAR OF PUBLICATION)	NUMBER OF PATIENTS	METHOD OF SCREENING	CORONARY ARTERY DISEASE (%)
Begg (1962)	198	Clinical history + ECG	19
DeWesse (1977)	103	Clinical history + ECG	34
Malone (1977)	180	Clinical history + ECG	58
Hughson (1978)	160	Clinical history + ECG	36
Szilagyi (1979)	531	Clinical history + ECG	38.5
Crawford (1981)	949	Clinical history + ECG	38
Hertzer (1981)	256	Clinical history + ECG	47
Vecht (1982)	100	Modified treadmill stress ECG	62
Hertzer (1984)	381	Angiography	90
Brewster (1985)	54	Dipyridamole stress-thallium imaging	63

*From Dormandy, J.A. and Mahir, M.S.: The natural history of peripheral atheromatous disease of the legs. In Vascular Surgery: Issues in Current Practice. R.M. Greenhalgh, C.W. Jamieson, and A.N. Nicolaides (eds.). New York: Grune & Stratton, 1986, p. 9.

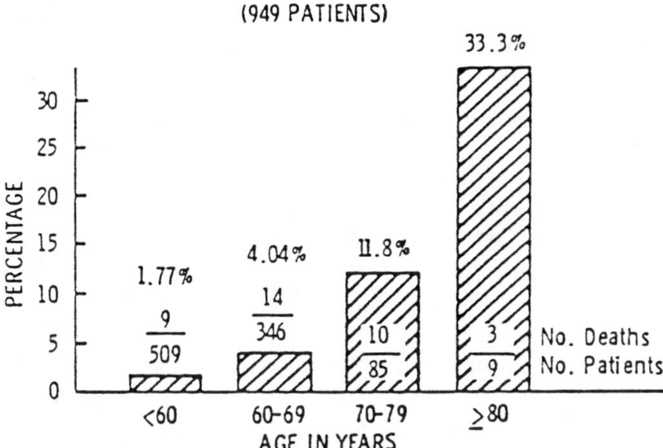

FIGURE 1.   Operative mortality rate according to age. From Crawford, E.S., Bomberger, R.A., Glaeser, D.H., et al.: Aorto-iliac occlusive disease: Factors influencing survival and function following reconstructive operation over a 25-year period. Surgery, 90:1056, 1981.

high as 33 percent. As you can see, these are not trivial procedures in the older patients.

If the surgery is not the therapeutic answer for the majority of patients with intermittent claudication, what can be done? Must we abandon our patients? The answer emphatically is NO. Probably the most important factor is the cessation of smoking. Hughson and colleagues[4] analyzed those patients who stopped smoking versus those patients who continued to smoke. They defined adverse events as death, amputation, onset of claudication in a previously asymptomatic limb, myocardial infarction, cerebrovascular accident, or the necessity of operation. Those patients who reduced or stopped smoking had an increased life expectancy, improved symptoms, and decreased amputation rate. The only correctable factor for symptom and outcome improvement was cessation of smoking.

In addition to cessation of smoking, it has been shown in multiple studies that patients should be started on exercise programs.[10,11] Ekroth and colleagues[10] followed patients for exercise tolerance changes as well as calf blood flow changes. They found that 88 percent of patients were able to improve total walking distance by 234 percent! Initially, 16 percent of the patients could only walk 1,000 meters; however, following the exercise program, greater than 40 percent could reach that distance. In addition, improvement appeared to be independent of the level of disease or the presence of diabetes mellitus.

Finally, there is the question of pharmacological treatment. Pentoxifylline has been compared in double-blind studies with placebo, and patients were then reevaluated subjectively. It works.[11,12] Pentoxifylline is not a direct vasodilator but would appear to increase both blood flow and tissue oxygenation by altering red blood cell rigidity. This new group of agents has been termed "hemorrheologic agents." It would appear that, by altering the red cell flexibility, erythrocytes have an increased ability to carry oxygen to tissues. Although this appears experimentally significant, further clinical investigation will need to be performed to outline its ultimate therapeutic role.

In review, when a patient with claudication comes to your office, it is first necessary to determine the onset and chronicity of the symptoms. For those patients who are over-weight and smoke, they should be encouraged to go on an exercise and weight-reduction program as well as to stop smoking. Successful anti-smoking and exercise programs will dwarf any other modes of therapy in ultimate efficacy.

If patients have more chronic or even progressive disease that is not disabling, they also should be followed conservatively and encouraged to stop smoking. For those patients who have significant disability that either alters their lifestyle or impairs their work, they should undergo arteriography. If they are found to have favorable anatomy, are not smokers, have good hearts and no evidence of diabetes mellitus, they should be offered the option of surgery. These are the patients who may actually benefit. The problem is that they are few and far between.

REFERENCES

1. Malone, J.M., Moore, W.S., and Goldstone, J.: Life expectancy following aorto-femoral arterial grafting. Surgery, 81(5):551–555, 1977.
2. Boyd, A.M.: The natural course of arteriosclerosis of the lower extremities. Angiology, 11:10–14, 1960.
3. Dormandy, J.A. and Mahir, M.S.: The natural history of peripheral atheromatous disease of the legs. In Vascular Surgery: Issues in Current Practice. R.M. Greenhalgh, C.W. Jamieson, and A.N. Nicolaides, (eds.). New York: Grune & Stratton, 1986, 3–17.
4. Hughson, W.G., Mann, J.I., Tibbs, D.J., Woods, H.F., and Walton, I.: Intermittent claudication: factors determining outcome. Br. Med. J., 1:1377–1379, 1978.
5. Kannel, W.B., Skinner, J.J., Schwartz, M.J., and Shurtleff, D.: Intermittent claudication: Incidence in the Framingham study. Circulation, 41:875–883, 1970.
6. Crawford, E.S., Bomberger, R.A., Glaeser, D.H., et al.: Aorto-iliac occlusive disease: Factors influencing survival and function following reconstructive operation over a 25-year period. Surgery, 90:1055–1067, 1981.
7. Juergens, J.L., Barker, N.W., and Hines, E.A., Jr.: Arteriosclerosis obliterans: Review of 520 cases with specific reference to pathogenic and prognostic factors. Circulation, 21: 188–195, 1960.
8. Darling, R.C., Brewster, D.C., Hallett, J.W., Jr., and Darling, R.C., III: Aorto-iliac reconstruction. Surg. Clin. North Am., 59(4), 565–579, 1979.
9. Greenhalgh, R.M., Laing, S., Ellis, M., et al.: How can we detect early subclinical disease? In Vascular Surgery: Issues and Current Practice. R.M. Greenhalgh, C.W. Jamieson, and A.N. Nicolaides, (eds.). New York: Grune & Stratton, 1986, 57–74.
10. Ekroth, R., Dahllof, A-G, Gundevall, B., Holm, J., and Schersten, T.: Physical training of patients with intermittent claudication: Indications, methods, and results. Surgery, 84:640–643, 1978.
11. Cronenwett, J.L., Warner, K.G., Zelenock, G.B., et al.: Intermittent claudication: Current results of nonoperative management. Arch. Surg., 119:430–436, 1984.
12. Bollinger, A.: Can drugs improve the circulation in arterial disease? In Vascular Surgery: Issues in Current Practice. R.M. Greenhalgh, C.W. Jamieson, and A.N. Nicolaides, (eds.). New York: Grune & Stratton, 1986, 29–35.

DEBATE XIV

Can White Cells Be Both Good And Bad?

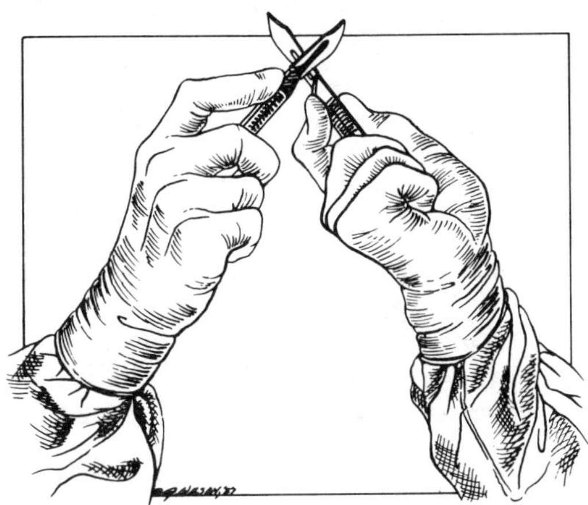

White blood cells serve as the body's circulating cellular defense mechanism. Somewhat surprisingly, only one percent of our white cells are intravascular. The white cell army is formidable—and almost all of it is in reserve. White cells can opsonize, phagocytize, and produce toxic oxygen-free radicals. When friendly, white cells provide essential and reassuring defense. However, Dr. Grosso argues that white cells, when provoked, can become ugly. He characterizes the white cell defenders as suicide pellets capable of metamorphosizing into a mindless, self-mutilating mob.

Much clinical research is subject to the vagaries of human investigation. Studies are not controlled. Conclusions are, at best, controversial. Not so with white cell studies, says Dr. Grosso. Human white cells can be explanted and specifically studied in elegantly precise fashion. No confusion here. White cells can be disruptive, dangerous, and detrimental.

Dr. Grosso catalogs a litany of *in vitro* investigations documenting microvascular lung injury by stimulated granulocytes. Even brief exposure of animal endothelial cells to autologous complement-activated white cells produces significant cytotoxicity. Indeed, the injury associated with oxygen toxicity, smoking, and even myocardial infarction arguably is mediated substantively by white cells. In addition, animal and clinical evidence overwhelmingly implicates white cells as mediators of both adult respiratory distress syndrome and multiple organ failure.

But, are neutrophils the whole, or even a major part, of the story? Dr. Patt says no.

Circulating blood is contained within an endothelial-lined vascular compartment. This endovascular endothelial lining should be the first line of defense against any blood-borne invasion. Indeed, endothelial cell damage is an early feature of adult respiratory distress syndrome and multiple organ failure. If neutrophils are essential culprits in these devastating clinical entities, then white cell depletion should eliminate, or at least attenuate, these syndromes. Dr. Patt presents full-blown ARDS in neutropenic patients following either bone marrow transplantation or chemotherapy. This is a severe blow to those who would incriminate the white cell as an essential mediator of endothelial cell injury.

The sole goal of animal studies is to permit extrapolation to human disease. Even the yuppies do not crusade against ARDS in rabbits. Dr. Patt critiques laboratory studies. She exposes investigations implicating neutrophils as non-physiologic either qualitatively or quantitatively. Examining pulmonary infiltrates following paraquat is like pitting Coppertone against a flame thrower. These extreme investigations are simply irrelevant. Even when it is feasible to mimic real human disease, the leap from a controlled but contrived basic laboratory animal preparation to a patient's bedside is a surreal leap of faith.

Dr. Patt then catalogs an imposing list of substances that can inflict endothelial damage directly without the aid of neutrophils. By documenting damage in neutropenic patients, reproducing end-organ failure by direct action of toxins, and assailing contrived laboratory studies as unrelated to clinical disease, Dr. Patt marshals a persuasive white cell defense. Perhaps the white cell is not guilty.

XIV-A: WHITE CELLS ARE DETRIMENTAL AND CONTRIBUTE TO DISEASE

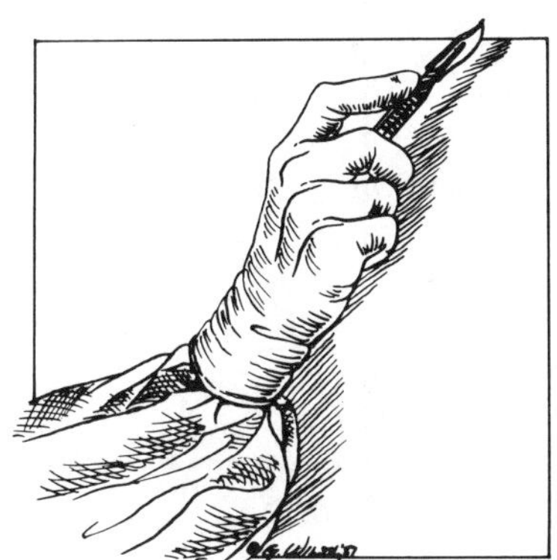

MICHAEL A. GROSSO, M.D.

Unlike most debates presented in this book, the question of whether white cells contribute to disease can be answered clearly and unambiguously. The answer is emphatically yes. Most clinical debates rely on research that is generated from patient populations. These studies, of necessity, have design flaws that impeach their conclusions. Clinical research cannot control most variables; the systems and model under study are exceptionally complex (the human organism), and the objective end points are often insensitive (i.e., mortality). Conversely, basic science research strives to control most, if not all, variables. In addition, the systems or model under study can be tightly controlled (i.e., isolated organ perfusion); and the results measured may be very specific (i.e., uptake of labeled serotonin).

The distinction between these two types of research is clear in this debate. The topic under discussion has been investigated under controlled laboratory conditions. Based on such rigorous investigation, we can definitively demonstrate that white cells contribute to disease.

The mechanisms by which white blood cells provide defense to the host have been elucidated. Two major mechanisms are known:

1. **Granule-associated.** This includes enzymes and cationic proteins plus myeloperoxidase.
2. **Granule-independent.** This involves uptake of oxygen by phagocytic cells and production of oxygen-free radicals including hydrogen peroxide, hydroxyl radical, singlet oxygen, hypochlorous acid, and chloramines.

Through these two mechanisms, the granule-associated and the granule-independent, white cells deliver lethal blows to invading organisms. It is now known, however, that, under some disease conditions, these same white cells can use both of these mechanisms to initiate and/or amplify autogenous cellular injury. Stimulated phagocytic leukocytes produce superoxide radicals that can be detected experimentally[1] (Figure 1). There is ample evidence to suggest that this is a major mechanism in the production of cellular injury by a patient's own white cells. Let us examine the

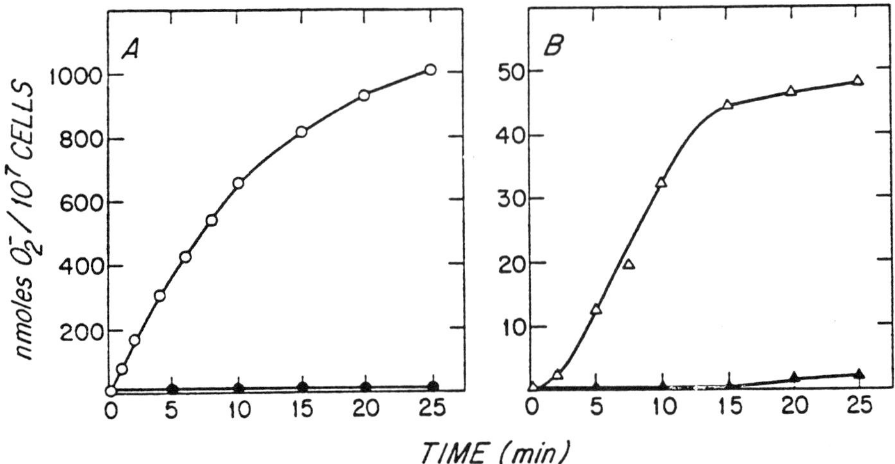

FIGURE 1.   Time-course of superoxide release by neutrophils. Each of the curves depicted is representative of the time-course of superoxide release by phagocytizing human blood neutrophils (A, ○) and elicited guinea pig peritoneal neutrophils (B, △). The corresponding closed symbols (● ▲) are for nonphagocytizing cells. Opsonized zymosan (3 mg/ml) served as the stimulating agent. From Badwey, J. and Karnovsky, M.: Production of superoxide by phagocytic leukocytes: A paradigm for stimulus-response phenomena. Curr. Top. Cell. Reg., 28:184, 1986.

evidence at two levels: (1) the organ level and (2) the organismal level—clinical disease states.

ORGAN DAMAGE *IN VITRO/IN VIVO*

Lung.   Studies[2,3] have shown that increases in microvascular permeability following injury by either microembolization (simulating pulmonary embolus) or by endotoxemia are granulocyte dependent. Measures of microvascular injury such as lung lymph flow and lung lymph protein clearance are significantly lower following granulocyte depletion. These studies[2,3] concluded that circulating granulocytes were obligate participants in the increased lung vascular permeability associated with microembolization or endotoxemia-induced injury.

Simon and colleagues[4] exposed rat alveolar epithelial cells to stimulated white cells. Cytotoxicity was measured by the amount of labeled chromium (51-Cr) released from 51-Cr labeled alveolar cells. They found a direct relationship between cytotoxicity (chromium release) and the total number of stimulated neutrophils exposed to the alveolar cells (Figure 2).

In a similar study,[5] cultured lung endothelial cells were exposed to complement-activated granulocytes; damage was measured by the chromium release assay. Brief exposure of the endothelial cells to the stimulated white blood cells (WBC) resulted in significant cytotoxicity (chromium release). This damage was inhibited appreciably by the oxygen radical scavengers superoxide dismutase (SOD) and catalase (Figure 3). These investigations concluded that white blood cells caused significant endothelial

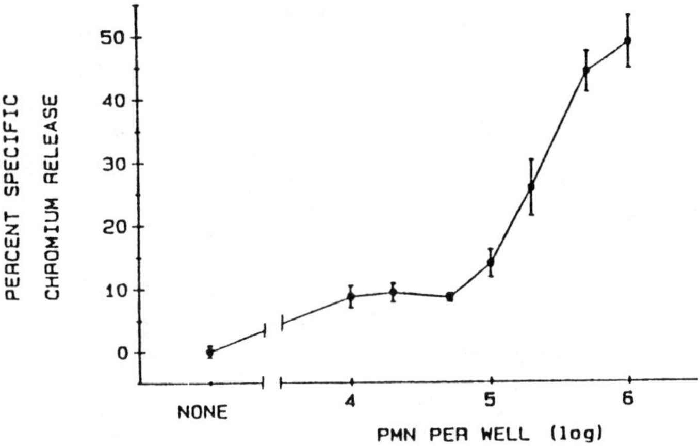

FIGURE 2. From Simon R.H., DeHart, P.D., and Todd, R.F., III: Neutrophil-induced injury of rat pulmonary alveolar epithelial cells. J. Clin. Invest., 78:1377, 1986.

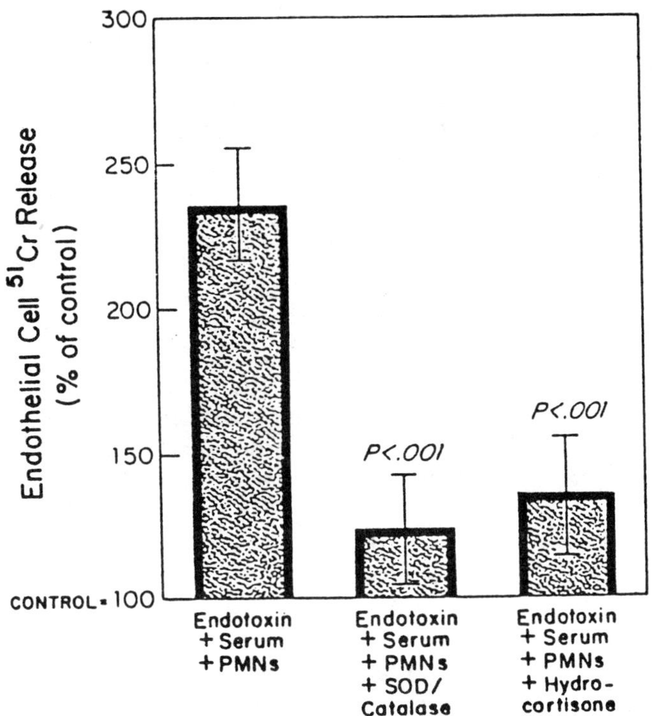

FIGURE 3. Effects of endotoxin on endothelial cells cultured from human umbilical veins and labeled with ^{51}Cr. Brief exposure to polymorphonuclear leukocytes (PMNs) and endotoxin damaged these cells, but this damage was appreciably inhibited by the toxic oxygen-radical dissipators, superoxide dismutase (SOD) and catalase, or by hydrocortisone (1 mg per milliliter). Similar amounts of endotoxin and serum, in the absence of polymorphonuclear leukocytes, caused no measurable damage. From Jacob, H.S., Craddock, P.R., Hammerschmidt, D.E., and Moldow, C.F.: Complement-induced granulocyte aggregation: An unsuspected mechanism of disease. New Engl. J. Med., 302:792, 1980.

cell damage via toxic oxygen metabolites. In fact, evidence exists that pulmonary oxygen toxicity may be mediated by white blood cells.[6] In rats exposed to hyperoxic conditions (100 percent O_2), pulmonary white blood cell lavage counts and the WBC chemotactic index of lavage supernatants correlated with the degree of exposure to hyperoxia.

An additional study by the same group[7] confirmed the initial observations. Rabbits exposed to 100 percent oxygen for 72 hours revealed increased lung water and increased albumin content in alveolar lavage fluids. These increases correlated with an increase in number of white cells recovered in lung lavages. Rabbits made neutropenic showed significantly reduced lung water, lavage albumin content, and mortality. This group concluded that white cells play a prominent role in the mediation of pulmonary oxygen toxicity.

An interesting study[8] recently revealed that white blood cells isolated from the lungs of smokers produce significantly greater amounts of superoxide radicals as compared to lung lavage white cells from non-smokers.

Liver. Keller and colleagues[9] isolated rat hepatocytes and quantitated cell function by the rate of protein synthesis as measured by H3-leucine incorporation. White cells were added to the isolated hepatocytes in the presence and in the absence of an endotoxin stimulus. Hepatocytes in the presence of endotoxin-stimulated white cells displayed a marked decrease in H3-leucine incorporation. These investigators concluded that stimulated white cells can induce hepatocyte injury.

The peripheral blood of patients with active liver disease, as well as peripheral blood of healthy controls, was exposed to chromium-labeled liver lipoprotein-coated erythrocytes; and cell toxicity was measured (chromium-release).[10] In this assay for target cells coated with human liver lipoprotein as compared to leukocytes from healthy controls, leukocytes from patients with active liver disease were markedly cytotoxic.

Kidney. Shah and colleagues,[11] using an hydroxy-proline release assay, measured the degradation of human glomerular basement membrane by stimulated neutrophils. They found that stimulated neutrophils produced significant release of hydroxyproline (cytotoxicity). This cytotoxicity could be decreased significantly by the addition of catalase (an oxygen radical scavenger) to the system. They concluded that the degradation of human glomerular basement membrane occurred by stimulated neutrophils via reactive oxygen metabolites.

In a rabbit model, antibody-induced glomerulonephritis could be reduced significantly by white blood cell depletion with anti-rabbit macrophage serum.[12]

Bowel. In a feline intestine model, Grisham and colleagues[13] utilized a three-hour ischemic injury followed by one hour of reperfusion using myeloperoxidase to monitor neutrophil accumulation and allopurinol and superoxide dismutase (SOD) to identify oxygen metabolite injury. They found that ischemia and reperfusion resulted in the accumulation of neutrophils and neutrophil-derived oxygen metabolites. White blood cells unequivocally mediated and exacerbated the intestinal ischemic injury.

Heart. A recent study investigated the role of leukocytes in acute myocardial infarction.[14] An acute coronary occlusion/reperfusion model was utilized in the open-chest dogs. Infarction was measured by the degree of arachidonic acid metabolite release. Treatment groups consisted of control animals and animals pretreated with hydroxyurea which induced neutrophil depletion. They found that the neutrophil-depleted group had a marked decrease in white blood cell infiltration into the injured myocardium, and this was associated with a dramatic decrease in total area infarcted.

A similar study by Romson,[15] again utilizing open-chest dogs with acute coronary occlusion, reperfusion, and white blood cell depletion (neutrophil anti-serum), yielded similar results. Infarct size as compared to area at risk was identified by the TTC/Evans Blue method. They found a marked reduction in leukocyte infiltration into the infarcted myocardium in treated (neutrophil-depleted) dogs. This was associated with a marked decrease in infarct size.

An overwhelming body of data exists implicating the WBC as an active participant in the initiation or amplification of cell or tissue destruction in clinically relevant animal models of human disease states.

CLINICAL STUDIES

Adult Respiratory Distress Syndrome—ARDS. Blood samples from two near-drowning patients were measured for toxic oxygen metabolites (lipid peroxides) in a recent study.[16] One patient developed acute pulmonary edema with hypoxemia. This patient with pulmonary insufficiency had marked increase in the serum level of lipid peroxides. Tennenberg and colleagues[17] looked at patients with frank ARDS, patients at risk for ARDS, and control patients and measured the degree of activated neutrophils in their serum. Patients with ARDS or patients at high risk to develop ARDS had significant evidence of complement-mediated neutrophil activation, indicating the presence of circulating stimulated white blood cells.

A recent review by Glauser[18] has summarized the current role of the neutrophil in ARDS:

1. Neutrophil numbers are increased in lung lavages of *animal models* and *patients* with ARDS.
2. Neutrophil function is abnormal in the blood of patients with ARDS (chemotaxis, complement activation).
3. Neutrophils accumulate in pulmonary capillaries in *animal models* and *human disease ARDS.*
4. Neutrophil-generated unstable oxygen radicals can produce endothelial cell damage. Scavengers of unstable oxygen radicals ameliorate increased alveolar capillary membrane permeability in animal models.
5. Neutrophil depletion blunts or eradicates increased alveolar capillary membrane permeability in animal models.

There is ample evidence to implicate the white cell as a mediator of pulmonary injury in animal models. There continues to grow supporting data in the clinical setting of ARDS.

Ischemia/Reperfusion—Heart, Bowel, Brain. A current review by Grisham and colleagues[13] has shown that circulating neutrophils appear to mediate and/or amplify tissue injury associated with an ischemic/reperfusion insult (Figure 4).

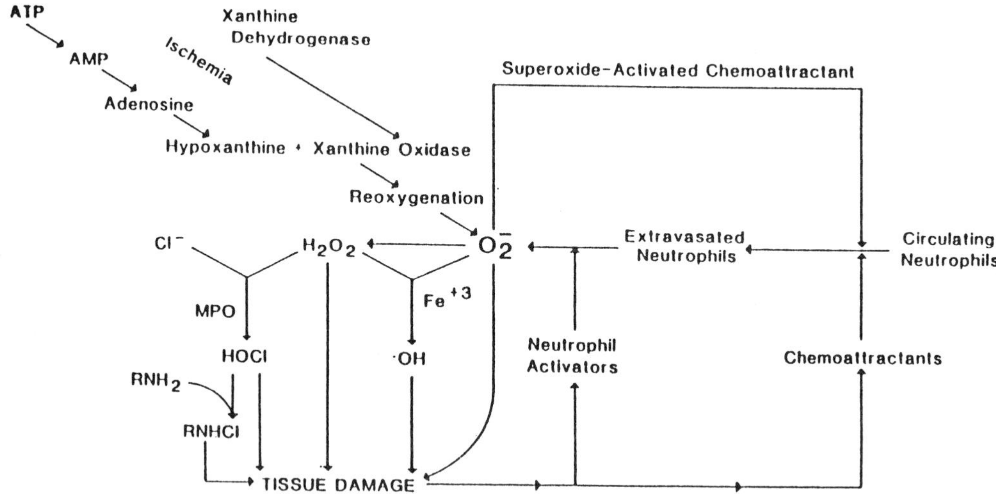

FIGURE 4. Proposed relationship between xanthine oxidase (XO)-generated superoxide (O_2^-), neutrophil infiltration, and mucosal injury. Reoxygenation of ischemic tissue leads to production of XO-generated O_2^-. Superoxide per se or reduced O_2 species derived from O_2^- may be cytotoxic to reperfused tissue. Injured cells release neutrophil activators and chemoattractants that recruit circulating leukocytes into tissues where they exacerbate cell necrosis. Alternatively, XO-generated O_2^- may not directly mediate cell injury; O_2^- may simply react with plasma lipoproteins to produce O_2^--activated chemoattractants. In this scheme, extravasated neutrophils directly mediate injury produced by reperfusion of an ischemic tissue. From Grisham, M.B., Hernandez, L.A., and Granger, D.N.: Xanthine oxidase and neutrophil infiltration in intestinal ischemia. Am. J. Physiol., 251:G573, 1986.

Although hypothetical, this schema continues to be supported overwhelmingly by animal model data; and evidence grows daily for its clinical applicability.

Hepatic Failure/Multiple Organ Failure (MOF). Nuytinck and colleagues[19] examined 71 patients with multiple trauma and measured daily blood samples for leukocytes, platelets, white blood cell enzymes, alpha-antitrypsin, protein, haptoglobin, albumin, fibronectin, and complement factors/activation. They found that the correlation between injury severity and multiple organ failure was best predicted by the human white blood cell enzyme levels, implicating the white blood cell as the mediator of MOF. Again, a recent review by Keller[20] delineates the macrophage-mediated modulation of hepatic function in multiple-system failure (Figure 5).

SUMMARY

There appears to be a large body of data in the *in vivo* and *in vitro* animal models that clearly supports the notion that white blood cells can either amplify and/or mediate destruction of autogenous cells and organs. Because of the complexity in the clinical situations, data to support the concept that white cells significantly contribute to human disease states in man has been slow to accumulate. However, data are accumulating. There is every reason to believe that the animal model systems of our clinical disease states are accurate representations; and, therefore, the white blood cell can and will be implicated as a mediator/amplifier of human disease states. Given

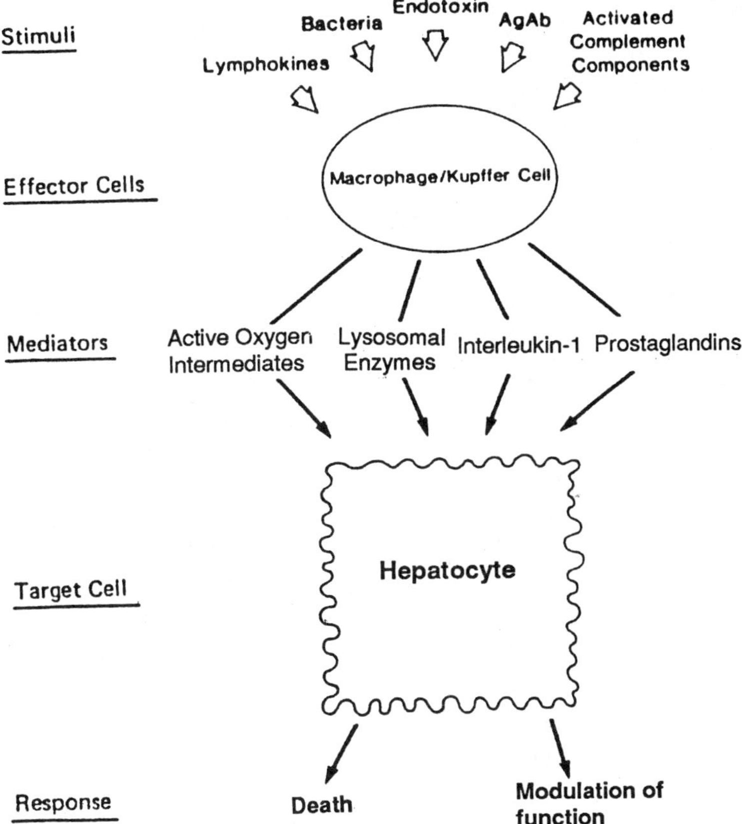

FIGURE 5. Macrophage/Kupffer-cell-mediated alteration of hepatocytes. A possible scheme for the mechanism of action of hepatic failure in patients with the MSOF syndrome is presented. Various stimuli occurring in septic or traumatized patients may cause the release of a number of potentially injurious mediators from macrophages or Kupffer cells. These mediators may result in an alteration of function or death of the adjacent hepatocytes. From Keller, G.A., West, M.A., Cerra, F.B., and Simmons, R.L.: Macrophage-mediated modulation of hepatic function in multiple-system failure. J. Surg. Res., 39:560, 1985.

this, specific therapies at inhibiting the destructive capacities of the white blood cell could lead to significant improvement in survival in such lethal conditions as adult respiratory distress syndrome, post-ischemic reperfusion injury following myocardial infarction, splanchnic ischemia, or stroke in addition to sepsis and multiple organ failure.

REFERENCES

1. Badwey, J. and Karnovsky, M.: Production of superoxide by phagocytic leukocytes: A paradigm for stimulus-response phenomena. Curr. Top. Cell. Reg., 28:183–208, 1986.

2. Flick, M.R., Perel, A., and Staub, N.C.: Leukocytes are required for increased lung microvascular permeability after microembolization in sheep. Circ. Res., 48:344-351, 1981.

3. Heflin, C.A., Jr., and Brigham, K.L.: Prevention by granulocyte depletion of increased vascular permeability of sheep lung following endotoxemia. J. Clin. Invest., 68:1253-1260, 1981.

4. Simon, R.H., DeHart, P.D., and Todd, R.F., III: Neutrophil-induced injury of rat pulmonary alveolar epithelial cells. J. Clin. Invest., 78:1375-1386, 1986.

5. Jacob, H.S., Craddock, P.R., Hammerschmidt, D.E., and Moldow, C.F.: Complement-induced granulocyte aggregation: An unsuspected mechanism of trauma. New Engl. J. Med., 302:789-794, 1980.

6. Fox, R.B., Hoidal, J.R., Brown, D.M., and Repine, J.E.: Pulmonary inflammation due to oxygen toxicity: Involvement of chemotactic factors and polymorphonuclear leukocytes. Am. Rev. Respir. Dis., 123:521-523, 1981.

7. Fox, R.B., Shasby, D.M., Harada, R.N., and Repine, J.E.: A novel mechanism for pulmonary oxygen toxicity: Phagocyte mediated lung injury. Chest, 80:3S-4S, 1981.

8. Bergstrand, H., Bjornson, A., Eklund, A., et al.: Stimuli-induced superoxide radical generation *in vitro* by human alveolar macrophages from smokers. J. Free Radicals Bio. Med., 2:119-127, 1986.

9. Keller, G.A., West, M.A., Cerra, F.B., and Simmons, R.L.: Modulation of hepatocyte protein synthesis by endotoxin activated Kupffer cells. Ann. Surg., 201:87-95, 1985.

10. Vogten, A.J.M., Hadzic, N., Shorter, R.G., et al.: Cell-mediated cytotoxicity in chronic active liver disease: A new test system. Gastroenterology, 74:883-889, 1978.

11. Shah, S.V., Baricos, W.H., and Basci, A.: Degradation of human glomerular basement membrane by stimulated neutrophils: Activation of a metalloproteinase(s) by reactive oxygen metabolites. J. Clin. Invest., 79:25-31, 1987.

12. Holdsworth, S.R., Neale, T.J., and Wilson, C.B.: Abrogation of macrophage-dependent injury in experimental glomerulonephritis in the rabbit: Use of an antimacrophage serum. J. Clin. Invest., 68:686-698, 1981.

13. Grisham, M.B., Hernandez, L.A., and Granger, D.N.: Xanthine oxidase and neutrophil infiltration in intestinal ischemia. Am. J. Physiol., 251:G567-574, 1986.

14. Mullane, K.M., Read, N., Salmon, J.A., and Moncada, S.: Role of leukocytes in acute myocardial infarction in anesthetized dogs: Relationship to myocardial salvage by anti-inflammatory drugs. J. Pharm. Exp. Therap., 228:510-522, 1984.

15. Romson, J.L., Hook, B.G., Kunkel, S.L., et al.: Reduction of the extent of ischemic myocardial injury by neutrophil depletion in the dog. Circulation, 67:1016-1023, 1983.

16. Bertrand, Y., Artoisenet, A., Allard, B., et al.: Lipid peroxidation and alpha-tocopherol during an acute respiratory failure after near drowning. Int. Care Med., 11:65-67, 1985.

17. Tennenberg, S.D., Jacobs, M.P., and Solomkin, J.S.: Complement-mediated neutrophil activated in sepsis- and trauma-related adult respiratory distress syndrome: Clarification with radioaerosol lung scans. Arch. Surg., 122:26-32, 1987.

18. Glauser, F.L. and Fairman, R.P.: The uncertain role of the neutrophil in increased permeability pulmonary edema. Chest, 88:601-607, 1985.

19. Nuytinck, J.K.S., Goris, R.J.A., Redl, H., et al.: Post-traumatic complications and inflammatory mediators. Arch. Surg., 121:886-890, 1986.

20. Keller, G.A., West, M.A., Cerra, F.B., and Simmons, R.L.: Macrophage-mediated modulation of hepatic function in multiple-system failure. J. Surg. Res., 39:555-563, 1985.

XIV-B: NEUTROPHILS ARE OVER-RATED AS MEDIATORS OF VASCULAR INJURY

ANITA PATT, M.D.

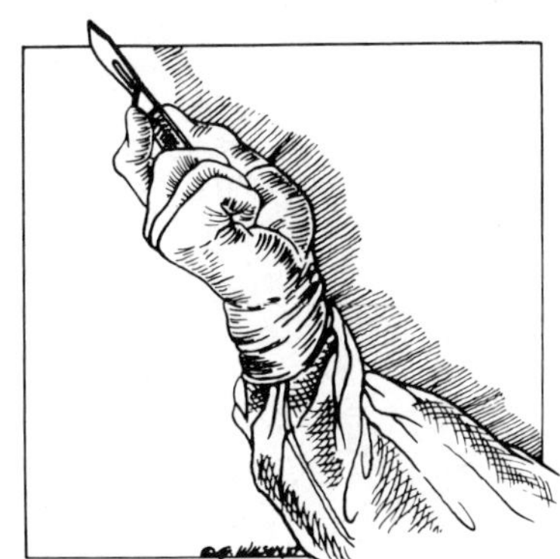

We know that endothelial cell damage and neutrophil accumulation are early features of many vascular permeability syndromes: ARDS, ischemia-reperfusion, and inflammatory diseases. However, the contention that neutrophils are the only primary or the most important mediator of endothelial cell injury in these syndromes is unproven.

There are at least four strikes against the contribution of neutrophils to vascular injury:

I. Endothelial cell damage occurs in the absence of neutrophil infiltration and activation.
II. Studies implicating neutrophils as mediators of endothelial cell damage are conducted in animal and *in vitro* models that do not reflect clinical disease accurately.
III. Many factors other than neutrophils can cause endothelial cell damage.
IV. Because neutrophils participate in host defense and healing, inhibiting neutrophil function would be detrimental.

Let us explore in greater detail the evidence supporting each of these premises.

I. Endothelial cell damage occurs in the absence of neutrophil infiltration and activation.

Two major observations support this statement. The first observation is that neutrophil depletion does not prevent endothelial cell injury. The most convincing and clinically relevant evidence supporting this observation is the many studies that have demonstrated that neutropenic patients develop ARDS. For example:

a. Nine patients following bone-marrow transplant[1,2]
b. Eleven patients with sepsis[3]
c. Eighteen bacteremic patients on chemotherapy[4]

231

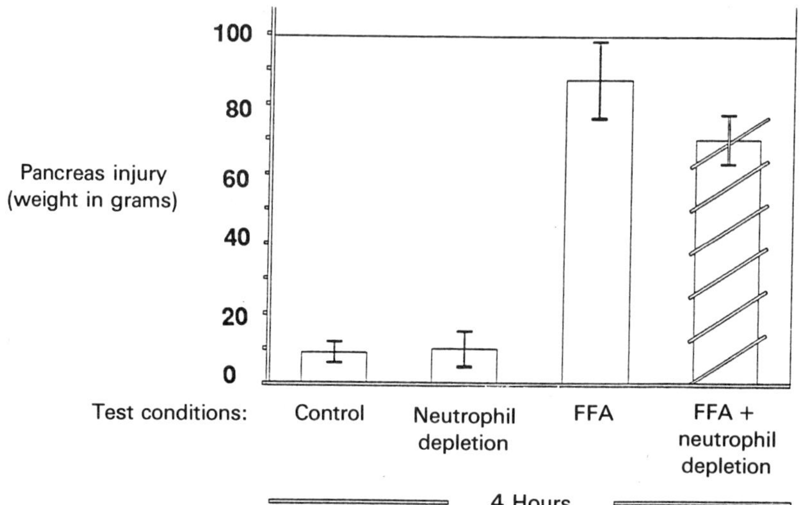

FIGURE 1. Neutrophil depletion does not decrease injury in acute pancreatitis. From Sarr, M.G., Bulkley, G.B., and Cameron, J.L.: The role of leukocytes in the production of oxygen-derived free radicals in acute experimental pancreatitis. Surg., 101:292–299, 1986.

In all cases, there was histologic evidence of ARDS; but no neutrophils were present. Therefore, in man, endovascular injury can occur *without* neutrophils.

Furthermore, there are many animal models in which neutrophil depletion does not decrease vascular injury; but I will present only two. The first is a study by Sarr and associates.[5] Following the infusion of free fatty acids into an *ex-vivo* blood-perfused canine pancreas, significant injury occurred. This injury did not decrease despite neutrophil depletion (Figure 1). Therefore, neutrophils do not contribute to acute pancreatitis.

In another example, neutrophil depletion did not decrease injury in hearts subjected to ischemia-reperfusion.[6] Following a 4-hour ischemic injury, 47 percent of tissue at risk infarcted. This area of infarction did not decrease despite neutrophil depletion (Figure 2).

The second observation that supports the statement that endothelial cell injury can occur in the absence of neutrophils is the alternative finding that neutrophil influx does not always cause endothelial injury. For example, neutrophil influx occurs without causing injury in mechanically ventilated lungs.[7] Snyder and colleagues found increased number of neutrophils in the bronchoalveolar lavage in dogs intubated and ventilated for six hours in the absence of lung injury (Figure 3).

In another example, Fowler and colleagues[8] showed that neutrophil influx, but not activation, occurs in lung lavages of ARDS patients. Although neutrophils are present early in ARDS lavages, there is no evidence that neutrophils are either activated or harmful:

a. No neutrophil elastase is present.
b. No increased alpha-1-antiprotease inactivation is found.

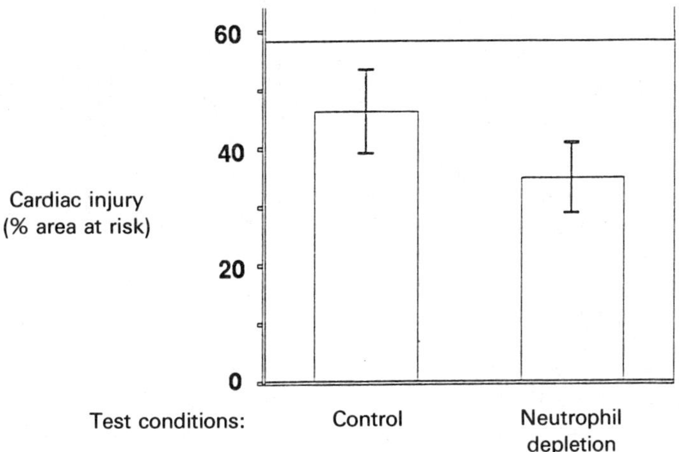

FIGURE 2. Neutrophil depletion does not decrease injury in hearts subjected to ischemia-reperfusion. From Jolly, S.R., Kane, W.J., Hook, B.G., et al.: Reduction of myocardial infarct size by neutrophil depletion: Effect of duration of occlusion. Am. Heart J., 112:682–690, 1986.

Therefore, although neutrophils are present, they are innocuous. In fact, they may be a marker of the injury already present.

II. Studies implicating neutrophils as mediators of endothelial cell damage typically are conducted in animal and *in vitro* models that do not reflect clinical disease accurately.

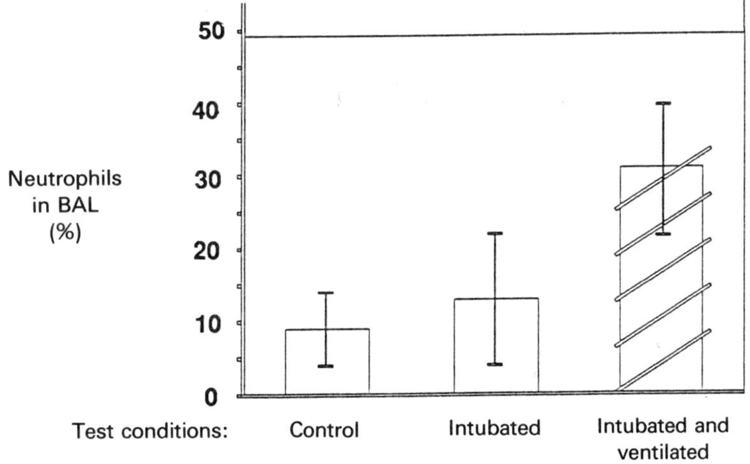

FIGURE 3. Neutrophil influx occurs without causing injury to mechanically ventilated lungs. From Snyder, R., Morgan, L., Glasgow, J., et al.: Mechanical ventilation causes neutrophil influx to the lung. Am. Rev. Resp. Dis., 125:98, 1982.

For example, experimental insults often are inappropriate in nature or delivery:

   a. Nonphysiologic agents are used, such as PMA, paraquat, beads, and glucose oxidase, all of which result in an exaggerated neutrophil response unlike anything in the physiologic state.
   b. When physiologic agents are used (e.g., C5a, ETX), excessively large doses are given—once again, unlike anything observed in the physiologic condition.[9]

Furthermore, species variability exists in the mechanisms of tissue injury by neutrophils:

   a. Sheep neutrophils do not contain elastase.
   b. Dog neutrophils produce less toxic oxygen metabolites (O_2^*).
   c. Rats, but not rabbits or dogs, develop tolerance to oxygen-free radicals.[10]

How can we extrapolate these animal experimental findings to human pathology when there are such great differences in neutrophil function among various species?

In addition, *in vitro* models oversimplify and give misleading results with respect to complex *in vivo* situations.

Figure 4 is a schematic representation of the isolated lung preparation. The lung is removed from the animal, placed in this system, and mechanically ventilated and perfused with balanced salt solution. The advantage of this system is that we have rigorous control of the variables. We can remove blood and focus on the mechanism of injury by individually adding single agents to the perfusate, in this case neutrophils.[11]

When PMA and neutrophils are added to the perfusate, significant lung injury occurs. Thus, investigators concluded that neutrophils cause ARDS. The flaw in this conclusion became apparent a year later when the same investigators added a small amount of red blood cells to the lung perfused with neutrophils and PMA and completely protected the lung against injury. This demonstrated that PMA-stimulated neutrophils cause lung injury in isolated lungs but this process is reversed with the addition of red blood cells[12] (Figure 5). How do we extrapolate this observation to ex-

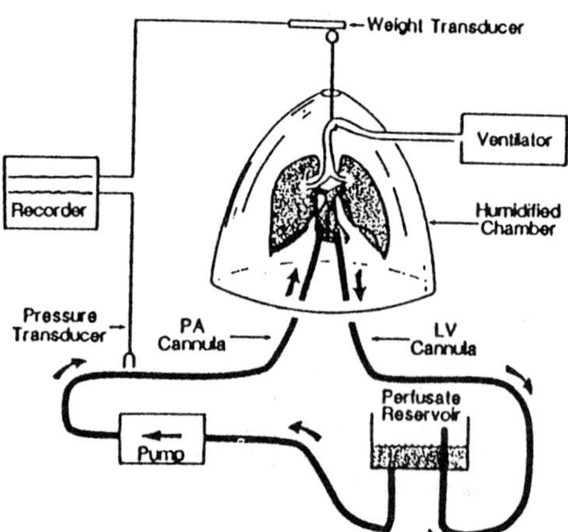

FIGURE 4. Schematic diagram of isolated lung model. From Repine, J.E.: Neutrophils, oxygen radicals, and the adult respiratory distress syndrome. In The Pulmonary Circulation and Acute Lung Injury. S.I. Said (ed.). New York: Futura Publishing Company, 1985, p. 265.

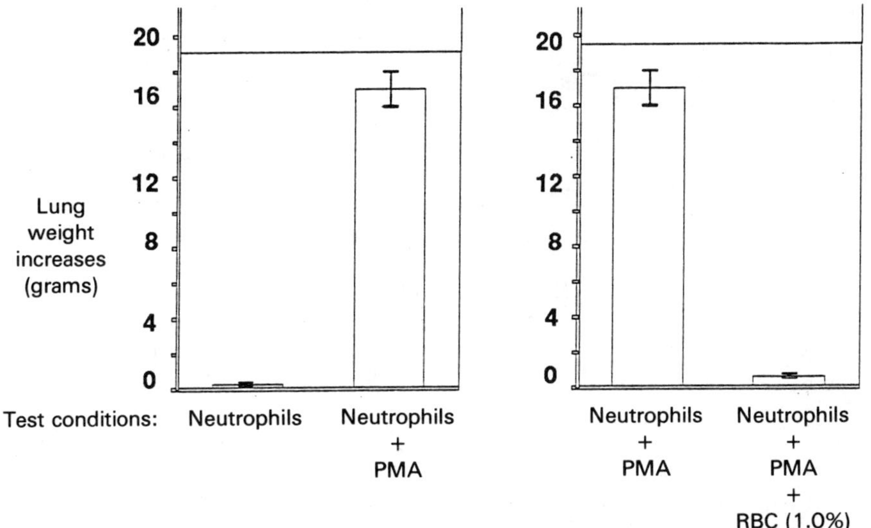

FIGURE 5.   PMA stimulated neutrophils cause lung injury in isolated lungs which is inhibited by RBC. From Toth, K.M., Clifford, D.P., Berger, E.M., White, C.W., and Repine, J.E.: Intact human erythrocytes prevent hydrogen peroxide-mediated damage to isolated perfused rat lungs and cultured bovine pulmonary artery endothelial cells. J. Clin. Invest., 74:292–295, 1984.

plain human pathology? Patients are loaded with red blood cells, but they still develop ARDS. Clearly, this example demonstrates that an isolated system is valuable in exploring the mechanism of injury of a single agent; but the observation cannot be directly extrapolated to complex human pathology.

III. Many factors other than neutrophils can cause endothelial cell damage.

Potential agents causing endothelial cell injury, which do not depend on neutrophils, include:

a. endotoxin
b. hyperoxia
c. paraquat
d. xanthine oxidase
e. arachidonic acid metabolites

f. platelets
g. oleic acid
h. macrophages
i. t-butyl hydroperoxide
j. glucose oxidase

. . . just to name a few.

There are many studies that demonstrate that agents other than neutrophils can cause endothelial cell injury, but I will present only three:

a. Endotoxin damages pulmonary endothelial cell monolayers in the absence of neutrophils[13] (Figure 6).

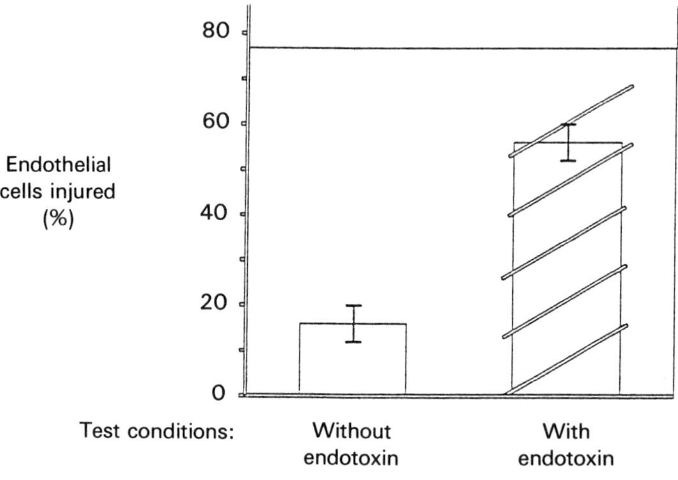

FIGURE 6. Endotoxin damages pulmonary endothelial cell monolayers. From Meyrick, B.O., Ryan, U.S., and Brigham, K.L.: Direct effects of E coli endotoxin on structure and permeability of pulmonary endothelial monolayers and endothelial layer of intimal explants. Am. J. Pathol., 122:140–151, 1986.

b. Hyperoxia and/or paraquat damages pulmonary endothelial cell monolayers in the absence of neutrophils[14] (Figure 7).

c. Xanthine oxidase damages isolated lungs—once again, in the absence of neutrophils[11] (Figure 8).

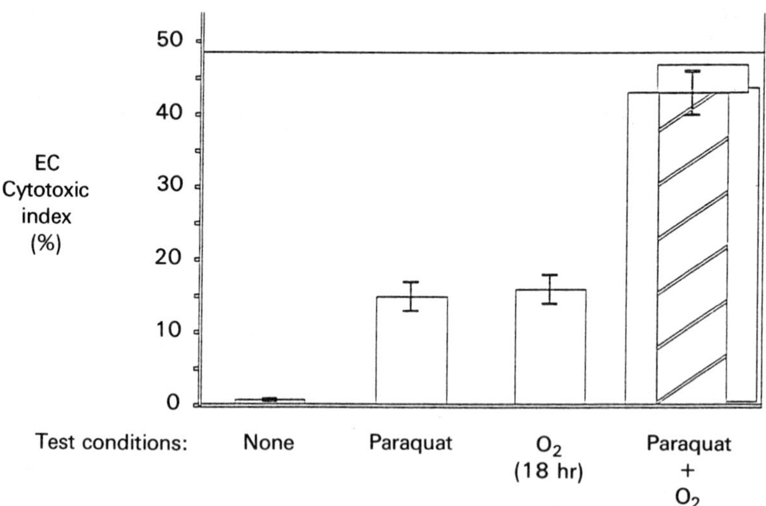

FIGURE 7. Hyperoxia and/or paraquat damages pulmonary endothelial cell monolayers. From Martin, W.J., Gadek, J.E., Hunninghake, G.W., and Crystal, R.G.: Oxidant injury of lung parenchymal cells. J. Clin. Invest., 68:1277–1288, 1981.

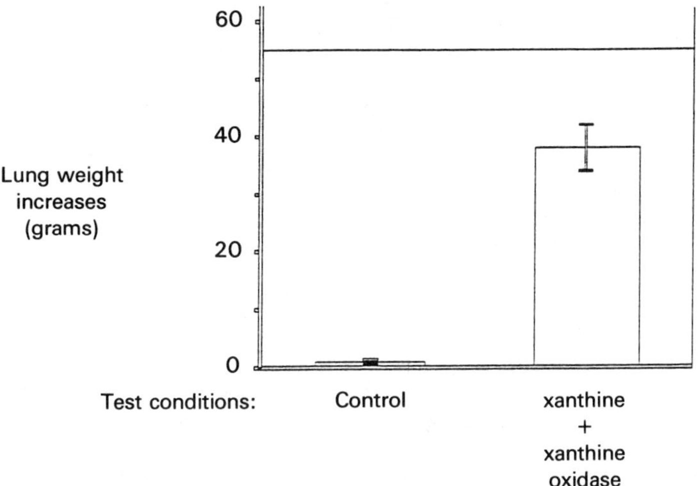

FIGURE 8. Xanthine oxidase damages isolated lungs. From Repine, J.E.: Neutrophils, oxygen radicals, and the adult respiratory distress syndrome. In The Pulmonary Circulation and Acute Lung Injury. S.I. Said (ed.). New York: Futura Publishing Company, 1985, pp. 249–281.

Thus, there are many, many studies that demonstrate that agents other than neutrophils can cause vascular injury.

IV. Because neutrophils participate in host defense and healing, inhibiting neutrophil function in sick patients would be both absolutely detrimental and ludicrous.

Many studies have shown that neutrophil dysfunction increases susceptibility to infection.[15] As a result, the following can occur:

a. recurrent bacterial infections
b. fungal infections
c. toxic shock syndrome
d. septic shock
e. multiple organ failure
f. superinfection.

Furthermore, neutrophils contribute to tissue repair. Neutrophils initiate repair of injured tissue in part by recruiting monocytes. For example, inhibition of neutrophil aggregation and activation decreases repair of infarcted heart tissue. Ibuprofen decreases infarct size; but, by inhibiting neutrophil aggregation and activation, the scar thickness is dangerously decreased[16] (Figure 9).

To repeat, there are four strikes against the contribution of neutrophils to vascular surgery:

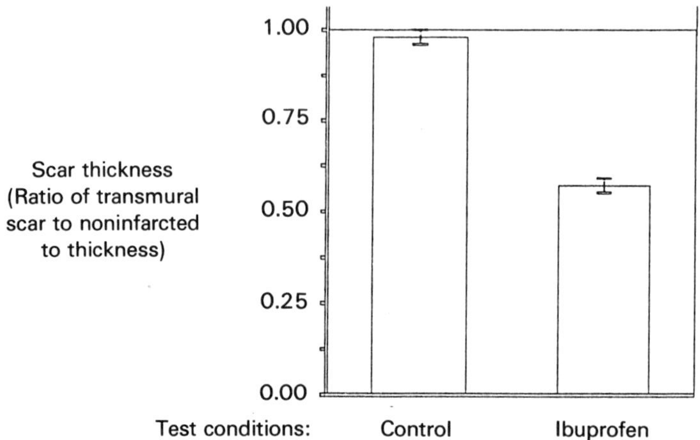

FIGURE 9. Inhibition of neutrophil aggregation and activation decreases repair of infarcted heart tissue. From Brown, E.J., Kloner, R.A., Schoen, F.J., et al.: Scar thinning due to ibuprofen administration after experimental myocardial infarction. Am. J. Cardiol., 51:877–883, 1983.

I. Endothelial cell damage occurs in the absence of neutrophil infiltration and activation.
II. Studies implicating neutrophils as mediators of endothelial cell damage are conducted in animal and *in vitro* models which do not reflect clinical disease accurately.
III. Many factors other than neutrophils can cause endothelial cell damage.
IV. Because neutrophils participate in host defense and healing, inhibiting neutrophil function would be detrimental.

In conclusion:

1. The presence of neutrophils and neutrophil products in vascular permeability syndromes may reflect rather than cause injury.
2. Once endothelial cells are injured by neutrophil-independent mechanisms, activated neutrophils may then enhance injury.
3. Treatments that alter the inflammatory cascade may be a double-edged sword.
4. Research should not focus on one mechanism in complex, multifactorial disease processes.

Therefore, neutrophils are clearly overrated as mediators of vascular injury.

REFERENCES

1. Braude, S., Apperley, J., Krausz, T., Goldman, J.M., and Royston, D.: Adult respiratory distress syndrome after allogeneic bone-marrow transplantation: Evidence for a neutrophil-independent mechanism. Lancet, 1:1239–1242, 1985.

2. Maunder, R.J., Hackman, R.C., Riff, E., et al.: Occurrence of the adult respiratory distress syndrome in neutropenic patients. Am. Rev. Respir. Dis., 133:313–316, 1986.
3. Ognibene, F.P., Martin, S.E., Parker, M.M., et al.: Adult respiratory distress syndrome in patients with severe neutropenia. N. Engl. J. Med., 315:547–551, 1986.
4. Laufe, M.D., Simon, R.H., Flint, A., and Keller, J.B.: Adult respiratory distress syndrome in neutropenia. Am. J. Med., 80:1022–1026, 1986.
5. Sarr, M.G., Bulkley, G.B., and Cameron, J.L.: The role of leukocytes in the production of oxygen-derived free radicals in acute experimental pancreatitis. Surgery, 101:292–299, 1986.
6. Jolly, S.R., Kane, W.J., Hook, B.G., et al.: Reduction of myocardial infarct size by neutrophil depletion: Effect of duration of occlusion. Am. Heart J., 112:682–690, 1986.
7. Snyder, R., Morgan, L., Glasgow, J., et al.: Mechanical ventilation causes neutrophil influx to the lung (abstract). Am. Rev. Respir. Dis., 125:98, 1982.
8. Fowler, A.A., Walchak, S., Giclas, P.C., et al.: Characterization of antiproteinase activity in the adult respiratory distress syndrome. Chest, 81(suppl):50S–51S, 1982.
9. Repine, J.E., Bowman, C.M., and Tate, R.M.: Neutrophils and lung edema. Chest, 81 (suppl)47S–50S, 1982.
10. Klebanoff, S.J. and Clark, R.A.: In The Neutrophil: Function and Clinical Disorders. Amsterdam, The Netherlands: Elsevier/North-Holland Biomedical Press, 1978, pp. 14–72.
11. Repine, J.E.: Neutrophils, oxygen radicals, and the adult respiratory distress syndrome. In The Pulmonary Circulation and Acute Lung Injury. S.I. Said (ed.). New York: Futura Publishing Company, 1985, pp. 249–281.
12. Toth, K. M., Clifford, D.P., Berger, E.M., White, C.W., and Repine, J.E.: Intact human erythrocytes prevent hydrogen peroxide-mediated damage to isolated perfused rat lungs and cultured bovine pulmonary artery endothelial cells. J. Clin. Invest., 74:292–295, 1984.
13. Meyrick, B.O., Ryan, U.S., and Brigham, K.L.: Direct effects of E coli endotoxin on structure and permeability of pulmonary endothelial monolayers and endothelial layer of intimal explants. Am. J. Pathol., 122:140–151, 1986.
14. Martin, W.J., Gadek, J.E., Hunninghake, G.W., and Crystal, R.G.: Oxidant injury of lung parenchymal cells. J. Clin. Invest., 68:1277–1288, 1981.
15. Tate, R.M. and Repine, J.E.: Neutrophils and the adult respiratory distress syndrome. Am. Rev. Respir. Dis., 128:552–559, 1983.
16. Brown, E.J., Kloner, R.A., Schoen, F.J., et al.: Scar thinning due to ibuprofen administration after experimental myocardial infarction. Am. J. Cardiol., 51:877–883, 1983.

Acknowledgment is extended to John E. Repine, M.D. for his assistance.

Index